Current Therapy Series

CURRENT THERAPY
IN
NEUROLOGICAL
SURGERY
1 9 8 5 • 1 9 8 6

DONLIN M. LONG, M.D., PH.D.

Professor and Chairman
Department of Neurological Surgery
The Johns Hopkins Hospital
Baltimore, Maryland

1985

B.C. DECKER INC. • Toronto • Philadelphia
THE C.V. MOSBY COMPANY • Saint Louis • Toronto • London

Publisher: **B.C. Decker Inc.**
3228 South Service Road
Burlington, Ontario   L7N 3H8

Publisher: **B.C. Decker Inc.**
P.O. Box 30246
Phildelphia, Pennsylvania   19103

North American and worldwide sales and distribution

The C.V. Mosby Company
11830 Westline Industrial Drive
Saint Louis, Missouri   63141

In Canada: **The C.V. Mosby Company, Ltd.**
120 Melford Drive
Toronto, Ontario   M1B 2X5

Current Therapy in Neurological Surgery   ISBN 0-941158-49-7

Library of Congress catalog card number: 85-071353

10 9 8 7 6 5 4 3 2 1

CONTRIBUTORS

KEITH ARONYK, M.D., F.R.C.S.(C)

Lecturer, Division of Neurosurgery, University of Alberta Faculty of Medicine, Edmonton, Alberta, Canada
Subdural Hematoma in the Adult

JAMES I. AUSMAN, M.D., Ph.D.

Chairman, Department of Neurological Surgery, Henry Ford Hospital, Detroit, Michigan
Transient Ischemic Attacks and Stroke from Carotid Artery Disease
Acute Carotid Occlusion and Related Progressive Stroke Syndromes

PERRY BLACK, M.D.

Professor and Chairman, Department of Neurosurgery, Hahnemann University School of Medicine, Philadelphia, Pennsylvania
Infection of the Spine

PETER McL. BLACK, M.D., Ph.D.

Associate Professor of Surgery, Harvard Medical School; Associate Visiting Neurosurgeon, Massachusetts General Hospital, Boston, Massachusetts
ACTH Tumors and Nelson's Syndrome

NIKOLAI BOGDUK, M.B., B.S., Ph.D.

Senior Lecturer, Department of Anatomy, University of Queensland; Visiting Medical Officer, Pain Clinic, Princess Alexandra Hospital, Brisbane, Australia
Greater Occipital Neuralgia

MARIO BONI, M.D.

Professor and Chairman, Orthopaedic and Traumatologic Clinic, University of Pavia, Pavia, Italy
Multiple Subtotal Somatectomy

CECIL BOREL, M.D.

Assistant Professor, Departments of Neurology, Neurosurgery, Anesthesiology, and Critical Care Medicine, The Johns Hopkins University School of Medicine; Co-Director, Neurosciences Critical Care Unit, The Johns Hopkins Hospital, Baltimore, Maryland
Monitoring the Critically Ill Patient

HENRY BREM, M.D.

Assistant Professor, Departments of Neurosurgery, Ophthalmology, and Oncology, The Johns Hopkins University School of Medicine; Attending Neurosurgeon, The Johns Hopkins Hospital, Baltimore, Maryland
Supratentorial Astrocytoma

RONALD BRISMAN, M.D.

Assistant Professor, Clinical Neurological Surgery, Columbia University College of Physicians and Surgeons; Assistant Attending Neurological Surgeon, Columbia Presbyterian Medical Center, New York, New York
Cerebrospinal Fluid Fistula

DEREK A. BRUCE, M.B., Ch.B.

Associate Professor of Neurosurgery and Pediatrics, University of Pennsylvania School of Medicine; Associate Neurosurgeon, Children's Hospital of Philadelphia, Philadelphia, Pennsylvania
Craniopharyngioma

JAMES N. CAMPBELL, M.D.

Associate Professor, Department of Neurosurgery, The Johns Hopkins University School of Medicine, Baltimore, Maryland
Painful Peripheral Nerve Syndrome

MICHAEL E. CAREY, M.D., M.S.

Professor of Neurosurgery, Louisiana State University School of Medicine in New Orleans, New Orleans, Louisiana
Brain and Spinal Wounds Caused by Missiles
Pyogenic Brain Abscess

BENJAMIN S. CARSON, M.D.

Assistant Professor of Neurosurgery and Oncology, The Johns Hopkins University School of Medicine; Attending Neurosurgeon, The Johns Hopkins Hospital, Baltimore, Maryland
Head Injury in the Child

LEONARD J. CERULLO, M.D.

Assistant Professor of Surgery (Neurosurgery), Northwestern University Medical School; Attending Physician, Northwestern Memorial Hospital, Chicago, Illinois
Foramen Magnum Meningioma

SHELLEY N. CHOU, M.D., Ph.D.

Professor and Head, Department of Neurosurgery, University of Minnesota Medical School—Minneapolis, Minneapolis, Minnesota
Neurological Deficit Comlicating Scoliosis

IVAN CIRIC, M.D.

Associate Professor of Clinical Surgery (Neurosurgery), Northwestern University Medical School, Chicago, Illinois; *Prolactin-Secreting Pituitary Adenoma*

ROBERT M. CROWELL, M.D.

Professor and Head, Department of Neurosurgery, University of Illinois College of Medicine, Chicago, Illinois *Cauda Equina Ependymoma*

BENJAMIN L. CRUE, Jr., B.S., M.D., F.A.C.S.

Clinical Professor of Neurosurgery and Director, Section of Algology, University of Southern California School of Medicine, Los Angeles, California; Director, New Hope Pain Center, Pasadena, California *Defining the Chronic Pain Syndrome*

FERNANDO G. DIAZ, M.D., Ph.D.

Director of Clinical Research, Department of Neurosurgery, Henry Ford Hospital, Detroit, Michigan *Transient Ischemic Attacks and Stroke from Carotid Artery Disease*
Acute Carotid Occlusion and Related Progressive Stroke Syndromes

CHARLES G. DRAKE, M.D., F.R.C.S.(C), F.A.C.S.

Professor of Surgery (Neurosurgery), University of Western Ontario Faculty of Medicine, London, Ontario, Canada *Giant Aneurysm of the Basilar Artery*

BERNARD J. D'SOUZA, M.D.

Associate and Chief in Pediatric Neurology, Duke University Medical Center, Durham, North Carolina *Brain Stem Glioma*

THOMAS B. DUCKER, M.D.

Professor of Neurological Surgery, The Johns Hopkins University School of Medicine and Clinical Professor, University of Maryland, Baltimore, Maryland; Consultant, Maryland Institute for Emergency Medical Service System, Annapolis, Maryland *Thoracic Fracture*
Herniated Thoracic Disc

GEORGE EHNI, M.D.

Professor of Neurological Surgery, Baylor College of Medicine; Senior Attending Physician, Methodist Hospital, Houston, Texas *Carpal Tunnel Syndrome and Ulnar Neuropathy at the Elbow*

HOWARD M. EISENBERG, M.D.

Professor and Chief, Division of Neurosurgery, University of Texas Medical School at Galveston, Galveston, Texas *Epidural Hematoma*

FRED J. EPSTEIN, M.D.

Professor of Neurosurgery, New York University School of Medicine; Director, Division of Pediatric Neurosurgery, New York University-Bellevue Medical Center, New York, New York *Spinal Cord Astrocytoma of Childhood*

JOSEPH A. EPSTEIN, M.D., F.A.C.S.

Clinical Professor of Neurological Surgery, State University of New York at Stony Brook Health Sciences Center School of Medicine; Attending Neurosurgeon, Long Island Jewish Hillside Medical Center; Attending Neurosurgeon, The North Shore University Hospital and Cornell University, New York, New York *Congenital and Acquired Spondylolisthesis*

MEL H. EPSTEIN, M.D.

Associate Professor of Neurosurgery and Director of Pediatric Neurosurgery, The Johns Hopkins University School of Medicine, Baltimore, Maryland *Hydrocephalus*

DONALD L. ERICKSON, M.D.

Associate Professor, Department of Neurosurgery, University of Minnesota Medical School—Minneapolis, Minneapolis, Minnesota *Cerebellar Hemorrhage*

CHARLES A. FAGER, M.D.

Assistant Clinical Professor of Surgery, Harvard Medical School; Former Chairman, Department of Neurosurgery, Lahey Clinic Medical Center, Boston, Massachusetts *Cervical Disc Herniation*

DAVID L. FILTZER, M.D.

Associate Professor, Department of Orthopaedic Surgery and Assistant Professor, Department of Neurosurgery, The Johns Hopkins University School of Medicine, Baltimore, Maryland *The Unstable Low Back*

BERNARD E. FINNESON, M.D.

Clinical Associate Professor of Surgery (Neurosurgery), Hahnemann University School of Medicine, Philadelphia, Pennsylvania; Director, Low Back Pain Clinic, Crozer-Chester Medical Center, Chester, Pennsylvania *Low Back Pain With or Without Sciatica*

ALLAN H. FRIEDMAN, M.D.

Assistant Professor of Neurological Surgery, Duke University School of Medicine, Durham, North Carolina *Spinal Injury Pain*

JOSEPH H. GALICICH, M.D.

Professor of Surgery, Cornell University Medical College; Chief, Neurosurgery Service, Memorial Sloan-Kettering

Cancer Center, New York, New York
Solitary Intracranial Metastasis
Spinal Metastasis With and Without Neurological Deficit

PHILIP H. GUTIN, M.D.

Associate Professor, Department of Neurological Surgery, University of California, San Francisco, School of Medicine, San Francisco, California
Clivus Chordoma

E. CLARKE HALEY, Jr., M.D.

Assistant Professor, Department of Neurology, University of Virginia School of Medicine, Charlottesville, Virginia
Subarachnoid Hemorrhage

DANIEL F. HANLEY, M.D.

Co-Director, Neuroscience Critical Care Unit and Assistant Professor, Departments of Neurology, Neurosurgery, Anesthesia, and Critical Care Medicine, The Johns Hopkins Hospital, Baltimore, Maryland
Monitoring the Critically Ill Patient

RUSSELL WILLIS HARDY, Jr., M.D.

Neurological Surgeon and Director, Center for the Spine, Cleveland Clinic, Cleveland, Ohio
Herniated Lumbar Disc

CHARLES M. HENDERSON, B.S., M.D., F.A.C.S.

Assistant Professor of Neurological Surgery, University of Maryland School of Medicine; Senior Attending, Neurological Surgery, University of Maryland Hospital and St. Agnes Hospital, Consulting Attending, Neurological Surgery, Kernan Hospital for Crippled Children, Baltimore, Maryland
Cervical Spur

ROBERTO C. HEROS, M.D.

Associate Professor of Neurosurgery, Harvard Medical School; Director of Cerebrovascular Surgery, Massachusetts General Hospital, Boston, Massachusetts
Giant Intracranial Aneurysm

JULIAN T. HOFF, M.D.

Professor of Surgery and Head, Section of Neurosurgery, University of Michigan Medical School, Ann Arbor, Michigan
Basilar Impression, Platybasia, Os Odontoideum, and Fracture of the Odontoid Process

HAROLD JOSEPH HOFFMAN, M.D., B.Sc(Med), F.R.C.S.(C)

Professor of Surgery, Division of Neurosurgery, University of Toronto Faculty of Medicine; Senior Neurosurgeon, Hospital for Sick Children, Toronto, Ontario, Canada
Myelomeningocele

JOHN A. JANE, M.D., Ph.D.

Professor and Chairman, Department of Neurological Surgery, University of Virginia School of Medicine, Charlottesville, Virginia
Craniosynostosis

PETER J. JANNETTA, M.D.

Professor and Chairman, Department of Neurosurgery, University of Pittsburgh School of Medicine, Pittsburgh, Pennsylvania
Cranial Rhizopathy

NEAL F. KASSELL, M.D.

Professor, Department of Neurosurgery, University of Virginia School of Medicine, Charlottesville, Virginia
Subarachnoid Hemorrhage

DAVID L. KELLY, Jr., M.D.

Professor and Head, Section of Neurosurgery, Department of Surgery, Bowman Gray School of Medicine of Wake Forest University, Winston-Salem, North Carolina
Choroid Plexus Papilloma and Other Tumors of the Lateral Ventricle

JOHN S. KENNERDELL, M.D.

Professor, Department of Ophthalmology, University of Pittsburgh School of Medicine; Eye and Ear Hospital, Pittsburgh, Pennsylvania
Optic Nerve Meningioma

DAVID G. KLINE, M.D.

Professor and Chairman, Department of Neurosurgery, Louisiana State University School of Medicine in New Orleans, New Orleans, Louisiana
Root and Nerve Injury

PAUL L. KORNBLITH, M.D.

Chief, Surgical Neurology Branch, National Institute of Neurological and Communicative Disorders and Stroke, National Institutes of Health, Bethesda, Maryland
Malignant Glioma

YOSEF KRESPI, M.D.

Associate Professor of Otolaryngology, Northwestern University Medical School; Attending Physician, Northwestern Memorial Hospital, Chicago, Illinois
Foramen Magnum Meningioma

SANFORD J. LARSON, M.D., Ph.D.

Professor and Chairman, Department of Neurosurgery, Medical College of Wisconsin, Milwaukee, Wisconsin
Spondylotic Myelopathy

EDWARD R. LAWS, Jr. M.D.

Professor of Neurologic Surgery, Mayo Medical School/ Mayo Clinic, Rochester, Minnesota
Growth Hormone-Secreting Pituitary Tumor

K. STUART LEE, M.D.

Resident, Section on Neurosurgery, Department of Surgery, Bowman Gray School of Medicine of Wake Forest University, Winston-Salem, North Carolina
Choroid Plexus Papilloma and Other Tumors of the Lateral Ventricle

JACK L. LE FROCK, M.D.

Professor of Medicine and Clinical Professor of Surgery, Hahnemann University School of Medicine, Philadelphia, Pennsylvania
Infection of the Spine

DONLIN M. LONG, M.D., Ph.D.

Head, Department of Neurological Surgery, The Johns Hopkins University School of Medicine, Baltimore, Maryland
Meningioma of Olfactory Groove and Planum Sphenoidale
Meningioma of the Visual Apparatus
Tumor of the Cerebellopontine Angle
Tumor of the Glomus Jugulare
Chronic Pain Syndrome

LEONARD I. MALIS, M.D.

Professor and Chairman, Department of Neurosurgery, Mount Sinai School of Medicine of the City University of New York; Neurosurgeon-in-Chief and Director, Department of Neurosurgery, The Mount Sinai Hospital, New York, New York
Spinal Arteriovenous Malformation

BERNARD L. MARIA, M.D.

Chief Resident in Pediatric Neurology, The Johns Hopkins University School of Medicine, Baltimore, Maryland
Brain Stem Glioma

JOSEPH C. MAROON, M.D.

Clinical Professor, Department of Neurosurgery, University of Pittsburgh School of Medicine; Director, Department of Neurosurgery, Allegheny General Hospital, Pittsburgh, Pennsylvania
Optic Nerve Meningioma

LAWRENCE F. MARSHALL, M.D.

Professor of Neurological Surgery, University of California, San Diego, School of Medicine; Chief of Neurosurgical Service, University of California Medical Center, San Diego, California
Closed Head Injury: Management Dilemmas

PAUL C. McAFEE, M.D.

Assistant Professor of Orthopedic Surgery and Assistant Professor of Neurological Surgery, The Johns Hopkins University School of Medicine; Chief of Orthopedic Spinal Reconstructive Surgery Service, The Johns Hopkins Hospital, Baltimore, Maryland
Thoracic Fracture

DAVID C. McCULLOUGH, M.D.

Professor, Neurological Surgery and Child Health and Development, George Washington University School of Medicine; Chairman, Department of Neurological Surgery, Children's Hospital National Medical Center, Washington, D.C.
Subdural Hematoma in the Pediatric Age Group

ROBERT L. McLAURIN, M.D.

Professor of Neurosurgery, University of Cincinnati College of Medicine; Neurosurgeon, Children's Hospital Medical Center, Cincinnati, Ohio
Posterior Fossa Ependymoma

NEIL R. MILLER, M.D.

Associate Professor, Neuro Ophthalmology and Orbital Surgery, The Johns Hopkins University School of Medicine, Baltimore, Maryland
Orbital Tumor

BLAINE S. NASHOLD, Jr., M.D., F.A.C.S.

Professor of Neurosurgery, Duke University School of Medicine, Durham, North Carolina
Spinal Injury Pain

RICHARD B. NORTH, M.D.

Assistant Professor, Department of Neurosurgery, The Johns Hopkins University School of Medicine, Baltimore, Maryland
The Failed Back Syndrome

HUMBERTO J. ORTIZ, M.D., Ph.D.

Professor of Neurosurgery, University of Puerto Rico School of Medicine; Attending Neurosurgeon, University Hospital/Puerto Rico Medical Center, San Juan, Puerto Rico
Granulomatous Abscess in the Brain
Parasitic Disease of the Brain and Spinal Cord

LARRY K. PAGE, M.D.

Professor, Department of Neurological Surgery, University of Miami School of Medicine, Miami, Florida
Medulloblastoma

JEFFREY E. PEARCE, M.D.

Resident in Neurological Surgery, Henry Ford Hospital, Detroit, Michigan
Transient Ischemic Attacks and Stroke from Carotid Artery Disease
Acute Carotid Occlusion and Related Progressive Stroke Syndromes

JOHN A. PERSING, M.D.

Assistant Professor, Departments of Neurological Surgery and Plastic Surgery, University of Virginia School of Medicine, Charlottesville, Virginia
Craniosynostosis

DAVID G. PIEPGRAS, M.D.

Associate Professor, Department of Neurologic Surgery, Mayo Medical School, Rochester, Minnesota
Convexity Meningioma

JOSEPH M. PIEPMEIER, M.D.

Assistant Professor of Surgery, Section of Neurosurgery, Yale University School of Medicine, New Haven, Connecticut
Cervical Fracture

MATTHEW QUIGLEY, M.D.

Resident, Neurosurgery, Northwestern University Medical School, Chicago, Illinois
Foramen Magnum Meningioma

HUBERT L. ROSOMOFF, M.D., D.Med.Sc.

Professor and Chairman, Department of Neurological Surgery, University of Miami School of Medicine; Medical Director, Comprehensive Pain Center, Miami, Florida
Nonoperative Treatment of the Failed Back Syndrome Presenting with Chronic Pain

EDWARD L. SELJESKOG, M.D., Ph.D.

Professor of Neurosurgery, University of Minnesota Medical School—Minneapolis, Minneapolis, Minnesota
Fracture of the Lumbar Spine

JOHN SHILLITO, Jr., M.D.

Professor of Surgery, Harvard Medical School; Associate Chief of Neurosurgery, Children's Hospital, Boston, Massachusetts
Cerebellar Astrocytoma

WILLIAM A. SHUCART, M.D.

Professor and Chairman of Neurosurgery, Tufts University School of Medicine; Chief of Neurosurgery, Tufts-New England Medical Center, Boston, Massachusetts
Hypothalamic and Thalamic Glioma (And Other Tumors of the Anterior Third Ventricle)

FREDERICK A. SIMEONE, M.D.

Professor of Neurosurgery, University of Pennsylvania School of Medicine; Chief of Neurosurgery, Pennsylvania Hospital, Philadelphia, Pennsylvania
Thoracic Spinal Cord Tumor (Meningioma and Neurofibroma)

BARRY H. SMITH, M.D., Ph.D.

Special Fellow, Neurosurgical Service, Memorial Sloan-Kettering Cancer Center, New York, New York
Solitary Intracranial Metastasis

ROGER D. SMITH, M.D.

Associate Professor, Department of Neurosurgery, Louisiana State University School of Medicine in New Orleans, New Orleans, Louisiana
Root and Nerve Injury

BENNETT M. STEIN, M.D.

Byron Stookey Professor of Neurological Surgery, Columbia University College of Physicians and Surgeons; Chairman, Department of Neurosurgery, The Neurological Institute of New York, New York, New York
Subarachnoid Hemorrhage From An Arteriovenous Malformation of the Brain or Spinal Cord

NARAYAN SUNDARESAN, M.D.

Assistant Professor of Surgery, Cornell University Medical College; Assistant Attending Surgeon, Memorial Sloan-Kettering Cancer Center, New York, New York
Solitary Intracranial Metastasis

THORALF M. SUNDT, Jr., M.D.

Cerebrovascular Research, St. Mary's Hospital; Department of Neurologic Surgery, Mayo Clinic, Rochester, Minnesota
Brain Stem Ischemia: Reconstructive or Bypass Surgery

GEORGE W. SYPERT, M.D.

C.M. and K.E. Overstreet Professor and Eminent Scholar, Departments of Neurological Surgery and Neuroscience, University of Florida College of Medicine, Gainesville, Florida
Craniofacial Neoplasia

NOEL B. TULIPAN, M.D.

Instructor, Department of Neurosurgery, The Johns Hopkins University School of Medicine, Baltimore, Maryland
Syringomyelia

JOHN M. VAN BUREN, M.D., Ph.D.

Professor of Neurological Surgery, University of Miami School of Medicine, Miami, Florida
Focal Epilepsy

JOHN C. VAN GILDER, M.D.

Professor and Chairman of Division of Neurological Surgery, University of Iowa College of Medicine, Iowa City, Iowa
Pituitary Chromophobe Adenoma

JOHN W. WALSH, M.D., Ph.D.

Associate Professor, Division of Neurosurgery, University of Kentucky School of Medicine, Lexington, Kentucky
Lipoma and Related Abnormalities Such As Dermal Sinuses

HENRY WANG, M.D.

Assistant Professor, Department of Neuroradiology, The Johns Hopkins Hospital, Baltimore, Maryland
Achondroplasia: Neuroradiological Investigation and Surgical Management of Craniocervical Junction and Pan-Spinal Stenosis

JOHN D. WARD, M.D.

Associate Professor of Neurological Surgery and Director

of Neuroscience Intensive Care, Chief, Pediatric Neurosurgery, Virginia Commonwealth University Medical College of Virginia School of Medicine, Richmond, Virginia
Closed Head Injury

CLARK WATTS, M.D.

Professor of Surgery, University of Missouri—Columbia School of Medicine; Chief of Neurosurgery, University of Missouri—Columbia Hospitals and Clinics, Columbia, Missouri
Sphenoid Wing Meningioma

BRYCE WEIR, M.D., F.R.C.S.(C)

Director of Neurosurgery, University of Alberta Faculty of Medicine, Edmonton, Alberta, Canada
Subdural Hematoma in the Adult

HAROLD A. WILKINSON, M.D., Ph.D.

Professor and Chairman, Department of Neurosurgery, University of Massachusetts Medical Center, Worcester, Massachusetts
Lumbar Adhesive Arachnoiditis

JEFFREY A. WINFIELD, M.D., Ph.D.

Assistant Professor of Neurosurgery, State University of New York, Upstate Medical Center, Syracuse, New York
Pineal Region Tumor

Achondroplasia: Neuroradiological Investigation and Surgical Management of Craniocervical Junction and Pan-Spinal Stenosis

JEFFREY H. WISOFF, M.D.

Instructor, Division of Pediatric Neurosurgery, New York University School of Medicine; Assistant Attending Physician, New York University, Bellevue Hospital Center, New York, New York
Spinal Cord Astrocytoma of Childhood

CHARLES J. WROBEL, M.D.

Resident, University of California Medical Center, San Diego, California
Closed Head Injury: Management Dilemmas

NICHOLAS T. ZERVAS, M.D.

Professor of Surgery, Harvard Medical School; Chief of Neurosurgical Service, Massachusetts General Hospital, Boston, Massachusetts
ACTH Tumors and Nelson's Syndrome

Intracerebral Hemorrhage

PREFACE

Why another text in neurosurgery? There are several authoritative and comprehensive works that provide detailed descriptions of neurosurgical disease, and a wide range of monographs on specific subjects are also available. However, there is no source where the interested practitioner can find a specific opinion by an expert which suggests an effective mode of therapy for an individual patient. *Current Therapy in Neurological Surgery* will fill this need. The topics have been chosen because of their clinical importance or the frequency of their occurrence; the authors have been chosen for their documented expertise in managing these specific problems, and because of their stature in the field of neurosurgery. The purpose of the book is to provide a ready reference for any physician who is confronted with a question of therapeutic management of a diagnosed neuro-surgical condition. Detailed discussion of etiology, pathophysiology, diagnosis, and natural history has been waived in order to sharpen the focus on therapy. For many of these conditions there are alternative techniques, but the descriptions in this book provide an effective treatment utilized and verified by an expert in the field.

The book is not all inclusive. There are topics which have been omitted deliberately. Some, fortunately a small number, were omitted owing to the pressures of the publication schedule. Undoubtedly some do not appear because of my own neglect. Still, the topics provide a broad overview of the most common and important neurosurgical problems.

I hope that the book will prove useful to those practicing neurosurgery, and that it will have special merit for residents and students confronted with neurosurgical problems during their training. The Current Therapy concept also provides a ready reference for the neurologist, internist, or other physician confronted with a patient with a neurosurgical disease. The management techniques are directly transferrable to individual patients with the assurance that a master of the field recommends a proven method of therapy.

I wish to thank the contributors of this volume for their compliance with my request for manuscripts and for the clarity and brevity of their contributions. Such authors make the editor's job both pleasant and educational. I also wish to thank Mr. Brian Decker and his outstanding staff. Their attention to detail and the quality of their work simplified my role as editor and expedited the publication of this volume. My secretary, Mrs. Shawne Tubinis, contributed greatly to the organization and record keeping of the enterprise.

Donlin M. Long, M.D., Ph.D.

CONTENTS

INTRACRANIAL TUMORS

MENINGIOMA OF OLFACTORY GROOVE AND PLANUM SPHENOIDALE

DONLIN M. LONG, M.D., Ph. D.

Meningiomas of the olfactory groove and planum sphenoidale are the most common basal meningiomas. Symptoms and signs are both subtle and insidious so that the tumors often grow to enormous size before they are found. The patient frequently notices an inability to smell or has a visual complaint. Headache may occur. Family members often notice personality change. Seizures are sometimes the presenting sign, and uncinate attacks are not unknown. There is a paucity of physical findings. Posterior extensions of these tumors are commonly associated with both unilateral and bilateral visual change. There is often a diminution in acuity, and a broad spectrum of field defects are present. There is nothing characteristic about the visual examination. The Foster-Kennedy syndrome has been described as typical for these tumors. In fact, the combination of ipsilateral optic atrophy associated with contralateral papilledema and anosmia is extremely rare and certainly cannot be considered diagnostic for these tumors.

The diagnosis is now made by CT scan, although angiography is still useful. Definition of the blood supply for possible embolization and the location of the major intracranial vessels in relation to the tumor are both important. A bolus scan now serves the latter purpose, but angiography is required to determine the location of the feeding vessels perforating the base of the skull and to determine whether embolization is a feasible adjunct. Our radiographers are prepared to carry out embolization at the time of angiography if it appears that the tumor can be significantly reduced by interrupting the blood supply.

The decision for surgery usually is based simply on the discovery of the tumor. However, there are circumstances in which removal of the tumor may not be indicated. The aged patient or one with serious intercurrent disease, which makes the surgical procedure unduly risky, may be followed expectantly with CT scan, and surgery is undertaken only for disabling symptoms. For most patients, surgery is the only answer and should be undertaken when the tumor is discovered. Growth of the tumor simply makes surgery more difficult, and any tumor that has become symptomatic should be treated. There is no alternative to surgical removal.

SURGICAL THERAPY

The surgical approach to these tumors depends on their location and size. If the tumor is largely unilateral, a unilateral frontal approach, carried to the midline, is required. Most are bilateral, however, requiring a bifrontal flap to allow complete exposure of the tumor. A coronal skin incision hidden behind the hairline is best, irrespective of the bony approach. Most of these tumors can be removed by simply elevating the frontal lobes, leaving the falx and sinus intact. An extremely large tumor requires division of the sagittal sinus at its most anterior extremity and section of the falx to allow adequate retraction of both frontal lobes and tumor removal. It is important to avoid injury to the large draining frontal veins during this maneuver.

The tumors are of two basic varieties. In one group the tumors are extremely firm, adherent to the base of the skull, and very difficult to remove by standard techniques. In the other group the tumors are soft and suckable; even conventional suction usually is adequate to remove them totally. The laser and ultrasonic suctions have greatly expedited the removal of all these tumors.

Three major technical problems confront the surgeon in the removal of such large frontal basal tumors.

1. The tumors may have a posterior extension that involves the anterior visual apparatus. The CT scan usually demonstrates this well. Even when symptoms are unilateral, the involvement is probably bilateral. At the posterior limits of the tumor, the surgeon must be prepared to dissect the tumor free from the optic nerves and chiasm.
2. The anterior cerebral arteries and the anterior portion of the circle of Willis are sometimes involved by this same posterior extension. This can be judged by the bolus CT scan or by the angiogram. Freeing these vessels from the posterior rim of tumor is a challenging exercise.
3. A major technical problem is the degree of involvement of the floor of the frontal fossa, particularly the ethmoid and sphenoid sinuses. When the sinuses are involved, a radical removal of bone and tumor from the sinuses with repair of the anterior fossa is required, if total tumor removal is to be achieved.

Patients undergoing removal of these tumors are virtually certain to become anosmic, even with tumors that are largely unilateral. Cerebrospinal fluid fistula is a risk when an extensive frontal fossa resection is undertaken. Injury to the anterior visual apparatus and anterior circle of Willis may occur. Bifrontal damage from

1

retraction or venous stasis and edema is possible. A rare but very real complication is progressive sinus thrombosis, secondary to an operative injury to the sinus or its major anterior tributaries. These patients usually awaken from surgery and do well for several days until subtle personality change signals the onset of difficulties. Their condition deteriorates to a state that verges on autism; they demonstrate quadriparesis and gradually lapse into coma. If the propagation continues far enough posteriorly, death from this complication is virtually certain.

OPTIC NERVE MENINGIOMA

JOSEPH C. MAROON, M.D.
JOHN S. KENNERDELL, M.D.

Once considered rare, optic nerve sheath meningiomas are now diagnosed with increased frequency owing primarily to the advent of high-resolution computed tomography. These tumors arise from the cap cells of the arachnoid villi of the optic nerve and may take origin at any site from the intracanalicular portion of the nerve to the globe.

The growth of these tumors may take one of three directions.

1. Most are located in the subdural space and extend axially anteriorly and posteriorly along the nerve.
2. Eventually the tumor may break through the dura and present as a combined exophytic and subdural mass.
3. Rarely the tumor may be primarily dural and extradural with very little if any subdural component.

The clinical presentation depends somewhat on the mode of growth of the tumor. As it expands within the subdural space, compression of the nerve occurs, and early progressive visual loss develops. With the chronic compression of the nerve and its blood supply, cilioretinal shunt veins develop which may be seen on the optic disc. These shunt vessels have been described as characteristic of optic nerve sheath meningiomas and are nicely demonstrated by fluorescein angiography. With progressive compression of the normal circulation and invasion of the optic nerve septa, secondary glaucoma may develop. When the mass is exophytic or is associated with progressive growth, proptosis may occur but almost always is preceded by visual impairment. The clinical triad of progressive visual loss, optic atrophy with edema, and optociliary shunt vessels is considered diagnostic of optic nerve sheath meningioma. For unexplained reasons, primary optic nerve sheath meningiomas occur predominantly in middle-aged women and are rarely encountered in children. It is suggested that when they do occur in children, the course is more aggressive. In our experience with over 35 cases, however, we have documented none under the age of 20.

The differential diagnosis includes primary optic nerve atrophy from vascular occlusive disease, primary optic nerve glioma, detached retina, multiple sclerosis, as well as many other conditions associated with the aforementioned findings. The diagnosis is established primarily by CT scanning. Although hypocycloidal polytomography and arteriography are occasionally used, they have been of little value. Ultrasonic scanning of the orbit may be helpful in eliminating other diagnostic possibilities. The CT scan characteristics include a tubular enlargement of the optic nerve or a bulbous appearance anywhere along the nerve sheath. Most commonly, the tubular enlargement contrasted with the normal optic nerve extends along the entire nerve. Detection of eccentric enlargements, however, is extremely important for therapy. On coronal sections of the nerve an area of hypodensity representing the nerve, surrounded by a more peripheral dense area, is considered diagnostic of primary perioptic meningioma.

The management of patients with primary optic nerve sheath meningioma is in a transitional phase. Formerly, radical surgical excision of the optic nerve and tumor at the time of suspected diagnosis was considered necessary. With a better appreciation of the growth characteristics of the tumor, the observation that they may be present for many years in a rather dormant state, and the capability of following their growth pattern with CT and now MRI scans, a less aggressive approach may be justified.

We have now treated over thirty cases of primary optic nerve meningiomas, and the form of treatment has been based primarily on the location of the tumor in the orbit, the status of frequent visual acuity examinations, and the informed consent of the patient after the various options of treatment are fully explained. If the tumor is located in the mid to anterior portion of the optic nerve and the visual acuity is stable and not seriously compromised, we usually elect to observe the patient with CT scans at 4- to 6-month intervals with CT scans once per year. If the tumor is thought to be located primarily in the mid to anterior portion of the nerve and there is documented progressive vision loss, we consider a lateral microsurgical approach to remove the tumor from its extradural as well as subdural location.

If the tumor is located in the apex and there is normal or near-normal vision, we follow the patient with serial checks of vision and CT scans. If the tumor is apical and there is progressive visual loss documented, we offer the patient radium therapy, 4000 to 5000 rads, as determined by the radiation therapist to interrupt the progressive vision loss. If there is a large apical tumor with intracranial extension, a craniotomy for tumor incision is performed without delay.

The lateral orbitotomy is performed through a 35- to 40-mm lateral incision. The lateral orbital wall is removed, and a specially designed self-retaining intraorbital retractor is used to obtain retraction of the lateral rectus muscles and the fat to allow visualization of the optic nerve. In the case of an anteriorly placed meningioma, a clear demarcation may be seen between the proximal nerve of normal diameter and the enlarged bulbous distal nerve with its encased tumor, which may or may not have broken through the dura. It is safe to open the optic nerve sheath on its lateral surface to expose the underlying normal arachnoid and a circumferential tumor. As in convexity meningiomas of the brain, these tumors indent the nerve, but usually have an investing arachnoidal plane between the tumor and the underlying pia. The plane is used to good advantage during removal of the tumor and the surrounding involved dura.

The operating microscope, the carbon dioxide laser, the CUSA ultrasonic aspirating device, and fine bipolar forceps are all surgical adjuncts which are quite helpful.

To expose the apex of the orbit and the optic nerve transcranially, we now use a fronto-orbital craniotomy. A minimal amount of hair is shaved to make a bicoronial skin incision. The frontal bone flap is then elevated and includes the orbital rim and orbital roof, which are removed in one piece with the frontal flap. This gives excellent exposure with minimal brain retraction of the apex of the orbit. The most direct surgical approach to the optic nerve is medially between the superior rectus and the levator muscles dorsally and the medial rectus muscle. This approach avoids potential trauma to the nerves passing through the oculomotor foramen. If one is dealing with a large optic nerve meningioma, it may be impossible to excise it intact without debulking with either the cavitron or the laser. After this, transection of the nerve at the globe as well as intradurally is carried out and the tumor is removed, if possible in one piece, by opening by annulus of Zinn. Frequently, however, there is tumor in the intracanalicular portion of the canal that spills in an en bloc fashion around the carotid artery and toward the tuberculum. Standard techniques are used to deal with this.

The primary complication associated with surgical attempts at removal is interference with the central retinal artery or the ophthalmic artery in the posterior medial third of the orbital compartment. In three patients on whom we operated via the lateral approach, we thought we obtained virtually complete removal only to find that we had interfered with the blood supply of the central retinal artery. Since the tumor is circumferential when it reaches the deep apex of the orbit, the central retinal artery must necessarily pass through the tumor prior to perforating the nerve. It is at this juncture that visual compromise occurs in surgical attempts at tumor removal.

The role of radiation therapy in orbital meningiomas is uncertain. However, our preliminary experience, as well as that of others, suggests that arrest of tumor growth, perhaps even with regression, may occur with appropriately administered radiation to these tumors. In patients with apical optic nerve meningiomas who have progressive loss of vision without CT scan evidence of intracranial spread, radiation therapy may be a reasonable consideration. In patients with large exophytic growths presenting with proptosis and preserved vision, we have performed primary debulking procedures for cosmetic purposes and then have given radiation therapy. The apparent arrest of growth in three patients thus treated and followed now for several years is notable. We also are using radiation therapy much more liberally in patients with evidence of recurrence of meningioma in the orbit or intracranially.

In summary, within the last 10 years we have seen incredible advances in imaging and surgical techniques. The CT scan, the operating microscope, the microsurgical instrumentation, and the laser have all resulted in a reorientation of our thinking concerning the management of optic nerve sheath meningiomas as well as many other tumors. On the horizon are magnetic resonance imaging, which may surpass computer tomography in the early detection of these lesions, and milliwatt lasers, which may provide a significantly higher degree of safety in the removal of such tumors. The role of radiation therapy also will unquestionably become better defined.

Supported in Part by a Grant from Allegheny-Singer Research Institute

MENINGIOMA OF THE VISUAL APPARATUS

DONLIN M. LONG, M.D., Ph. D.

Most meningiomas occurring in the base of the skull, except those of the distal clivus, have the potential for involving the visual apparatus. Any of the four principal meningiomas occurring in the anterior skull base routinely present in the chiasmal area. *Tumors of the planum and olfactory groove* may extend posteriorly to compress one optic nerve or the chiasm. Fortunately, these tumors usually carry with them a small amount of arachnoid and brain tissue so that it is possible to dissect the tumor free from the optic nerve and chiasm without great difficulty. *Tumors of the medial sphenoid wing* commonly involve one or both optic nerves as well. Again, these tumors often carry compressed arachnoid, which makes their separation from optic nerve and carotid artery easier. That particular medial tumor which arises in the cavenous sinus is a greater problem. These often surround the carotid artery and are intimately adherent to the optic nerve, even extending into the optic canal. *Tumors of the upper third of the clivus* may extend anteriorly and compress the optic chiasm from beneath or laterally with compression of the optic tracts. These tumors characteristically surround the basilar artery and its branches, making surgical removal hazardous. The classic tumor that affects the anterior visual apparatus is the *tuberculum meningioma*. This tumor is usually spherical, located beneath the chiasm, and affects both optic nerves.

SYMPTOMS AND SIGNS

The cardinal symptom is painless, progressive visual loss. This always suggests a compressive lesion. Visual acuity is usually diminished, at least in one eye, and a multiplicity of unusual field defects are also present. Pain in the eye, proptosis, chemosis, pituitary and hypothalamic insufficiency, amaurosis fugax, and diplopia all occur in conjunction with these tumors. Large olfactory groove tumors may produce anosmia. Medial sphenoid wing tumors can present with seizures and contralateral hemiparesis. The upper clival tumors characteristically produce weakness of one or both sides of the body, coupled with fourth and sixth nerve palsies.

DIAGNOSIS

The diagnosis of these tumors is now made by CT scan. Noncontrast and contrast scans usually suggest that the lesion is a meningioma. Rapid infusion techniques delineate the vascular anatomy. Angiography may be used if there is a suspicion of aneurysm and will locate the carotid arteries. With small tumors, this is not important, but with larger tumors, particularly those of the medial sphenoid wing, it is necessary to know the location and status of the carotid. Embolization of feeding vessels may be helpful, and the neuroradiologist should be alerted to the nature of the tumor before angiography is carried out.

Careful neuro-ophthalmologic examination with determination of acuity, fields, and color fields is important to detail the visual loss and to determine whether the problem is unilateral or bilateral. A prognosis can usually be established, and the examination provides a baseline for monitoring improvement.

TREATMENT

The treatment of all of these lesions is surgical. Once visual symptoms begin, progression to blindness is inexorable. Smaller tumors are much simpler to remove than large ones, and there is little to be gained by waiting, except with those tumors originating in the cavenous sinus and infiltrating bone. Since total surgical removal is rarely possible with sinus tumors, it is reasonable to wait and be certain that a progression of symptoms dictates partial removal.

The surgical approach may be either unilateral or bilateral. A coronal skin incision, coupled with a bifrontal exposure, is useful for large tumors arising on the planum. A unilateral approach suffices for virtually all other tumors. The tuberculum meningioma can be approached by a unilateral subfrontal route or down the sphenoid wing. It is important to remember that even when symptoms are unilateral, there is bilateral involvement of the optic nerve and chiasm in over two-thirds of cases, and both carotid arteries are involved with almost equal frequency. The goal of surgery should be cure with preservation or restoration of normal vision. Total surgical removal is frequently possible now. Vision can nearly always be stabilized. Restoration of vision depends on the damage done by the tumor and is not always possible. In our series of 30 patients, 70 percent were improved or stabilized after surgery, and 30 percent worsened. No eye that was blind improved, but several patients with markedly impaired vision made dramatic improvements to the functional level. Serious permanent damage to a functional nerve is uncommon, occurring only 10 percent of the time in our series. Most patients who are worsened by surgery eventually improve, and a permanent decrease in vision occurred in only 3 eyes in our surgical series.

The laser and cavitron with microsurgical techniques have greatly improved the surgery of meningiomas of the chiasm. Gross total removal is frequently possible. When it is not, radiation or brachytherapy is a consideration. There is not yet enough information to be certain of the value of x-ray therapy for residual tumor. Irradiation of recurrent tumor does seem to improve the patient's symptoms.

ORBITAL TUMOR

NEIL R. MILLER, M.D.

Tumors that originate in, or invade, the orbit produce symptoms and signs by compression, infiltration, and/or infarction of the orbital structures. In some cases, they may act simply as mass lesions, producing only proptosis and generalized limitation of eye movement. Most tumors, however, eventually produce neuro-ophthalmologic symptoms and signs through their effects on the optic nerve, the ocular motor nerves, the orbital branches of the ophthalmic division of the trigeminal nerve, and, rarely, the nerve supply to the iris sphincter and dilator muscles.

GENERAL CONSIDERATIONS

Proptosis

Most orbital tumors produce some proptosis, although the degree of proptosis is not always impressive and may be overlooked during the initial examination. Optic nerve sheath meningiomas, which take up little room within the orbit, usually produce minimal proptosis. Similarly, vascular tumors, which have a soft consistency, may become quite large before they produce significant proptosis. On the other hand, gliomas that involve the orbital portion of the optic nerve usually produce more impressive protrusion of the eye as do firm tumors such as neurinomas and tumors of the lacrimal gland. Tumors located within the extraocular muscle cone (e.g., hemangioma, optic nerve glioma, meningioma) are more likely to produce axial proptosis (the eye is pushed directly forward), whereas tumors outside the muscle cone (dermoid cyst, neurinoma, lacrimal gland tumor) tend to push the eye out and in a direction opposite that of the lesion. Thus, both the amount and direction of proptosis may be helpful in identifying the nature of an orbital process.

Although proptosis is usually caused by orbital processes, lesions outside the orbit, particularly those in the cavernous sinus, may impair venous outflow from the orbit and produce proptosis. In such cases, however, other signs of cavernous sinus disease are usually present, and the use of computed tomography or magnetic resonance imaging is sufficient to allow the correct diagnosis.

Optic Neuropathy

Tumors within the orbit may compress the optic nerve, producing one of three classic syndromes. In some cases, there is progressive visual loss associated with proptosis and swelling of the optic disc. However, many patients retain good visual acuity despite substantial optic disc swelling. This is particularly true in patients with optic nerve gliomas and optic nerve sheath meningiomas. Other tumors that may produce a similar picture are hamartomas (hemangioma, lymphangioma), choristomas (dermoid cyst), and malignant neoplasms (carcinoma, lymphoma, sarcoma, multiple myeloma). In such patients, careful testing of color vision may reveal subtle defects even when visual acuity is thought to be normal. There may occasionally be an afferent pupillary defect. The visual field of the involved eye generally shows only enlargement of the blind spot, although slight peripheral field constriction may also be present. When other signs of orbital disease (proptosis, limitation of ocular motility, orbital congestion) are absent, these patients may be thought to have unilateral "papilledema" from increased intracranial pressure. Nevertheless, while it is obvious that patients with slowly progressive, unilateral visual loss and proptosis associated with optic disc swelling should undergo evaluation for a possible orbital tumor, patients with "isolated" optic disc swelling without visual loss should also undergo such an evaluation as well, particularly when they have no systemic or neurologic symptoms or signs suggestive of increased intracranial pressure. The most common cause of unilateral optic disc swelling without visual loss is orbital disease.

A second form of presentation of orbital tumors is that of unilateral, transient visual loss. The visual loss occurs only in certain positions of gaze and immediately clears when the direction of gaze is changed. It has been assumed that either direct pressure on the optic nerve or interruption of blood supply is the explanation for this phenomenon.

Finally, in many patients with chronic compression of the intraorbital (and intracanalicular) portion of the optic nerve, a specific clinical triad develops: (1) loss of vision, (2) optic disc swelling that resolves into optic atrophy, and (3) the appearance of optociliary shunt veins. Optociliary shunt veins are vessels that overlie the optic disc and shunt blood between the retinal and choroidal venous circulations. The common denominator in patients with this triad appears to be prolonged compression of the optic nerve with gradual compression and obstruction of the central retinal vein. The normal route of retinal venous blood flow is through the central retinal vein directly to the cavernous sinus. Chronic obstruction of the central retinal vein presumably results in dilation of a previously existing system that shunts blood to the choroid, allowing it to leave the eye via the vortex veins. These veins drain directly into the superior and inferior ophthalmic veins that anastomose with the facial and angular veins and with the pterygoid venous plexus. Thus, an outlet is provided for retinal venous blood other than via the central retinal vein to the cavernous sinus. This clinical picture has been described most frequently in patients with spheno-orbital meningiomas, but it may also occur in patients with optic nerve gliomas as well as in patients with other types of chronic optic nerve compression.

Ocular Motor Nerve Paresis

All three of the ocular motor nerves enter the orbit through the superior orbital fissure. Each of these nerves may be damaged by enlarging orbital tumors, resulting in varying degrees of diplopia. Patients may complain of double vision that is horizontal, vertical, or both. Such patients usually have some degree of proptosis, but this is by no means always the case. Tumors that are located at the orbital apex may involve the ocular motor nerves early, before they are large enough to produce proptosis. Thus, such patients may present with a partial oculomotor nerve, abducens nerve, or, rarely, a trochlear nerve paresis. The ophthalmoparesis that is produced by orbital tumors is indistinguishable from that produced by intracranial lesions. The appropriate diagnosis can only be made clinically by the presence of other signs of orbital disease. Often, it is made only when computed tomography or magnetic resonance imaging is performed. The most common orbital tumor that produces diplopia is metastatic carcinoma or lymphoma, although optic nerve gliomas, neurinomas, hemangiomas, and lymphangiomas can also produce it.

It is important to realize that since some orbital tumors may infiltrate or compress one or more of the extraocular muscles, preventing them from functioning properly, the diplopia produced by orbital tumors may be neurogenic or myogenic and is occasionally a combination of both. In such cases, several tests may be used to determine whether a mechanical restriction of ocular motion is present. Mechanical limitation can be inferred if intraocular pressure increases substantially when the patient attempts to look in the direction of gaze limitation. The intraocular pressure measurements are most easily performed by means of a pneumatic tonometer, although any instrument may be used.

Mechanical limitation of motion can also be detected with forced duction (or traction) testing. In such tests, an attempt is made to move the eye forcibly in the direction(s) of gaze limitation. This test is performed as follows. The cornea is anesthetized with several drops of a topical anesthetic such as proparacaine or tetracaine hydrochloride. The conjunctiva is further anesthetized by holding a cotton swab or cotton-tipped applicator soaked with 5 to 10 percent cocaine against it for about 30 seconds. The conjunctiva is then grasped with a fine-toothed forceps near the limbus on the side opposite the direction in which the eye is to be moved. The patient is instructed to try to look in the direction of limitation, and an attempt is made to move the eye in that direction (i.e., opposite that in which mechanical restriction is suspected). If no resistance is encountered, the motility defect is not restrictive; however, if resistance is encountered, then mechanical restriction does exist. In some patients, particularly those who are cooperative and have substantial limitation of movement, the forced duction test can be performed simply by asking the patient to look in the direction of limitation and then attempting to move the eye by placing a cotton-tipped applicator stick against the eye on the opposite side just posterior to the limbus.

Pain

As a general rule, neoplasms that involve the orbit are not painful; however, when pain is present, the tumors are likely to be malignant. Tumors that spread to the orbit from the paranasal sinuses are usually associated with late pain. In some cases, however, pain may be the earliest sign of a tumor involving the orbital apex and cavernous sinus. The pain is severe, continuous, and associated with facial dysesthesia. It has been described as chronic, burning, and intermittently stabbing, and it involves one or more divisions of the trigeminal nerve. When this type of pain is present, it is evidence of intraneural infiltration by neoplastic cells, usually from basal cell, squamous cell, or nasopharyngeal carcinoma. When the pain is combined with involvement of one or more ocular motor nerves, it reliably predicts neural infiltration within the cavernous sinus.

Pupillary Abnormalities

Since both parasympathetic and sympathetic nerve pathways pass through the superior orbital fissure to reach the eye, it is theoretically possible that patients with an orbital tumor could develop either a Horner's syndrome from damage to the oculosympathetic pathway that supplies the iris dilator muscle or a tonic pupil from damage to the ciliary ganglion or short ciliary nerves that supply the iris sphincter muscle. In fact, such abnormalities rarely occur in isolation, probably because tumors that produce them are usually so extensive that they produce oculomotor nerve palsy with pupillary involvement as well. Thus, if there is separate damage to either the sympathetic or parasympathetic fibers, it is usually masked by the oculomotor nerve palsy.

SPECIFIC ORBITAL TUMORS

Because of the many technical advances in orbital surgery, most orbital tumors, even those located in the superior orbit, are outside the province of the neurosurgeon. Such lesions can be more easily and safely managed by the ophthalmic surgeon using any one of a number of approaches. The transcutaneous, transseptal approach is used for palpable tumors within the confines of the anterior orbit. The transcutaneous, extraperiosteal approach is used for palpable tumors thought to lie between the bone and its periorbital covering. A lateral orbitotomy is used for virtually all nonpalpable tumors within the muscle cone as well as for lacrimal gland tumors. Medial orbital tumors can be reached through a transconjunctival approach that is usually combined with a lateral orbitotomy that allows appropriate manipulation of the eye. In addition, there are several tumors that are of concern to the neurosurgeon, and their removal may require a craniotomy with unroofing of the orbit.

Neurinoma

Neurinomas may arise from branches of the ocular motor or trigeminal nerves. They usually begin intracranially, often within the cavernous sinus. Thus, when they involve the orbit, it is usually by extension through the superior orbital fissure. In such cases, a craniotomy or a combined craniotomy-lateral orbitotomy approach is used.

Optic Nerve Glioma

Optic nerve gliomas account for about 3 percent of all orbital tumors. Seventy-five percent of cases of optic nerve glioma present in the first decade of life, and 90 percent are diagnosed by the age of 20 years. The peak incidence is at age 2 to 6 years. Females are affected slightly more often than males. It seems clear that there is a relationship between optic nerve (and chiasmal) gliomas and neurofibromatosis. Among reports of optic nerve gliomas, the incidence of neurofibromatosis varies from 12 to 38 percent. The clinical presentation of optic nerve gliomas falls into two patterns, depending on whether the tumor is primarily orbital or intracranial. Patients with optic nerve gliomas that are primarily intracranial usually present with monocular loss of vision associated with a normal or pale optic disc, and patients with intraorbital optic nerve gliomas usually present with strabismus, proptosis, and optic disc swelling. Pain is unusual. Visual field defects are variable and range from central scotomas to peripheral constriction. With the increasing use of screening computed tomographic scanning and magnetic resonance imaging in patients with neurofibromatosis, more and more asymptomatic optic nerve gliomas are being identified.

The clinical diagnosis of optic nerve glioma can be confirmed by means of either computed tomographic scanning or magnetic resonance imaging. Within the orbit, the tumor is seen as a fusiform enlargement of the optic nerve that is often, but not invariably, associated with enlargement of the optic canal. In view of the excellent imaging techniques currently available, biopsy of such lesions simply to establish the diagnosis is unnecessary.

The management of optic nerve gliomas remains one of the most controversial topics involving ophthalmologists, neurologists, and neurosurgeons. It has been the practice of many physicians to recommend an attempt at complete removal of the tumor as soon as it is diagnosed in an effort to prevent its spread to adjacent structures such as the optic chiasm, the opposite optic nerve, and/or the hypothalamus. In recent years, however, it has been suggested that these tumors have a self-limited growth pattern and behave more like benign hamartomas than true neoplasms. If this were the case, there would certainly be no need to excise them immediately, particularly if there were still vision remaining in the involved eye. It has been my experience that, indeed, many of these lesions show no clinical or radiologic evidence of growth over many years. Some of these tumors, however, clearly possess the ability to expand and spread to adjacent structures. For this reason, I recommend that once a diagnosis of optic nerve glioma is made with relative certainty, the patient be followed closely with respect to both clinical and radiologic parameters. I examine such patients every 6 months and obtain some type of scan every year. Each patient is told to contact me immediately should he or she develop any further loss of vision or other neurologic symptoms. If and when useful vision is lost or there is evidence of tumor growth, I recommend surgical excision via either a transcranial route (if the tumor clearly extends intracranially or if the optic canal is enlarged) or a lateral orbitotomy (if the tumor is clearly confined to the orbit).

Although most optic nerve gliomas are benign, malignant optic nerve gliomas do exist. They usually occur in middle-aged males, producing progressive visual loss, often associated with pain. These tumors are highly invasive and extend along the subpial portion of the nerve compromising its blood supply. The tumor may progress toward the globe, where it produces swelling of the optic disc and subsequent occlusion of the central retinal artery and/or vein. At the same time, the tumor often extends to involve the optic chiasm, the opposite optic nerve, and the hypothalamus. The course is rapid. Most patients are completely blind within 2 to 4 months, and all die within 6 to 9 months. There is at present no surgical or radiotherapeutic treatment for this lesion.

Meningioma

Meningiomas of the orbit may be primary, originating from the sheath of the intraorbital or intracanalicular optic nerve, or secondary, originating along the sphenoid wing or in the basofrontal region and subsequently invading the orbit through bone or foramina. Secondary meningiomas are much more common than are primary intraorbital meningiomas and are usually managed by a combined craniotomy-orbitotomy approach.

In any large series, intraorbital optic nerve sheath meningiomas comprise about 5 to 7 percent of primary orbital tumors. They occur more often in females than in males and usually present in the fourth and fifth decades of life. Patients with optic nerve sheath meningiomas that originate in the orbit usually complain initially of a vague feeling that their vision is abnormal. When such patients are evaluated, they may be found to have normal visual acuity associated with optic disc swelling. Whereas some of these patients can be shown to have color vision defects and/or an afferent pupillary defect in the involved eye, other patients have virtually no clinical visual abnormalities. In such patients, the diagnosis is made only after a computed tomographic scan or magnetic resonance imaging is obtained. By means of such techniques, the orbital optic nerve can be seen to be diffusely thickened. When coronal views of the optic nerve are obtained, the nerve can often be seen to be surrounded by the tumor.

Because these tumors are virtually always located within the subdural space of the optic nerve (between the dura and the pia-arachnoid) and are wrapped completely around the nerve at the time of diagnosis, in most instances, they cannot be removed without sacrificing vision. Occasionally, such tumors are located anteriorly and may be peeled away, but this is a rare phenomenon. Thus, as with optic nerve gliomas, the optimum management of patients with optic nerve sheath meningiomas has not been determined. If there is no evidence of intracranial extension, the patient can be followed until

he or she loses vision, at which time the nerve and tumor can be removed together. However, some physicians suggest immediate surgery in the hope that subsequent intracranial extension can be prevented. At the Johns Hopkins Hospital, we have decompressed the optic canal and opened the intracanalicular dural sheath in eight patients with optic nerve sheath meningiomas. In all patients, the progression of visual loss stopped over a period of follow-up ranging from 3 to 7 years. However, the effect of this procedure on subsequent intracranial spread of the tumor is not yet clear. Similarly, the value of radiotherapy in the treatment of optic nerve sheath meningiomas has not been determined.

HYPOTHALAMIC AND THALAMIC GLIOMA (AND OTHER TUMORS OF THE ANTERIOR THIRD VENTRICLE)

WILLIAM A. SHUCART, M.D.

Over the past several years there has been a resurgence of interest in the diagnosis and treatment of neoplasms involving the thalamus, the hypothalamus, and the anterior third ventricle. The reasons for this are the increasing sophistication in imaging techniques plus refinements in surgical technique and instrumentation, which allow definition of, and access to, these areas with relative safety. Thalamic gliomas will be dealt with specifically and tumors of the hypothalamus and anterior third ventricle dealt with as a group in this chapter.

THALAMIC GLIOMAS

These uncommon tumors comprise a small percentage of all supratentorial gliomas and for years were considered hopeless, certainly in regard to any possibility of resection. They now require increased neurosurgical attention, not because the curability of gliomas has improved, but because it is clear that the unconfirmed diagnosis of glioma is often incorrect; in some reports as many as 30 to 40 percent of lesions diagnosed as thalamic gliomas have turned out to be other, and usually more readily treatable, lesions.

By far the most common presenting sign in thalamic tumors is hemiparesis. On occasion there are sensory abnormalities located in the same distribution, and less commonly, abnormal movements and tremors may be seen in the contralateral extremity similar to those seen in disorders of the basal ganglia. Headaches usually are not part of the symptomatology until there is compromise of

the foramen of Monro, causing hydrocephalus. The presence of a hemiparesis suggests some element of infiltration of the underlying neural structures as opposed to a pedunculated lesion with only a small attachment to the thalamus. On occasion, subtle changes in mentation are noted which are not related to hydrocephalus, and these may occur at a time when the hemiparesis is mild and not of concern to the patient. Unfortunately, we do not usually see these patients until the hemiparesis is obvious.

Computerized tomography is the best widely available way to define these lesions. This technique, utilizing contrast material and reconstruction in both the sagittal and coronal planes, allows excellent appreciation of the origin and extent of the lesion. Arteriography can be useful in further defining the nature of the lesion, but is perhaps most helpful when a craniotomy is planned, for it defines the blood supply to the lesion, displays the vascularity (or lack of it) of the lesion, and demonstrates the vascular supply and drainage of the hemisphere involved, which can affect the surgical approach.

Astrocytomas of varying grade are the most common lesions involving the thalamus, but abscesses, hamartomas, inflammatory lesions, metastatic tumors, etc. have all been reported. The practice of giving radiation therapy without a tissue diagnosis, which was done for many years, is no longer appropriate. The remarkably safe and accurate use of CT-assisted stereotactic biopsies now makes these lesions susceptible to at least a needle biopsy. The stereotactic biopsy can be done under local anesthesia, generally requires only 24 hours of hospital stay, and provides a rational basis for therapy.

If diagnostic studies (CT scan with and without contrast and probably arteriography) are strongly suggestive of an infiltrating glioma, a stereotactic biopsy is done. If the tumor has a heterogeneous appearance on CT scan, biopsies are taken from at least two different areas to better sample the nature of the lesion. A concern with stereotactic biopsy is the possibility of hemorrhage in the biopsy site, which seldom happens. If hemorrhage were to occur, the anticipated consequence would be a worsening of the already present hemiparesis and, very much less likely, some obstruction to CSF pathways by the blood. The latter potential complication is much more theoretical than real. If the biopsy shows a grade I or grade II astrocytoma, our current practice is continued clinical observation, with CT scans done at 6-month or yearly intervals. If there is evidence of growth of the lesion or an increase in the patient's deficit, radiation therapy is instituted. There have been several long-term survivals with these low-grade astrocytomas. If the biopsy shows a grade III or grade IV astrocytoma, the patient is treated according to our current protocol for malignant astrocytomas. This includes conventional radiation therapy to the tumor and an area of 5 cm around the tumor periphery. This is followed with chemotherapy. If the tumor is well demarcated, interstitial implantation of radioactive material to provide a 6000-rad tumor boost to the tumor itself will be given. If the tumor is poorly demarcated, its growth is followed on CT scan; if there is evidence of regrowth, consideration is given to the use of intra-arterial chemotherapeutic agents. The complication we have seen with interstitial implantation of radioactive material is an increase in the hemiparesis. The outlook for the grade III and grade IV astrocytomas is poor, with survival data being no different from those of malignant astrocytomas elsewhere in the brain.

If the CT scan is suggestive of a lesion other than an astrocytoma, arteriography is always done. If the mass appears pedunculated, primarily extra-axial, or has a discrete blood supply suggesting that it may be excisable, a craniotomy is performed. I use primarily a transcallosal approach to the lateral ventricle, which provides an excellent view of the thalamic area regardless of ventricular size. Complications related to the approach through the corpus callosum have been very uncommon; most are related to the location of the lesion and the surgery in that area. Again, the most likely complication is worsening of the hemiparesis. We have removed abscesses, through a formal craniotomy as well as by means of stereotactic aspiration, and have not had any evidence of clinically significant ventriculitis. Ependymomas, hamartomas, and metastatic tumors have all been removed by means of this approach. The small risk of complications is greatly outweighed by the ability to both diagnose and occasionally remove and cure some lesions.

If the diagnosis is uncertain, a stereotactic biopsy is done, and if this shows what should be a resectable lesion, surgery is carried out. In some cases, I was certain that the tumor was malignant astrocytoma, only to have it turn out to be an area of infarction or focal encephalitis, or one of the aforementioned lesions. Given the current sophistication of diagnostic techniques and the safety and low morbidity of stereotactic biopsy, treatment without a tissue diagnosis is no longer appropriate.

TUMORS OF THE THIRD VENTRICLE

These tumors are confusing to categorize because relatively few are solely in the third ventricle; many arise in the paraventricular region and have some component extending into the ventricle. In this chapter, except for the hypothalamic glioma, only tumors that arise solely within the third ventricle will be discussed.

Hypothalamic Gliomas

These tumors are seen primarily in young children, but can occur in any age group. Distinction between a glioma arising in the hypothalamus and one arising in the optic chiasm can be difficult, and as they often have the same symptomatology and treatment plan there is little benefit in attempting a sharp distinction. The clinical symptomatology in these lesions is usually subtle and slowly progressive. The earliest changes, both in children and in adults, may be a change in behavior and personality. In adults, particularly, some disturbance in recent memory is common. Obvious endocrine and optic abnormalities may not occur until late in the course of the disease. Particularly in children in whom visual field defects may not be noticed until they are well advanced, these tumors may be of significant size before being discovered. The only specific syndrome described in hypothalamic gliomas has been the so-called "diencephalic syndrome" (hyperkinesis and alertness associated with emaciation) which is seen in infants. Probably the earliest endocrine abnormality would be some alteration in growth hormone activity, but other expected abnormalities such as diabetes insipidus usually do not occur until late in the course of the disease, if at all. In adults, depending on the growth characteristics of the tumor, visual field disturbances may be the earliest abnormality noted.

In both adults and children, the hypothalamic lesion is usually an astrocytoma and often low-grade (grade I or II). These lesions are not resectable, making the primary purpose of surgery the establishment of tumor type. The prognosis for the low-grade astrocytomas in this area is surprisingly good; many patients survive for several years.

Preopertive CT scanning and arteriography help to establish the nature of the lesion. As in other areas, if the lesion appears to be an astrocytoma, a stereotactic biopsy is likely to be done. The risks of biopsies in this area are minimal. If the lesion appers to be more chiasmatic than hypothalamic, it is safer to perform a craniotomy to allow selection of a biopsy site which will not compromise the optic pathways. If the lesion is a low-grade astrocytoma, the patient is followed with close clinical observation and serial CT scans. If there is evidence of tumor growth or clinical deterioration, radiation therapy is given. If the astrocytoma is grade III or IV, radiation therapy is given. The prognosis for the more malignant astrocytomas is poor, with survival of more than one year being uncommon.

Other Third Ventricular Tumors

Other lesions which occur in the anterior third ventricle include ependymomas, choroid plexus papillomas, choroid plexus carcinomas, meningiomas, hamartomas, and colloid cysts. On rare occasions a craniopharyngioma may arise solely within the third ventricle. Several of these lesions are curable with surgery.

The clinical symptomatology of third ventricular tumors is variable. Because the major portion of these lesions is within the ventricular cavity, there may be no infiltration of surrounding structures to cause localizing signs. The vagueness of the symptoms, plus the fact that these lesions have to be large or strategically placed to cause hydrocephalus, allows them to become sizable before they are clinically detected.

A so-called "ventricular syndrome" is talked about in association with tumors of the third ventricle. This syndrome is thought to be reflective of intermittent acute obstruction of CSF flow, giving rise to episodes of increased intracranial pressure associated with severe headaches. These are said to be brought on and relieved by changes in position. I have rarely seen this particular syndrome and doubt that it is any more common than the evanescence of other headaches associated with increased intracranial pressure. More commonly, the symptomatology secondary to increased intracranial pressure is one of continuous headaches, which may be intermittent initially, becoming progressively more frequent and severe.

Third ventricular lesions give rise to hydrocephalus and increased intracranial pressure nearly 100 percent of the time in children and somewhat less often in adults. Seizures are uncommon; endocrine deficits are uncommon; visual defects are uncommon and may be related to ventricular enlargement rather than to actual involvement of the optic pathway by tumor. Mental changes may be a prominent part of the symptomatology. In children, this can be manifested by irritability and restlessness associated with increased intracranial pressure. In infants, an enlarging head secondary to the hydrocephalus may be the only clinical sign. In adults, changes in recent memory and behavior (particularly increasing apathy) may occur in the absence of increased intracranial pressure, or the signs and symptoms of increased intracranial pressure may be paramount. "Drop attacks", in which the patient suddenly has his legs give out from under him without any associated loss of consciousness, have also been reported with third ventricular lesions, but I have rarely seen this. The reason to suspect the presence of one of these lesions generally revolves around the appearance of increased intracranial pressure without lateralizing hemispheral signs, or a change in behavior, mentation, or memory function in the absence of associated neurological signs.

Plain skull films may be helpful if they show changes secondary to increased intracranial pressure, focal calcifications, and, in children with chiasm-hypothalamic gliomas, the "J-shaped" sella; a normal study does not rule out the possibility of a third ventricular or hypothalamic lesion. The diagnosis of these various lesions is best made by CT scanning, particularly with sagittal and coronal reconstructions. Arteriography is helpful to further elucidate the nature of the lesion and, if relevant, the source of its blood supply.

Because some lesions that occur solely within the third ventricle are benign, curable by resection, and resistant to radiation therapy, it is most rational to obtain a biopsy and, if appropriate, excise these lesions as the preferential form of treatment. If there is no associated visual field defect, we approach these lesions through the corpus callosum and gain access to the third ventricle either through a dilated foramen of Monro, by separating the fornices, or by going subchoroidally in the space between the thalamus and the body of the fornix. Complications of surgery for these lesions have primarily been related to the surgery of the tumor itself and rarely to the approach to the tumor. Although the complications are uncommon, they include significant memory loss, akinetic mutism, hyperthermia, diabetes insipidus, and, on occasion, gastrointestinal bleeding. These complications are generally seen with infiltrative lesions, but can be seen with any surgery in the area of the anterior third ventricle. Most of these deficits would appear with continued growth of the lesion.

The only lesion lying solely within the third ventricle which sometimes is not approached directly is the colloid cyst of the third ventricle (a benign, resectable lesion). In situations in which the patient is a poor operative candidate or has strong objections to surgery, I have inserted a ventriculo-peritoneal shunt to relieve the hydrocephalus and followed the size of the colloid cyst with serial CT scans. Some of these patients have remained asymptomatic for several years with no evidence of cyst growth. The disadvantages of having a shunt in place as opposed to removing the tumor are an increased likelihood of infection and greater susceptibility to serious sequelae from minor head trauma because of the presence of the shunt. If there is any question about the diagnosis, surgery is indicated.

Stereotactic biopsies are also useful in lesions of the third ventricle to determine whether surgical removal is possible.

FORAMEN MAGNUM MENINGIOMA

LEONARD J. CERULLO, M.D.
MATTHEW QUIGLEY, M.D.
YOSEF KRESPI, M.D.

The insidious onset of vague, often migratory, symptoms and confusing neurologic signs usually delays the diagnosis of foramen magnum meningioma until cerebral compensatory mechanisms have been exhausted and decompensation has begun. Although they are uncommon (15% of spinal meningiomas and 1.2 to 3% of all meningiomas) tumors, their successful surgical removal is gratifying to operator and operated. The older age of the patient population (51 years), preoperative neurological deterioration, and location (60% anterior, 20% lateral, and 20% posterior to the spinal cord) render the surgery technically difficult and demanding. Certainly, high-resolution CT scanning and MRI are the tools of choice in terms of establishing the diagnosis. Myelography is becoming of historical interest. Preoperative evaluation should include vertebral angiography because the most frequent site of origin is at the foramen rim adjacent to the entrance of the vertebral artery, and encasement or involvement of this vessel should be appreciated preoperatively. In addition, transverse and sigmoid sinusography may be helpful in determining whether surgical sacrifice of this channel, if indicated, would be feasible.

The surgical approach should offer the following advantages: (1) immediate access to tumor with minimal retraction of already compromised neurologic tissue; (2) minimal thermal and mechanical trauma coincident with tumor removal, (3) preservation of normal arterial and venous anatomy to avoid vascular compromise at the site of the lesion or distal to it; (4) maintenance of craniovertebral stability; (5) avoidance of cranial nerve sacrifice; and (6) complete removal.

The direction of surgical approach is mandated by the location of tumor, its extent, and the preoperative status of the patient. For tumors located directly posterior or posterolaterally, a midline or para-midline vertical incision with exposure of the occiput to include the horizontal portion of the occipital bone and the arch of C1 is performed in routine fashion. At our institution, the operation is performed with the patient in the sitting or prone position while appropriate attention is given to the anesthesiologic considerations. Continuous monitoring of both sensory and brain stem-evoked response is considered mandatory. We prefer craniotomy to craniectomy because of the potential to reconstruct the posterior skull and the ability to thereby improve cosmetic results and comfort. Careful attention is paid to identification and preservation of the vertebral artery as the dissection continues laterally toward the lateral mass of C1 on the side of the tumor. Similarly, dural opening is mandated by the exact location of the lesion, and the configuration of the opening must consider the occipital sinus. Generally, the standard Y-shaped midline incision extended inferiorly into the upper cervical region is adequate. The first step in tumor removal, following exposure, with all meningiomas is the identification and separation of the arachnoidal plane. This isolates the tumor from surrounding, often engulfing, neurovascular structures. Maintenance of this plane between tumor on the one hand and an arachnoid/nervous tissue on the other is essential in preventing damage to these tissues. If the lesion extends significantly into the spinal canal, laminectomy must be appropriately extended. Section of the upper dentate ligaments may allow the neural tissue to retract away while the tumor bulges into the operative exposure. Internal decompression of tumor is done at our institution using the carbon dioxide laser to minimize thermal and mechanical trauma. Bipolar cautery is essential for controlling arterial bleeding from the tumor, although venous and sinusoidal tumor ooze are easily dealt with by aspirating blood from the field while vaporizing in slightly defocused fashion beyond bleeding points. The consistency and vascularity of the tumor dictate the most efficient tool for its internal decompression. The more firm and fibrous the tumor, the more helpful the laser. On the other hand, the more gelatinous the tumor, the more useful is regulated suction or ultrasonic aspiration. Once a significant portion of tumor has been so removed, attention is paid to the capsule. Capsule shrinkage is an effective way to allow the tumor to dissect itself away from surrounding neural and vascular structures. This is performed either with bipolar cautery or with defocused CO_2 laser. By alternating between exenteration (internal decompression) of tumor and shrinkage of the capsule, the neoplasm can be dissected away from the surrounding tissues and its site of origin determined. Throughout, preservation of the arachnoidal plane and maintenance of this space with moist cotton is essential. Although eleventh nerve section has been recommended and is occasionally mandatory, it is usually possible to preserve this structure by removing the tumor from within rather than attempting to dissect it away en bloc. Upon removal of the tumor, dural closure is performed in a watertight fashion, and the occipital bone is replaced. Closure is routine. Since no points of stabilization of the craniovertebral junction have been disrupted, postoperative orthoses are not required. The patient is ambulated as soon as anesthesiologic and medical considerations allow.

Tumors located at the lateral aspect of the foramen magnum are approached through a more lateral exposure. The skin incision is midway between the inion and the mastoid process. It is generally vertical, but superiorly can be extended laterally and anteriorly into the temporal region if the situation warrants. Occipital craniotomy to the foramen magnum and upper cervical laminectomy is performed as indicated. The sigmoid and transverse sinuses are dissected from under the bone, and the bony exposure is extended out laterally into the mastoid air cells and superiorly above the transverse sinus as the tumor location mandates. Similarly, inferior decompression and exposure may mandate removal of the lateral arch and lateral mass of C1, taking care to isolate and protect the vertebral artery. The vessel is surrounded by a venous plexus at this level, but bipolar cautery should be sufficient to ensure hemostasis without injury to the adventitial wall of the vertebral artery. The dural opening is vertical with horizontal extensions or oblique extensions superiorly and inferiorly to allow for maximum exposure of tumor and minimal uncovering of CNS. The sigmoid sinus may be ligated, if necessary, to improve exposure, assuming that preoperative sinusography indicated this to be feasible. The tumor removal follows the same steps as previously outlined. The additional caution, however, is that extreme care must be exercised in skeletalizing the vertebral artery and its major branches. Postoperative care is routine.

Tumors located at the anterior rim of the foramen magnum and extending superiorly or inferiorly pose the greatest challenge. Although the transoral route has been recommended, we find this too confining in terms of surgical exposure and prefer the transmandibular approach. The patient is placed supine. A tracheostomy is performed through the second or third tracheal ring. A horizontal neck incision is made 3 fingerbreadths below the mandible. The incision is extended to the mastoid tip posteriorly and to the submental region anteriorly. After the platysma muscle is divided the dissection is carried beneath the submandibular gland. The digastric tendon and the stylohyoid muscle are released from their attachment and reflected superiorly with the submandibular gland. The sternocleidomastoid muscle is retracted laterally to expose the carotid sheath. The jugular vein and the common carotid artery are identified. The internal and external carotid arteries are followed toward the skull base deep to the posterior belly of the digastric. Initially, a suture ligature is placed around the external carotid artery at a point distal to the superior thyroid artery, thus diminishing blood loss. The hypoglossal, vagus, and spinal accessory nerves are identified and preserved. The incision is then carried toward the lower lip. A midline lip-splitting incision is made in a staggered fashion, exposing the anterior portion of the mandible. The gingival and labial mucosa are incised. The mucoperiosteum is elevated, and the lower lip is pulled away from the midline to expose the anterior portion of the mandible.

Prior to mandibulotomy, four drill holes are made for wire fixation and immobilization of the mandibular segments for later closure. An oscillating power saw can be used to divide the mandible stepwise between the drill holes. The tongue is retracted to the opposite side, and the floor-of-the-mouth mucosa is divided. The supporting musculature, the myohyoid, the hypoglossus, and the anterior belly of the digastric are divided. The postganglionic fibers from the lingual nerve to the submandibular gland are transected. The lingual nerve is identified and may be preserved. The hemimandible may be retracted further after splitting the floor of the mouth. This exposes the parapharyngeal space and its structures. To increase exposure, the neck incision is deepened in the suprahyoid region until it is continuous with the oral cavity incision. For maximal mandibular retraction laterally, the external carotid artery distal to the lingual artery must be divided. This allows greater access to the infratemporal fossa and the parapharyngeal space. The intraoral incision is extended upward onto the palate and pterygoid plates. The resultant mucoperiosteal incision is extended along the hard palate 1 cm medial to the gingival margin. The hemipalatal flap may then be elevated by sacrifice of the greater palatine artery and nerves on the side of the dissection. With blunt dissection, a surgical space is created behind the superior and middle constrictor muscles above the hypoglossal nerve. The dissection is extended superiorly between the prevertebral fascia and the constrictor muscles. The styloglossus and the stylopharyngeal muscles, as well as the glossopharyngeal nerve, are divided. Incision of these structures allows retraction of the oral pharynx to the contralateral side, consequently widening the retropharyngeal dissection plane. To detach the nasopharynx from the skull base without tearing its mucosa and musculature, the eustachian tube and both palatine muscles must be divided. This is performed under direct vision. This maneuver maintains the integrity of the tube and detaches the nasopharynx from the skull base. The nasopharynx and oral pharynx are now retracted across the midline to the opposite side. This exposes the upper cervical spine, foramen magnum, clivus, and midline compartment of the skull base.

A high-speed drill is then used to bur down the mid to lower clivus as far as the foramen magnum. Inferior exposure is made by removal of the arch of C1, the dens, and, if necessary, the body of C2. Further inferior dissection can be obtained by removing appropriate vertebral segments. The dura is opened in an I-shaped fashion and reflected laterally. This affords excellent access to tumor anterior to the brain stem. It also allows considerable lateral excursion through the wide surgical field. Again, tumor removal is as previously outlined. Closure of the dura can be performed either primarily or with a fascial graft. The dura can be maintained in position either with direct suturing or with hemoclips. An alternative is the use of CO_2 laser for gentle welding of the structure. The dural closure should be watertight. Unless the dissection has been carried out laterally to involve one or both occipital condyles, stabilization is not necessary. If sufficient C1-C2 dissection has been performed, a posterior cervical fusion may be required at a subsequent sitting. The closure of the nasal and oral pharynx reattaches the superior constrictor muscles to paraspinal muscles at the skull base. A nasogastric tube is inserted for postoperative nutrition. Cricopharyngeal myotomy is mandatory prior to the pharyngeal closure. The palatal flap is approximated in a single layer by suturing the mucosa. A palatal splint may be applied to obtain adherence of the flap to the hard palate. The lateral floor of the mouth incision is closed with simple one-layer nonabsorbable sutures. The anterior floor of the mouth is best prepared after the mandible has been wired together. A lingual splint is wired around the premolar teeth to reinforce the mandibular closure. Intermaxillary fixation is not required. The floor-of-the-mouth suture line is supported by approximation of the myohyoid and the digastric muscles. A large soft suction catheter is placed along the carotid sheath extending upward to the nasopharynx. The catheter exits from a separate stab incision in the lower neck. Lip incision is closed in three layers taking care to approximate the vermilion border accurately. The platysma and neck skin are closed in the usual fashion. Our experience has demonstrated that contamination of the surgical field is not a concern if prophylactic antibiotic coverage is begun preoperatively and con-

tinued for 72 hours postoperatively. The transcervical transmandibular surgical technique provides wide field exposure and access to the midline compartments of the skull base.

The foregoing surgical approaches should offer a total access to lesions at the foramen magnum. Naturally, the anatomy of each individual lesion mandates the optimal surgical approach. The surgery, often extensive, is gratifying in terms of patient outcome because of its emphasis on exposure, minimal retractor, preservation of neural and vascular anatomy, and minization of trauma.

CONVEXITY MENINGIOMA

DAVID G. PIEPGRAS, M.D.

Cerebral convexity meningiomas are relatively common, but less so than those arising from the midline falx or sphenoid wing, the majority being located anterior to the rolandic fissure. As pointed out so clearly by Cushing, tumors arising close to the rolandic fissure and hence the primary sensory-motor areas of the brain are apt to make their presence known relatively earlier and at a smaller size than tumors located more anteriorly or posteriorly. In the pararolandic areas, convexity meningiomas typically present with focal seizure phenomena, or with a slowly progressive contralateral paresis, or with a combination of these. With dominant hemisphere tumors, aphasia may be present as well. In the more silent areas, especially frontal, the tumors may attain large proportions before causing nonspecific mental disturbances including dementia or symptoms and signs of increased intracranial pressure without focal deficits. Currently, recognition of such symptoms and signs leads to a computerized tomographic (CT) examination of the head, which is certainly the single most definitive test in detecting and diagnosing cerebral convexity meningiomas. It is important to realize, however, that even large tumors may escape detection unless scanning is carried out with intravenous contrast augmentation, which tends to enhance the tumor in a striking fashion compared to the surrounding brain. Also, particularly when the clinical picture suggests a high-convexity lesion, as with progressive spastic paresis affecting one lower extremity, the CT cuts should be carried to the very top of the cerebral hemisphere. Occasionally, in elderly patients undergoing scanning for other reasons, small and even moderate-sized tumors may be identified which are, in fact, asymptomatic, and in these situations no specific treatment for the meningioma is usually indicated.

In large tumors, plain films of the head may show

characteristic changes of convexity meningioma, including increased vascular markings and hyperostosis of the inner table of the skull. For surgical planning, carotid angiography, usually with selective external and internal carotid studies, is manditory to demonstrate the exact site of tumor origin as well as its blood supply from meningeal and cerebral vessels. Particularly in cerebral convexity meningiomas, meningeal branches of the external carotid artery constitute the primary tumor supply, although there are often contributions from scalp and cerebral arteries as well.

The treatment of symptomatic cerebral convexity meningiomas consists of complete excision of the tumor with its dural attachments and removal of any involved overlying bone. Preoperative treatment with steroids is desirable inasmuch as these tumors may induce considerable edema in the adjacent cerebral tissue. Perioperative anticonvulsant prophylaxis should be considered in all cases, especially pararolandic tumors, and is manditory in patients who have experienced overt seizures. In the latter cases it is necessary to continue anticonvulsant therapy for 6 to 12 months postcraniotomy and indefinitely if seizures recur thereafter.

Excision of the tumor is accomplished through a craniotomy designed to expose the entire circumference of the tumor. The dura is opened around the margins of the tumor and, where necessary, left attached to the tumor to minimize operative bleeding. Smaller tumors may be reflected away from the underlying brain tissue and removed in a single specimen, whereas larger tumors should be internally debulked and the shell of the remaining tumor then elevated away from the brain, taking care to disturb the cerebral tissue and vasculature, especially the surface-draining veins, as little as possible. Internal decompression may be adequately achieved by traditional methods of sharp dissection and electrocautery cutting loops or by newer instrumentation such as ultrasonic fragmentation of the tumor. Reduction of the tumor may also be accomplished with CO_2 laser, but this technique is rarely necessary in convexity tumors, which are readily accessible to surface dissection. Usually total removal of the tumor is possible, and recurrence is uncommon except for those rare cases of malignant or mitotically active meningioma, which may actually invade the adjacent brain. In the latter cases, multiple reoperations and even local radiation therapy may be necessary.

Postoperative care, as with all craniotomy cases, requires close observation for neurologic deterioration secondary to intracranial hematoma, cerebral edema, and seizures. The advisability of perioperative steroid administration and anticonvulsants has already been mentioned. Although cortical vein thrombosis is uncom-

mon, it may produce devastating hemorrhagic infarction should it develop; meticulous operative technique to protect major surface veins adjacent to the tumor is most important in its prevention, but adequate hydration and head elevation after operation may also be beneficial. The impression of widely experienced surgeons that postoperative meningioma patients are at increased risk for deep venous thrombosis and pulmonary embolus may lack statistical foundation, but should incline today's neurosurgeons toward appropriate prophylactic measures short of anticoagulation.

SPHENOID WING MENINGIOMA

CLARK WATTS, M.D.

Sphenoid wing meningiomas are actually meningiomas arising on the sphenoid ridge, a curvilinear bony structure which begins medially at the anterior clinoid and ends laterally at the pterion, separating the anterior fossa from the middle fossa. Its medial two-thirds is composed of the inner wing of the sphenoid bone, and the outer third the flaring margin of the greater wing of the sphenoid.

Cushing, in his major treatise on meningiomas, divided sphenoid wing meningiomas into three groups, based on their location on the sphenoid ridge. The clinoidal meningiomas were found on the medial third of the sphenoid ridge, the alar group on the middle third, and the frontoparietal or pterional on the outer third. I believe it is now more appropriate to divide these tumors into a medial location corresponding to Cushing clinoidal tumors and a lateral location, which would encompass the lateral two-thirds of the sphenoid ridge. This division is appropriate, and is based on presentation of the patient, requirements of evaluation procedures, and complications and results. There is a third group of related tumors, presenting much less frequently than the 18 percent of meningiomas which are located on the sphenoid ridge proper. These tumors are found extremely laterally, confined to the lateral dura in the region of the pterion, arising in an en plaque configuration in contradistinction to those found on the sphenoid ridge proper, which primarily are globular in presentation.

PRESENTATION

The clinical presentation of the tumor depends on its location. Although the tumor may arise on the crest of the ridge, theoretically it may grow more into the middle fossa or into the frontal fossa, or it may project directly superior and posterior into the region of the Sylvian fissure separating the frontal and temporal lobes.

Characteristically, the medial sphenoid wing meningiomas arise in the angle formed by the clinoid and the area of the cavernous sinus. These begin very early to involve the structures in this area, producing fairly characteristic and potentially devastating neurological deficits. The optic nerve may be involved early, producing unilateral amblyopia or, with involvement of the optic chiasm, a homonymous hemianopsia. Involvement of the structures entering the supraorbital fissure, including the third, fourth, and sixth cranial nerves, may result in unilateral ophthalmoplegia. The fifth nerve, especially the ophthalmic division, may be involved early, resulting in corneal hypesthesia. Compromise of venous drainage in the area may produce venous engorgement and exophthalmos. In addition, if the tumor should grow primarily superiorly and frontally, the ipsilateral olfactory nerve may be compromised. The location of the tumor is such that the medial posterior basilar portion of the frontal lobe and the medial aspect of the temporal lobe may be disturbed, producing so-called "uncinate" fits among other symptomatology. The patient may have seizures with an aura of a disturbance of smell, which is described in many ways. Often described is a pungent, disagreeable smell of burnt oil or other such odors. The tumor often displaces the proximal portion of the internal carotid artery. Rarely, it may actually encompass the artery, producing constriction and resulting in initial complaints that suggest transient ischemic episodes such as transient amblyopia, hemiparesis, and, if on the left side, speech disorders.

The lesions on the outer two-thirds of the sphenoid wing are comparatively much quieter. They can become quite large, causing chronic complaints of only mild headache. If the tumor should produce marked hyperostosis of the sphenoid wing and the adjacent orbit, the patient may note exophthalmos of a chronic nature and decreased vision. The symptoms may be present for several years; reports of 20 to 30 years in the older literature are not uncommon. The tumor may grow superiorly and posteriorly into the Sylvian fissure, producing temporal lobe disturbances manifested by seizures.

The more laterally placed en plaque meningioma is usually seen as a thin layer of tumor involving the dura with marked overlying hyperostosis. Some of these tum ors appear to be extremely aggressive, invading not only the bone, but also the overlying temporalis muscle. The hyperostosis may extend anteriorly into the lateral wall of the orbit producing—as with the outer, more globular, sphenoid wing meningioma—visual compromise and exophthalmos.

DIAGNOSIS

The diagnostic procedure of choice today for any patient suspected of having a brain tumor is computerized tomography (CT scan), and this is no less true of sphenoid wing meningiomas. Even the smaller tumors, if large enough to produce objective neurological deficits, can be seen on most unenhanced scans, but they are seen more clearly on the enhanced scan. The location of the lesion, coupled with the chronicity of the neurological symptoms and signs, should lead one to strongly suspect a meningioma. However, depending on the location, the diagnostic work-up should not stop at that point. Most of these tumors should not be surgically approached without an arteriogram. Certainly the inner-third tumors, because of their propensity to compromise in some manner the internal carotid artery, should be so investigated. However, these tumors, because of their dural involvement, should be investigated angiographically also for the external carotid artery component of their blood supply. The lateral globular meningiomas and the en plaque meningiomas, are especially richly supplied by branches of the external carotid artery, particularly the middle meningeal artery. It may be wise for the surgeon to attack this blood supply either by ligating the external carotid artery directly or by the use of more peripherally placed emboli with intravascular catheter techniques prior to an intracranial approach.

Patients with clinoidal meningiomas should have baseline visual acuity and visual field examinations. This information may later be of value to the surgeon or personal physician in observing the patient for evidence of recurrence. Of lesser importance, but probably of some use, would be electroencephalographic examination of patients with seizure disorders. It is my feeling that any such patient who presents with seizures, who develops seizures after surgery, or who has EEG evidence of spike foci should be placed on anticonvulsants until either he or she has been seizure-free for one year or no EEG evidence of potential seizure activity is recorded.

SURGICAL CONSIDERATION

These tumors, like all meningiomas, grow at variable speeds but usually quite slowly. The location of the tumor will determine the rapidity with which the patients neurological signs and symptoms progress and, therefore, the urgency for surgery. The clinoidal tumors cause symptoms relatively early and therefore at a smaller size.

This presents a major dilemma for the surgeon and the patient. Early the neurological signs are potentially reversible. However, because of the location of the tumor, even microsurgical techniques do not militate against significant neurological damage as a result of surgery. The longer the decision is delayed regarding surgery, the greater the potential for irreversible neurological deficit produced by the tumor and the greater the surgical difficulty in removing the tumor, irrespective of the potential for surgically manipulated deficits. Thus it is imperative that the patient have more than just adequate informed consent about the potential risks and benefits of surgical versus nonsurgical care.

There is no other uniformly accepted therapy for these tumors. Some investigators report promising results with high-energy forms of radiation therapy for this tumor, but none have recommended, based on well-studied experience, substituting irradiation for surgery. Although the blood supply is often well demonstrated angiographically, this supply comes through numerous small branches of the external carotid artery at the base of the tumor, none of which are suitable for definitive embolization. To date there is no demonstrated efficacy of chemotherapy, hyperthermia, or other experimental modes of brain tumor therapy in this group of tumors.

As already noted, the lateral group of global tumors tend to present early with headache and perhaps temporal lobe seizures. Now that CT scan is used in diagnosing these patients, the tumors are being noted earlier. In evaluating the decision to operate, one must consider that these tumors may be present many years without causing significant deficits. Their progress can be followed closely with little risk and cost to the patient by periodic CT scan. If the seizure disorder, which may not be corrected by surgery, is controlled with anticonvulsants, one might wish to simply observe the patient over time. This is especially true if the patient is in the later decades of life. My own personal bias is to remove the tumor as soon as it is diagnosed if the patient is at all symptomatic and otherwise a respectable surgical candidate. Although it is acknowledged that there is a 5 to 10 percent recurrence rate for meningiomas that are "completely" excised, the unpredictable possibility that these meningiomas may spontaneously hemorrhage and the probability of greater cortical damage with time and therefore a more severe seizure disorder lead me to believe my approach to be reasonable.

I especially believe that this approach is reasonable with the en plaque meningioma. Cushing described several of these cases, which presented with huge bony and soft tissue defects that resulted from lateral, rather than intracranial, growth of the tumor. This type of presentation is now less likely to be seen because of the relative medical sophistication of the general public and the ease of diagnosis with CT scans. Therefore, we should see these tumors at a much earlier period in their neoplastic life. The larger the tumor, the more difficult it is to excise and the greater the cosmetic deficit produced by the excision. Therefore, I believe it worthwhile to remove these tumors when they are found, given the aforementioned caveat regarding surgical candidacy.

Whereas the outer, more globular, sphenoid wing meningiomas, especially those that do not attain great size, are certainly approachable by most trained and experienced neurosurgeons today, removal of the clinoidal meningioma and the en plaque meningiomas should be carried out by surgeons who have special experience and expertise in these specific areas. Removal of the clinoidal tumors requires significant expertise in microsurgical technique. Removal of en plaque meningiomas requires an understanding of the surgical approaches to the lateral and, particularly, the basal skull in the temporal and frontal area, to include the orbit, and the reconstruction of these areas following excision of the tumor.

For the en plaque meningioma and the more laterally placed outer sphenoid wing meningioma, I prefer a straight vertical incision and a free bone flap centered in the pterional region. This permits the surgeon to cut away, with a rongeur, the involved sphenoid wing or the lateral roof of the orbit. The involved dura can be incised and replaced with suitable galea, with fascia lata, or with frozen cadaver dura. I do not use the artificial dural substitutes because of an increased occurrence of CSF leaks with this material.

For the clinoidal tumors, I prefer a frontotemporal bone flap. This permits either a frontal or a more temporal approach, depending on the presentation of the tumor and the progression of the surgical resection. As previously noted, when the angiogram shows extensive external carotid artery vascularization of the more laterally placed tumor, I encourage the neuroradiologist to assist me in embolizing specific large feeding vessels. These are usually branches of the middle meningeal, superficial temporal, or internal maxillary artery.

Although I plan a total resection for virtually every tumor I see, rarely do I place the patient at significant risk for operative neurological deficit by attempting more than a subtotal removal. The surgeon, the referring physician, and the patient should know the skills and limitations of the surgeon, and the procedure should follow only after a frank discussion of the significant risks and the impact of these risks, should they be translated into actual complications, on the life style of the patient. Although symptoms seem to appear earlier with each recurrence, these tumors do grow rather slowly. Fifteen years of gradually decreasing vision and oph-thalmoparesis, punctuated by two or three operative procedures, may be much better for the patient than 15 years of blindness and complete ophthalmoplegia without recurrence following a single radical surgical procedure.

COMPLICATIONS

It is not difficult to imagine the complications that are associated with surgical procedures for these tumors if one just visualizes their location, the anatomy, and the presenting neurological signs and symptoms.

Injury to the carotid artery during the removal of a clinoidal meningioma is, unfortunately, not a rare report in the literature. Removal of these tumors can lead to misadventures which result in injury to the optic chiasm; ophthalmoplegia may occur following injury to the third, fourth, and sixth cranial nerves, and corneal hypesthesia from injury to the first division of the trigeminal nerve. Blindness may result from injury to the optic nerve or from injury to the ophthalmic artery, the first intracranial branch of the internal carotid artery. Carotid injury may result in cerebral infarction, or in fatal hemorrhage if the cavernous sinus is injured.

Except for the attendent general risks of general anesthesia and craniotomy, namely, idiosyncratic reactions to drugs, technical errors in oxygen supply, disorders that are the result of the positioning of the patient (e.g., peripheral nerve compressions), and infection and CSF leak following craniotomy, removal of the lateral or outer sphenoid wing meningiomas is relatively uncomplicated. Because of the presentation, however, cortical injury to the frontal and temporal lobes may occur during dissection of the tumor within the Sylvian fissure. This may lead to new or increased seizure activity and, on the left side, to disorders of speech, especially of the expressive, nonfluent, or Broca's type. Because of the relatively extensive involvement of bone by the en plaque meningioma, the subsequent surgical cosmetic result may be devastating to the patient, especially the young person. This removal often requires extensive bone removal and, occasionally, removal of temporalis muscle and the lateral wall of the orbit. With extensive infiltration of the wall of the orbit, injury to the orbital contents, including the rectus muscles, the globe, and the optic nerve, may occur during surgery.

CHOROID PLEXUS PAPILLOMA AND OTHER TUMORS OF THE LATERAL VENTRICLE

K. STUART LEE, M.D.
DAVID L. KELLY, Jr., M.D.

A tumor arising in the ventricular system is one of the most challenging problems in neurosurgery. These tumors are often slow-growing and many are benign; hence, their removal often leads to a cure or at least a prolonged period of tumor-free existence. However, the successful removal of tumors in the ventricular system requires careful preoperative planning and meticulous surgical technique. The relative rarity of these tumors means that many neurosurgeons lack experience in their management.

CHOROID PLEXUS PAPILLOMAS

Tumors of the choroid plexus account for 0.4 to 0.6 percent of all brain tumors. Although choroid plexus papillomas have been reported in patients from birth to the eighth decade of life, about half of these tumors occur in patients younger than 20 years. In adults, choroid plexus papillomas are most common in the fourth ventricle; in children, they are most common in the lateral ventricles. They have a propensity for the left lateral ventricle, and the atrium of the lateral ventricle is the usual site of origin. Choroid plexus papillomas rarely occur in the third ventricle.

The symptoms of choroid plexus papillomas are usually those of increased intracranial pressure. Most patients have headache, nausea, vomiting, dizziness, and diplopia as presenting symptoms. The headache may be positional and is often worse early in the morning. Occasionally, tumors arising in the fourth ventricle are manifested by ataxia, nystagmus, and cranial nerve palsies. The symptoms in an infant are often those of hydrocephalus, as well as failure to thrive and irritability.

Several mechanisms have been proposed as the cause of hydrocephalus related to choroid plexus papillomas. There may be an increased production of cerebrospinal fluid (CSF) in very large tumors; the CSF pathways may be obstructed by tumor; or recurrent hemorrhages from the tumor may obstruct the CSF pathways. Finally, there is the rare patient who presents with a symptom complex similar to that of a subarachnoid hemorrhage and who has an intraventricular hemorrhage with acute hydrocephalus secondary to the hemorrhage.

The treatment of choroid plexus papillomas is surgical excision. For the rare choroid plexus papilloma of the third ventricle, surgery is accomplished through either a transcallosal or a transcortical-transventricular approach, just as is any other tumor of the anterior third ventricle. Removal of choroid plexus papillomas of the fourth ventricle is accomplished through a standard midline suboccipital craniectomy, just as is any other lesion occurring in the fourth ventricle. Tumors of the fourth ventricle often extend through the foramen of Luschka or may be attached to the floor of the fourth ventricle so that their total removal is impossible. The surgical management of choroid plexus papillomas of the lateral ventricle will be discussed in the section entitled *Treatment of Intraventricular Tumors.*

INTRAVENTRICULAR MENINGIOMAS

Intraventricular meningiomas account for 0.5 to 2 percent of all intracranial meningiomas. Female patients are affected twice as often as male patients. The incidence in relation to age is similar to that of other meningiomas, the peak incidence being in the fifth to sixth decade. Most intraventricular meningiomas are located in the lateral ventricle, but occasionally one is found in the fourth ventricle or the anterior third ventricle. Of the lateral ventricular meningiomas, 85 to 90 percent arise in the trigone of the lateral ventricle, with the other 10 to 15 percent arising in the anterior horn near the foramen of Monro. In early articles, it was reported that the left lateral ventricle was affected more often than the right, but some recent articles report the incidence to be about the same. Some authors classify meningiomas of the lateral ventricle into those arising from the glomus of the choroid and conforming to the shape of the ventricle and those arising from the velum interpositum and assuming a different configuration. Others dispute this classification.

The symptoms of an intraventricular meningioma are due to obstruction of CSF pathways or to pressure on surrounding brain tissue, and may be quite nonspecific. Most patients with intraventricular meningiomas have headache accompanied by nausea and vomiting; personality changes are relatively common, as are visual symptoms, motor deficits, and seizures. Visual field deficits are often the most common physical findings, with motor and sensory deficits being somewhat less common in most series. Ataxia and incoordination are also relatively common. Speech difficulties may be produced by a tumor located in the dominant hemisphere.

The treatment of intraventricular meningiomas is surgical excision. Many of these tumors are large when diagnosed, and their surgical excision can be difficult. The surgical techniques are to be discussed.

GLIOMAS OF THE LATERAL VENTRICLE

Gliomas occurring in the lateral ventricle include astrocytomas and ependymomas. Astrocytomas in the ventricular system are relatively uncommon, and tend to arise in either the midbody or frontal horn of the lateral ventricle.

Ependymomas account for approximately 5 percent of all gliomas, and the average age of a patient with an ependymoma is approximately 23 years. About half of all ependymomas arise in the fourth ventricle, the lateral ventricles being the next most common sites. Within the lateral ventricles, they appear to have no one characteristic location, although some articles record a higher frequency at the temporoparietal-occipital junction. These tumors often adjust their shape to the ventricle and grow into adjacent brain tissue by a process of expansion rather than infiltration.

The presenting symptoms of gliomas of the lateral ventricles are nonspecific, approximately 80 percent of patients having headache and usually nausea and vomiting. Ataxia and vertigo are also common; seizures are relatively common. Physical findings include papilledema, focal neurologic deficits such as paresis or sensory deficits, and visual field deficits.

Treatment of gliomas of the lateral ventricles consists of surgical excision followed by radiation therapy. Often their total surgical removal is not possible. The operative approach should allow access for biopsy, since histologic identification of the tumor may aid in the decision regarding further resection. Radiation therapy plays an important role in the management of these tumors, especially for the ependymoma, which is second only to medulloblastoma in its radiosensitivity. All ependymomas tend to seed through CSF pathways, although those of the fourth ventricle seed most commonly. Due to this tendency for CSF seeding, irradiation of both the cranial and the spinal contents is advocated for ependymomas. Ependymoblastomas are malignant, and they tend to metastasize rather than to seed.

OTHER TUMORS OF THE LATERAL VENTRICLE

Angiomas of the choroid plexus can occur in the lateral ventricle, but are extremely rare. The presenting symptom of these tumors is usually a spontaneous intraventricular hemorrhage. Teratomas are usually midline tumors, but they can occur in the lateral ventricle. Epidermoid and dermoid tumors are also usually midline tumors and only rarely occur in the lateral ventricle. Sarcomas are usually found on the surface of the brain connected to the meninges, but an occasional sarcoma of a lateral ventricle has been reported.

DIAGNOSIS OF INTRAVENTRICULAR TUMORS

Because the symptom complex of intraventricular tumors is nonspecific, ancillary studies are necessary for diagnosis. Skull roentgenograms may show evidence of increased intracranial pressure in the child. There may be calcification of the tumor, especially of choroid plexus papillomas, two-thirds of which in some series have been reported to be calcified. Electroencephalography (EEG) may be useful in patients with seizure disorders, since intraventricular tumors that have infiltrated adjacent brain may have focal signs. However, the EEG findings are nonspecific and often are normal.

Computed tomography (CT) of the head is the best way at present to diagnose an intraventricular tumor. Hydrocephalus may be seen with any of the intraventricular tumors and is a nonspecific finding. On noncontrast CT, a choroid plexus papilloma is usually a well-defined, smoothly marginated mass of increased density. With infusion of contrast, the tumor enhances intensely and usually homogeneously. An intraventricular meningioma is also of increased density before infusion and often enhances homogeneously after infusion of contrast. However, the meningioma is less likely to be confined to the ventricle, and it may be very large by the time a CT scan is obtained. The age difference in patients with lateral ventricle meningiomas versus those with choroid plexus papillomas is helpful in making the diagnosis. Ependymomas are often isodense or hypodense before infusion and may have punctate areas of calcification. Ependymomas enhance with infusion of contrast, but not homogeneously. Astrocytomas of the ventricle are usually isodense or hypodense and do not enhance greatly. By considering the patient's age, as well as the location and degree of enhancement of the tumor, one can diagnose many types of intraventricular tumors from noninfused and infused CT scans.

Arteriography is also important in the diagnosis of an intraventricular tumor, as well as in preoperative planning. Many of these tumors, especially the choroid plexus papilloma and the intraventricular meningioma, are supplied by the anterior or posterior choroidal arteries, and identification of a tumor's major blood supply is essential in the planning of the operative approach.

TREATMENT OF INTRAVENTRICULAR TUMORS

The treatment of these lesions is surgical excision if possible. Preoperation care of the patient includes the use of steroids and anticonvulsants. Some patients require preoperative CSF diversion in the form of either an external ventricular drain or a shunt.

One aspect of intraventricular tumor surgery that is applicable to all the various approaches is use of the route that allows the best access to the tumor and its blood supply while avoiding damage to functional areas. Retraction on the hemispheres should be minimal to avoid postoperative neurological deficits.

The most common site for lateral ventricle tumors is the trigone region, and most choroid plexus papillomas and intraventricular meningiomas occur in this region. Several approaches to the atrium of the lateral ventricle have been introduced, but none are completely satisfactory. A cortical incision in the lateral temporoparietal region is useful in that there is little brain tissue between the cortical surface to the tumor and the atrium of the ventricle. However, the anterior and posterior choroidal arteries are hidden by the bulk of the tumor in the ventricular system. If a highly vascular lesion, such as a choroid plexus papilloma, is removed en bloc by this approach, extensive manipulation of the tumor is required which could result in damage to adjacent brain. Piecemeal removal of such a tumor could lead to uncontrollable blood loss due to the inability to see feeding vessels. Postoperative language deficits may be present if the operation is carried out in the lateral temporoparietal region on the dominant side.

An incision in the posterior part of the middle temporal gyrus allows the surgeon to be close to the tumor and to deal with blood supply of the tumor early in the procedure, since the choroidal arteries enter the lateral ventricle in the medial and inferior aspect of the ventricle. However, postoperative language deficits are also possible when this approach is used in the dominant hemisphere. The trigone region of the lateral ventricle can also be approached through an incision in the occipital lobe or through an occipital lobectomy, but both approaches make it difficult to control the blood supply to the tumor early in the resection, and both commonly result in postoperative visual field deficits.

It should be stressed that choroid plexus papillomas should not be removed in a piecemeal fashion since, especially in children, this may result in uncontrollable blood loss. These tumors should be removed en bloc after the main feeding artery to the tumor has been divided. Because intraventricular meningiomas are often as large, it may be necessary to remove them piecemeal, but again that should be done only after occlusion of the feeding vessels in order to avoid excessive bleeding.

Since no one approach for excision of tumors of the trigone is adequate for all tumors, it is important that the surgeon be familiar with all approaches, and that his or her selection of the approach be based on the individual patient's CT scan and arteriogram. It may also be necessary to combine more than one approach in a single patient.

Tumors of the midbody of the lateral ventricles are often extremely difficult to approach and remove. They tend to be present in both lateral ventricles by the time the patient seeks medical attention. A lateral transcortical incision, which would allow the surgeon to traverse little brain tissue before reaching the tumor, cannot be used because the midbody of the ventricle lies just below the motor and sensory cortices. When the tumor occurs in just one lateral ventricle and obtains its blood supply from the anterior choroidal artery, a cortical incision made in the middle frontal gyrus on the side of the tumor and carried down to the ventricle may be used. However, for tumors that occur in both midbodies, a transcallosal approach is probably most appropriate. This approach involves a craniotomy at the level of the coronal suture. An arteriogram must have been obtained preoperatively to define the anatomy of the venous drainage of the superior sagittal sinus, and the bone flap should be placed on the side that requires the sacrifice of the fewest veins. The right frontal lobe is retracted laterally, and the corpus callosum is identified. A longitudinal incision is made in the corpus callosum and the lateral ventricle is entered. The pericallosal arteries should be preserved.

Tumors of the frontal horn are usually ependymomas or astrocytomas, as already noted, but approximately 10 percent of intraventricular meningiomas occur in the frontal horn near the foramen of Monro. For a tumor in the frontal horn of one lateral ventricle, a cortical incision in the middle frontal gyrus can be used. After a frontal craniotomy, the middle frontal gyrus is identified, and a 2- to 3-cm cortical incision is made in the posterior aspect of the middle frontal gyrus and carried down to the ventricle. Once the ventricular wall is identified, it is opened and the tumor can usually be identified. The blood supply to these tumors may be some bleeding early on except on the surface that is being resected. Glial tumors are usually attached to the ventricular wall, and when this attachment is encountered, the main feeding vessels can be cauterized at that time. Meningiomas in this region are usually attached to the choroid plexus, and here too the choroid plexus can be identified and the blood supply controlled as the resection continues.

POSTOPERATIVE CARE

Results of intraventricular tumor surgery vary, depending on the type of tumor removed. The mortality for choroid plexus papillomas ranges from 15 to 40 percent, with the high rates having been seen in earlier series. Overall mortality for intraventricular meningiomas ranges from 15 to 22 percent, again with the higher figures having occurred in the earlier series.

Postoperative care of the patient with intraventricular tumor surgery is the same as that following any craniotomy. The patient should be maintained on steroids, which can be tapered over the first postoperative week. The patient should also be maintained on adequate doses of anticonvulsants since seizures are common with all surgical approaches except the transcallosal approach. A ventricular drain may be necessary postoperatively. Not all patients with hydrocephalus preoperatively have their hydrocephalus resolved by removal of their tumors, and thus some require a permanent shunt.

Certain complications are common after intraventricular surgery. Because brain tissue must be traversed in order to reach these tumors, there may be new neurologic deficits. Intraventricular hemorrhage, either intraoperatively or postoperatively, is a major problem and a source of morbidity and mortality in patients undergoing surgery of the ventricular system. Postoperative cerebral edema can be a problem and is usually due to retraction of brain tissue during removal of the tumor. The cortex may collapse postoperatively, and subdural hygromas or hematomas are relatively common. Progressive hydrocephalus may be a problem postoperatively.

CLIVUS CHORDOMA

PHILIP H. GUTIN, M.D.

PATHOLOGY

Chordomas occur along the pathway of the primitive notochord. In human embryos, the notochord extends from the retrosellar basisphenoid (dorsum sellae) to the coccyx. At the level of the basisphenoid it is ventral, almost touching the pharynx. Lower, at the level of the basiocciput, the notochord migrates dorsally to lie close to the dura at the foramen magnum. The clivus chordoma arises in the bone of the dorsum sellae and midline clivus from remnants of the notochord.

Chordomas are multilobulated tumors that occur extradurally and may vary in consistency from soft to cartilaginous and may contain incompletely resorbed bone. Chordomas are pseudoencapsulated by the periosteum or dura against which they press. Rarely, more invasive chordomas may penetrate the dura. Metastasses are also rare, particularly from cranial chordomas.

Chordomas arising from the dorsum sellae may invade the pituitary fossa and the parasellar structures, including the cavernous sinus and Meckel's cave. They can also invade beneath the sella to fill the sphenoid sinus or push up through the diaphragma sellae into the suprasellar region. Chordomas arising lower on the clivus can grow either symmetrically or asymmetrically in an anterior-posterior, lateral, or craniocaudal direction.

The typical chordoma contains cord-like rows of distended vacuolated (physaliferous) cells. A variant, the chondroid chordoma, has distinctly chondroid elements and, as a rule, is less invasive. None of the usually encountered histopathologic features of chordomas (cellularity, pleomorphism, mitoses) seems to be related to invasiveness and rate of growth.

CLINICAL FEATURES

The diagnosis of clivus chordoma cannot be made on the basis of clinical features alone. The symptoms at onset, usually headache and intermittent diplopia, are so vague and insidious that the appropriate diagnosis is often delayed, and this (usually) slow-growing tumor can grow to a large size, locally invading bone. Gradually, headache (lesions of the upper clivus) and neck pain (lesions of the lower clivus) become more persistent. Superiorly situated clivus chordomas that expand laterally and superiorly can cause visual failure, diplopia, and hypopituitarism in addition to headache as the pituitary fossa is invaded, compression of the optic apparatus as the suprasellar area is invaded, and third, fourth, and sixth cranial nerve palsies as the cavernous sinus is invaded. Facial numbness or facial pain can occur as tumor enters Meckel's cave.

Tumors arising in the lower clivus that grow beyond their initial stages cause, in addition to increasing headache and neck pain, unilateral or bilateral lower cranial nerve (sixth through twelfth) palsies as tumor progressively obliterates the cerebellopontine angles, compression of the brain stem as they grow dorsally, and nasopharyngeal obstructive symptoms as they grow ventrally. Commonly, the sixth nerve is affected because it is vulnerable to lower clival tumors in its subarachnoid course and to upper clival tumors in the cavernous sinus.

Tumors in the differential diagnosis include basal meningioma and schwannoma, nasopharyngeal carcinoma, pituitary adenoma, and craniopharyngioma. Usually, radiographic studies distinguish between these tumors and clivus chordomas.

RADIOLOGY

The location of clivus chordoma and its almost invariable tendency to destroy bone can be identified readily on radiographs. The calcification seen in many chordomas represents partially destroyed bone or primary tumor calcification. Computed tomography (CT) scans provide the best visualization of cranial chordomas, both for diagnosis and for planning the surgical approach. A soft tissue mass that destroys basal midline bone of the skull and sometimes extends into the sphenoid sinus and/or nasopharynx strongly suggests the diagnosis. Bone windows may help to identify areas in which bone has been destroyed by tumor. Results of contrast studies of these tumors are variable, and enhancement usually is not as dramatic as that seen with meningiomas.

Early experience with the use of magnetic resonance imaging (MRI) for the diagnosis of chordomas has been encouraging. The tumor can be visualized dramatically in the sagittal view. However, because bone cannot be visualized on MRI, it should be used with CT scans to establish the diagnosis.

SURGICAL APPROACHES TO THE CLIVUS

Surgery is obligatory to obtain tissue for histopathology, to reduce the size of the tumor in order to enhance the effectiveness of subsequent radiation therapy, and to improve the patient's clinical condition. A favorable effect on headaches, cranial nerve palsies, and signs of compression of the brain stem can be anticipated if a major portion of the tumor has been resected. A variety of approaches to the skull base have been developed. In many instances, only the surgeon's preference dictates which approach is used. For lesions of the upper clivus that are primarily in the sella and/or sphenoid sinus and are confined to the extradural space, I prefer a transsphenoidal approach. Transdural extensions of upper clivus chordomas into the interpeduncular cistern must be resected via a transcranial subtemporal approach. Because exposure is limited and tumor may be tough and may adhere to vital structures, the carbon dioxide laser is valuable for decompression at or near the brain stem. The transcranial intradural approach must be used for chordomas high on the dorsum sellae, a region that is difficult to expose transsphenoidally. Intradural approaches are difficult, of course, because cerebral arteries and cranial nerves in the basal cisterns must be protected.

For chordomas of the lower clivus, a transoral approach is the most direct route and offers the widest exposure. When the operative microscope is used with this approach, excellent decompression of the brain stem can be obtained. Important surgical adjuncts include the C-arm fluoroscope for intraoperative localization and the Cavitron Ultrasonic Surgical Aspirator (CUSA) (Cooper Lasersonics, Inc., Santa Clara, CA) for rapid, atraumatic tumor removal. A potential serious complication of the transoral approach is a cerebrospinal fluid leak caused by injury of the dura. Care should be taken to protect the dura and to preserve pharyngeal mucosa for a strong closure.

For large clival tumors that extend superiorly toward the dorsum sellae and/or inferiorly to involve the upper cervical spine, a wider exposure than can be gained through the conventional transoral approach may be necessary. Splitting the tongue and mandible in the midline provides a wide field through which the microscope can be positioned inferiorly enough to adequately visualize the cervical spine and to provide a better angle for a view superiorly toward the more rostral clivus. Occasionally, a combination of surgical approaches must be used to achieve effective decompression of large tumors.

RADIATION THERAPY

Postoperatively, patients should have radiation therapy with the expectation of obtaining palliation only. Although higher doses may delay the recurrence, no more than 6000 rads can be administered because of the limitations of brain tolerance. In common practice, the tumor volume and some margin of surrounding tissue are irradiated to 5000 to 5500 rads.

There is evidence that irradiation of chordomas with charged particles may be superior to conventional irradiation with photons from linear accelerators. Because of the Bragg effect, charged particles can be localized very precisely to the tumor volume deep within tissue while sparing interposed structures. The geometry of the volume to be irradiated can be determined by a computer to irradiate precisely the volume of tumor seen on a CT or MRI scan. Some of charged particles used for treatment have a higher relative biological effectiveness—they kill tumor cells more efficiently—than conventional x-ray photons. Unfortunately, in the United States, charged particle accelerators that can be used to treat patients are available only in Berkeley and Boston.

Early results obtained with hyperfractionated radiation therapy (multiple small fractions given daily) using conventional, readily available equipment are encouraging. This approach may allow the delivery of higher total doses that may provide better control of tumor.

TREATMENT OF RECURRENT TUMORS

After subtotal tumor resection and conventional external beam irradiation, cranial chordomas recur in a large percentage of patients. The only currently available treatment for previously irradiated chordomas is reoperation, which may produce survivals of 5 to 10 years. Obviously, repeat surgery becomes more difficult because postoperative adhesions and recurrent tumor distort the normal anatomic landmarks. Occasionally, sacral chordomas can be reirradiated with conventional techniques, but cranial chordomas cannot. On an experimental basis, we have treated several multiply recurrent basal chordomas with interstitially implanted iodine-125 sources for local irradiation of these tumors. There is no known effective chemotherapy for chordoma.

OUTLOOK

Because surgical techniques have reached a plateau of sophistication and efficacy, results obtained by resection of the invasive cranial chordoma are not likely to improve outcome dramatically. Irradiation with charged particles or with conventional x-ray photons on multiple daily fractionated schedules offer the most promise for more effective treatment of clivus chordomas.

TUMOR OF THE CEREBELLOPONTINE ANGLE

DONLIN M. LONG, M.D., Ph. D.

The principal tumors of the cerebellopontine angle are the acoustic neuroma and the meningioma. Cholesteatomas are also relatively common. Cerebellar gliomas, brain stem gliomas, metastatic tumors, lipomas, arteriovenous malformations (AVMs), and primary tumors of the petrous bone all may present with cerebellopontine angle masses. However, all of these tumors are rare, and the acoustic neuroma is the most common lesion found in this location.

SYMPTOMS AND SIGNS

The cardinal symptom of the cerebellopontine angle tumor is hearing loss. Patients commonly discover they are unable to hear in a crowded room when multiple persons are talking or that they cannot hear well on the telephone. Tinnitus is also common. Dizziness is a frequent complaint. An ipsilateral seventh nerve palsy may develop and may occasionally be the presenting symptom. These tumors may grow to enormous size before producing symptoms. Meningiomas are much less likely to involve hearing early and commonly are very large before symptoms occur. As the tumor increases in size, palsies of cranial nerves IX, X, and XI may develop. Brain stem compression can lead to hydrocephalus, with headache and some symptoms of personality change or mild dimentia. Hemiparesis from brain stem compression may progress, but significant brain stem signs are unusual, even with very large tumors. Extension of the tumor upward produces deficits in function of the fifth cranial nerve; the corneal reflex is diminished, numbness in the face, paresis of the muscles of mastication, and occasionally trigeminal pain may occur. Pain is more commonly present with meningiomas than with acoustic neuroma.

DIAGNOSIS

At one time, it was important to carefully define the hearing loss with tests that were sensitive to the sensorineural hearing loss produced by these tumors. The CT scan has changed the evaluation of these tumors completely. Virtually all lesions of the petrous bone and cerebellopontine angle can be delineated with CT scan. Occasionally, with small tumors, it may be necessary to outline the porus and its contents with a small amount of air in order to be certain about the presence or absence of a mass. The CT scan usually can differentiate meningioma from acoustic neuroma. The configuration of the meningioma is irregular, and frequently the porus is not enlarged. The acoustic neuroma is much rounder and smoother, and porus enlargement is virtually certain. Lipomas and cholesteatomas can be identified by their CT numbers. Most destructive tumors involving the bone and intrinsic tumors of cerebellum and brain stem can be easily identified. Angiography is not necessary, except in unusual situations. One must always remember that very small tumors of the petrous bone may mimic an acoustic neuroma. Cholesteatoma is the most common; a small cholesteatoma can easily be confused with an air cell and overlooked.

TREATMENT

The treatment for acoustic neuroma is surgical. Since the natural history of the tumor is to grow, and since the treatment of the small acoustic tumor is much simpler than the treatment of the large tumor, it is important that the tumor be removed before it attains a size large enough to produce brain stem compression, in which circumstance removal of the tumor may not be wise. A tumor that produces a few symptoms in an elderly patient may be observed until it is certain that symptoms warrant surgery. A very small tumor in a

young patient with reasonable hearing may be observed until it is certain that hearing will be impaired and the tumor is growing. As techniques improve, and it becomes possible to save hearing routinely, this philosophy may change.

At present, there are three surgical options for the treatment of the acoustic neuroma: the tumor may be approached through the middle fossa, by the translabyrinthine route, or through the posterior fossa.

Middle Fossa Approach

This approach to acoustic tumors has fewer adherents than the other routes available. It does allow removal of a small tumor with the possibility of salvage of hearing, but the need to retract the temporal lobe and the relatively restricted exposure have limited the popularity of this technique.

Translabyrinthine Route

When the tumor is small and hearing is seriously impaired, the translabyrinthine approach provides a simple and safe way to remove the acoustic tumor. Hearing must be sacrificed, but the cerebellum is scarcely exposed. My colleagues in otolaryngology and I carry out these operations under general anesthesia with the patient in the park-bench position. A small curvilinear incision behind the ear is all that is required, and only a small patch of hair must be shaved. The petrous bone is drilled away to expose the seventh nerve, which is followed to the auditory canal. The tumor is easily identified in the canal and separated from the nerve. If necessary, the exposed posterior fossa dura can be opened, and it is possible to remove tumors of considerable size by this route. However, it is more difficult to remove the large tumors in this way, and we reserve the translabyrinthine route for smaller tumors.

Posterior Fossa Route

This approach may be utilized for tumors of all sizes. We employ it for all larger tumors and for small tumors when hearing is intact and an effort will be made to preserve audition. These procedures are also carried out under general anesthesia with the patient in the park-bench position. A unilateral retromastoid incision is made. A posterior fossa craniectomy is carried out and the dura opened to expose the cerebellopontine angle. This approach allows the cranial nerves to be identified prior to tumor removal in the case of the smaller lesions and certainly facilitates dissection of adherent blood vessels from the capsule. With larger tumors, the posterior fossa approach gives better exposure of the tumor and increases the chance for total removal with preservation of cranial nerve functions.

Meningiomas of the cerebellopontine angle can be approached by the posterior fossa or by a radical translabyrinthine resection of bone and tumor. Tumors with major intracranial extensions should be approached through the posterior fossa. When there is extensive involvement of the petrous bone, a two-stage operation may be used whereby removal of the intracranial portion of the tumor is followed in a few weeks by radical removal of the temporal bone. When the tumor is isolated to the temporal bone and intracranial extension is small, the radical translabyrinthine approach is all that is necessary.

Most other lesions of the cerebellopontine angle are best approached through the posterior fossa. Small irritative lesions, such as cholesteatomas of the petrous bone, may be treated by transpetrous exposure and removal.

CHOICE OF APPROACH

Our surgical philosophy for dealing with these tu mors can be summarized in the following way. When the tumor is small and hearing is seriously impaired, the translabyrinthine approach offers a safe way to deal with these tumors. When hearing is preserved with small tumors, the posterior fossa approach with an attempt to save useful hearing is preferred. The middle fossa approach can accomplish the same thing, but is less well known and utilized less commonly. Moderate-sized tumors with impaired hearing may be removed by either the posterior fossa or the translabyrinthine route. The posterior fossa approach is more familiar for most neurosurgeons. Salvage of hearing in the face of a moderate or a large tumor is unlikely, but the posterior fossa route does offer this possibility. For large tumors, the posterior fossa approach is preferable. Skilled translabyrinthine surgeons can successfully treat tumors of all sizes, but most surgeons prefer the posterior fossa approach for the larger tumors. The translabyrinthine surgery still has a part to play with large tumors. Some elderly patients have very large tumors which cannot be approached for cure. Internal decompression via the translabyrinthine route can relieve pressure on the brain stem and provide real symptomatic improvement for these individuals.

RESULTS OF SURGERY

There has been a dramatic improvement in our ability to deal with tumors of the cerebellopontine angle over the past 10 years. With small and moderate acoustic tumors, preservation of all cranial nerve function except hearing is the rule. In a few reported cases, hearing has been preserved or improved. At present, this is the major surgical challenge with these smaller tumors. Although temporary seventh nerve paralysis may occur following removal of one of these tumors, anatomic continuity of the nerve is virtually never disrupted now, and recovery of seventh nerve function is the rule. Patients must be warned of the possibility of paralysis beforehand, but most recover within 3 to 6 months, even when postoperative paralysis is complete. The larger tumors are still a formidable challenge. There is a very real risk to life and function. It is virtually never possible to preserve hearing with larger tumors, but the other cranial nerves can usually be saved. A permanent seventh nerve paralysis rarely occurs with current surgical techniques. Even when the seventh nerve is disrupted in the course of total tumor removal, it is usually possible to obtain a primary anastomosis of the ends or interpose a graft with satisfactory recovery.

Total removal of acoustic tumors, no matter what the size, is now the rule. All cranial nerves, except VIII, can be salvaged routinely. The next surgical challenge is the preservation or restoration of hearing.

There are special circumstances regarding acoustic tumors which require discussion. Rarely, these tumors are bilateral. In this situation, it is my philosophy to approach these tumors surgically only when symptoms are unequivocal and seriously distressing. Usually the tumors are asymmetrical, one being large and the other small. The large tumor routinely produces first symptoms and should be approached first. It is clear that, with current techniques, the second tumor, even when small, cannot be removed with a high probability that hearing will be preserved. For this reason, I usually defer the second surgical procedure, allowing the patient to function with hearing as long as possible. The patient should be instructed in lip reading and made acquainted with all of the assistance available for the deaf. Then, when it becomes necessary to remove the second tumor, the patient will be prepared for the deafness which will probably ensue. As techniques for preserving hearing improve, this philosophy may change, and it may be possible to attack small tumors before they have seriously injured hearing.

Total removal of small and moderate-sized acoustic neuromas has now become routine. Cranial nerve preservation is now commonplace, and the master surgeons of the angle are now attempting to save hearing. Large tumors remain a major surgical challenge, but total removal with preservation of seventh nerve function is still possible most of the time.

When the seventh nerve does not recover its function, reinnervation to provide a symmetrical face is possible. During the time that one awaits reinnervation, the face may be stimulated with a small muscular stimulator to provide good muscle tone. I like to use the sternocleidomastoid branch of the eleventh nerve and bring it up to make an anastomosis with the seventh nerve just where it exits from the stylomastoid foramen. The entire eleventh nerve may be used, but the resulting shoulder droop is a disability for some patients, particularly heavy laborers. The twelfth nerve may be used, but the resultant hemiatrophy of the tongue is distressing to many.

MENINGIOMAS

The surgery of meningiomas of the cerebellopontine angle is generally very satisfactory. Utilizing the cavitron ultrasonic dissector or laser, it is possible to obtain total removal of most of these tumors with preservation of cranial nerve function. Hearing routinely improves following tumor removal. When the petrous bone is heavily infiltrated, radical removal is necessary for tumor cure. In this circumstance, hearing is virtually always lost prior to surgery from the bone involvement. Cholesteatomas can be removed with preservation of cranial nerve function in most instances. The other tumors occurring in this area present varying problems unique to their particular location and biology.

TUMOR OF THE GLOMUS JUGULARE

DONLIN M. LONG, M.D., Ph. D.

Tumors of the glomus jugulare are unusual but curable, and it is important that they be recognized promptly and treated effectively. Symptoms and signs relate to the tumor's location in the jugular foramen. Hoarseness is a common first symptom. Patients may complain of difficulty in swallowing. Pain in the shoulder from weakness secondary to eleventh nerve involvement is also a common complaint. The tumors may grow large enough to involve the seventh and eighth nerves with resultant disturbance of hearing, dizziness, or facial weakness. The twelfth nerve can be involved, producing weakness of the tongue and dysarthria. Occasionally, these tumors have an extension that is visible in the middle ear. More commonly, the diagnosis is suggested only by the unilateral cranial nerve dysfunction.

The diagnosis is confirmed by CT scanning. Plain films of the skull are unnecessary because CT reveals the characteristic destructive lesion of the jugular bulb area. Coronal sections are useful in delineating intracranial extension. The differential diagnosis includes meningioma, malignant tumor of the bone, and metastatic tumor.

It is important to obtain an angiogram. These tumors are extremely vascular, and the surgery may be simplified when significant feeding arteries can be embolized at the time of angiography. It is wise to alert the neuroradiologist to the fact that embolization may be necessary before the diagnostic study is carried out. It is important to determine involvement of the carotid artery, and the venous anatomy must be understood as well. Occasionally, one of these tumors grows in the lumen of the jugular vein. Since the sinus will have to be ligated on the side of the tumor, it is necessary to be certain of the venous drainage of the brain before the ligation is carried out. This usually is not a problem because the tumor has obstructed the jugular vein and multiple collateral channels for venous drainage have developed. However, it may be important to be certain that these are preserved during surgery. They must be carefully identified, and the venous anatomy understood before surgery begins.

The definitive treatment of these tumors is surgical. A two-stage approach offers an excellent way to obtain a surgical cure with minimal neurological deficit. The first stage is to isolate the tumor and provide a new false dural surface to prevent cerebrospinal fluid fistula. The procedure is carried out under general anesthesia with the patient in the park-bench position. A small posterior fossa craniectomy is utilized to expose the jugular bulb and the tumor. Simultaneously, a graft of fascia lata is obtained. The tumor, which is virtually always extradural, is identified and all of the cranial nerves and vessels freed from its surface. Of course, the ninth, tenth, and eleventh cranial nerves enter the tumor, but they are isolated to their entrance. The fascia lata graft is then fashioned to completely cover the tumor and provide adequate margins on all sides to allow an extradural removal of the tumor to take place at a second stage. Slits are cut in the graft to go around the nerves, and the all important vessels are placed medial to the new dura. When the dural graft is in place, the wound is closed. No attempt is made to remove the tumor from the intracranial route. At a second stage, 10 to 14 days later, the wound is reopened and extended down into the neck along the course of the carotid artery and jugular vein. During the first operation, the junction of the transverse and sigmoid sinus was isolated to facilitate ligation at the second stage, and the petrous vein was coagulated and divided. The jugular vein can now be isolated in the neck and the sinus above the tumor. Following venous ligation, the bleeding from the tumor is greatly reduced. The tumor can then be removed totally. The cavitron or laser is very helpful. It is rarely possible to dissect the cranial nerves through the tumor, but they can be isolated extracranially and the intracranial stump can frequently be found. This allows grafting to take place, and the patient should always be prepared for the acquisition of a suitable nerve graft. The false dura previously placed provides a watertight seal so that bone removal can be as radical as necessary to obtain a surgical cure.

When the tumor cannot be totally removed, two courses of action are possible. These tumors are usually slow-growing and do not recur quickly. It may be feasible to (1) simply observe the tumor with regular CT scanning and carry out additional surgery as indicated by recurrence, or (2) give x-ray therapy, particularly when the tumors are highly vascular.

MALIGNANT GLIOMA

PAUL L. KORNBLITH, M.D.

Malignant gliomas constitute one of the most difficult therapeutic challenges in neurosurgery. Recent advances in diagnostic techniques, coupled with some new therapeutic tools, have made prospects a bit brighter for patients with this group of diseases.

Included in the adult category of "malignant gliomas" are astrocytomas of the higher grades (II, III, and IV), malignant oligodendrogliomas, and malignant ependymomas. Of these, the astrocytic group is by far the most common. Oligodendrogliomas are often mixed with astrocytic elements, and it is the astrocytic component that is most likely to behave aggressively. Ependymomas are less common and often benign, but even when malignant, they tend to be indolent.

In children, medulloblastoma is the most common malignant CNS tumor, and although there is some debate about its cellular origin, it is best considered as a malignant glioma. Astrocytomas in children are usually of less malignant potential except for those of the brain stem region. Only infrequently are optic nerve gliomas of a highly malignant type, and there is question as to their real natural history as tumors. In many cases these tumors remain quiescent for long periods.

All of the malignant gliomas are invasive and infiltrate the surrounding brain. They rarely metastasize outside the CNS. Medulloblastoma in particular often seeds the neuraxis, and secondary deposits in the spinal canal are common.

DIAGNOSIS

In the history of a patient with a malignant tumor of the CNS, the most notable problem is increasing headache, most severe in the morning. Seizures are a common presenting symptom. As intracranial pressure increases, nausea, vomiting, and somnolence occur. Focal motor, sensory, cranial nerve findings develop in patients with lesions in the corresponding anatomic regions. Often focal findings occur later in the disease course. In the prototype lesion, the malignant astrocytoma, the course is distinctively rapid, relentlessly progressive, and the interval between the first symptoms and definitive diagnosis may be as short as one month.

The neurological picture in a patient with malignant glioma depends on the location of the lesion and its size at the time of presentation. Of importance are the findings of papilledema when increased intracranial pressure is present and of visual field deficits when the optic pathways are involved. Careful motor and sensory testing can aid in localization of the lesion. In brain stem gliomas and in medulloblastomas, cranial nerve findings are more common. The majority of adult astrocytomas are supratentorial, and therefore motor, sensory, and visual findings predominate. Because of the edema surrounding the tumor mass, the findings may reflect a fairly large area of brain involvement.

In establishing the diagnosis of the malignant gliomas, the key measure is the CT scan. This test has completely changed the approach to diagnosis of these lesions. The CT scan without contrast can detect areas of calcification as in an oligodendroglioma, the low density of peritumoral edema, or a lower grade tumor. With contrast enhancement, the full extent of the tumor is apparent. Detection of a mass by CT scan approaches 95 percent or even higher, but one cannot be absolutely sure of its histology without pathologic verification. Posterior fossa masses are somewhat harder to detect by CT, but it is still the most useful radiologic test.

Angiography is a useful adjunctive study or may be used if CT is not available. It can show distinctive vascular patterns with early appearance of draining veins as typical features. Since angiography by the transfemoral route carries real risks, it is not necessarily a routine measure.

A radioisotopic brain scan may be helpful in diagnosis and in "three-dimensional" location of the lesion. It is risk-free, but has a lower rate of detection than CT scan.

The use of lumbar puncture in the initial diagnosis of brain tumor is to be discouraged as there is a real risk of herniation by rapid drainage of CSF. However, lumbar puncture may be used in following patients with medulloblastomas who may have spinal spread. Millipore studies of the CSF should reveal tumor cells when spinal spread has occurred. The elevated protein in CSF in brain tumor patients is also accompanied by increases in other biological compounds such as polyamines. These features may be of value in following patients or their therapy, but are not worth the risk of doing a "diagnostic" lumbar puncture.

EEG findings of slowing over a tumor or of spikes over an active focus can be of interest, but the use of an EEG as a screening tool has been supplanted by CT scan.

Pneumoencephalography and ventriculography, so valuable in the pre-CT scan era, are now rarely if ever used. There are two newer neuroradiologic tools which have potential significance for management. The MRI scan (magnetic resonance imaging) should allow frequent, completely safe follow-up of patients with tumors and serial evaluation of the quantitative effects of therapy. The PET scan (positron emission tomography), using ^{18}FDG, follows the course of a positron emitting isotope (fluorine) bound to a form of glucose which is metabolically trapped in the cells. These PET scans have proved valuable in grading the lesions as to their malignancy and also in distinguishing tumor recurrence from radiation-induced necrosis. In the future, the fate of therapeutic agents and their effects on the tumor may be visualizable by means of newer approaches in PET and MRI.

NATURAL HISTORY

In the patient with an untreated malignant astrocytoma, one can expect a fairly rapid progression from focal deficits through coma to death in an average of 6 months from the time of initial diagnosis. Oligodendroglial elements in a tumor improve survival by about 1 to 2 years. Ependymomas have a highly variable course.

There is much concern regarding the grading of astrocytomas and the prognosis. In the grade I lesion, long-term survival is possible—5 to 10 or even 20 years. In the so-called "anaplastic astrocytoma", grades II to III, 1 to 2 years may be achieved. In the (grade IV) glioblastoma multiforme, the 6-month figure is unfortunately the standard.

In predicting the natural history of these patients, certain variables have been found to be critically important. The age of the patient plays a major role, the younger patient having a significantly better outlook. The condition of the patient from a functional standpoint is another helpful factor; the patient who is intact has a much better chance than the one who is disabled. The development of a 1 to 100 scale of performance (Karnofsky rating) has been of use in quantitating the pre- and posttherapy status. The location of the lesion is also important. As might be expected, frontal and occipital lesions are more favorable than those of the deeper structures or the dominant parietal lobe.

THERAPEUTIC OPTIONS

For the malignant astrocytoma, there are three primary therapeutic choices, surgery, radiation, and chemotherapy.

Surgery has several key roles. It is essential in virtually all surgically accessible cases to establish the exact histologic diagnosis. Thus biopsy is at the very least critical. It only takes one patient who is found to have a lesion other than a presumed malignant astrocytoma to make the case for such histologic verification. The advent of CT scan-guided stereotactic biopsy makes all but deep brain stem and midline lesions at least theoretically accessible. In patients with a lesion in the frontal, temporal, or occipital lobe, without evidence of spread to the contralateral hemisphere or adjacent parts of the ipsilateral hemisphere, lobectomy is a worthwhile consideration. Unfortunately, many patients do not have lesions in these areas, and a decompression with a less than subtotal removal is the usual maximum surgical goal. In surgical resection, use of the operating microscope, microsurgical instruments, the ultrasonic suction devices, and the high-energy laser can make for greater care and safety in tumor removal. Even with all the technical advances, surgery alone can only be considered as the first step in therapy, as the extensive tumor infiltration is rarely amenable to microscopically proven total resection.

The use of radiation therapy is the second option. It is clear that radiation is useful in extending patient survival. The program found to be most useful encompasses 4500 rads of whole brain radiation and 1500 rads of local tumor boost. When radiation is combined with surgery, the life expectancy improves to about 9 months from the 6 months noted with surgery alone. Some newer techniques of radiotherapy may prove applicable for certain patients. Interstitial radiotherapy using ^{125}I or other implantable isotopes shows promise for localized smaller lesions (generally those of a less malignant type). To date, radiosensitizers and hyperthermia have not proved to be of consistent value.

The third therapeutic option is chemotherapy. A wide variety of agents have been studied, but at present the only agents to measure up under careful phase III study are the nitrosoureas, especially BCNU. In practice one can expect to achieve a 30 to 40 percent response rate with either BCNU or CCNU, given every 6 weeks at a dose of 110 mg/m^2. This response rate leads to about an additional 3 months of survival on the average, thus reaching about a 12-month interval.

Other agents that are promising include AZQ (aziridinylbenzoquinone) and cisplatin, but as yet these are still in phase II study. AZQ in particular shows promise inasmuch as it appears to achieve a 30 to 40 percent response rate even in patients who have failed on nitrosoureas. A relatively recent development, the use of intra-arterial therapy, is intriguing. This approach permits a high-dose local delivery with less systemic exposure to the drug. Most work so far has been with BCNU, and this agent has apparent CNS toxicity which may limit its efficacy. With highly selective catheter delivery and possible removal of drug before systemic exposure, the intra-arterial route may be of future value.

Immunotherapy is a fascinating approach, but for malignant gliomas, there is much to learn before it is a clinically relevant option.

For medulloblastoma, complete gross surgical resection followed by craniospinal radiation is clearly indicated. This may then be followed by PCV chemotherapy (procarbazine, CCNU, and vincristine) to achieve the best overall results. There are some who would defer the PCV until the time of recurrence rather than use it initially.

CHOICE OF THERAPY

Although it is clear that no therapy for malignant glioma is really achieving "cures", the palliation achieved by combined modality therapy is significant to the patient. As the current plan, surgical resection, if possible, or biopsy, if not, should be followed by 6 weeks of radiotherapy and then CCNU chemotherapy on a 6-week cycle. CCNU has better patient acceptance as it is given orally and is easier for the patient and family. Its potency is sufficiently close to that of BCNU to make it preferable.

In patients with medulloblastoma, the most effective plan is surgical resection and craniospinal radiation, to be followed by PCV chemotherapy. One must be careful to allow the bone marrow to recover from the effects of marrow-suppressing spinal radiation before starting the chemotherapy.

POTENTIAL COMPLICATIONS

Certain problems are clearly more common in patients with malignant gliomas. The most common is the occurrence of thrombophlebitis and pulmonary emboli, which result from the apparently abnormal clotting system in these patients.

The complications of surgical therapy include damage to vital structures, the infrequent postoperative hematoma or infection, and the all too common urinary infection.

Radiation therapy results in loss of hair, and there may be subtle but detectable long-term effects on cerebral function in patients who survive long enough to have these changes documented.

The major toxic effect of nitrosourea chemotherapy is on the bone marrow, especially on platelet formation. Thus frequent blood counts are essential in planning therapy.

Other effects of nitrosoureas include hepatic necrosis, pulmonary fibrosis, and teratogenic effects. These are all infrequent in the patient with a malignant glioma, owing perhaps to the short life expectancy.

Effective treatment of malignant gliomas is still limited. Earlier and more effective diagnosis and new therapy modalities may gradually turn the tide in the patient's favor.

SUPRATENTORIAL ASTROCYTOMA

HENRY BREM, M.D.

Of the approximately 12,000 new brain tumors that occur each year, about one-half are primary glial tumors. Of these, approximately 30 percent are low-grade astrocytomas. Although astrocytomas are more common in males, there is no difference in outcome between the sexes. The peak incidence occurs between ages 20 and 50. The survival with a low-grade astrocytoma is highly variable. There is an 87 percent 15-year survival in "good" patients, i.e., those who are young, present with a seizure, do not have a pre- or postoperative deficit or headache, and do not have an altered level of consciousness. In contrast, the 15-year survival is 16 percent in those who do not have these characteristics, i.e., they present at an older age, start off with neurological deficits or change in mental status, and are unable to have their tumors totally resected.

As with most intracranial lesions, the symptoms of low-grade astrocytomas are caused either by focal neurological deficits due to the mass or by diffuse increased intracranial pressure. Signs and symptoms of increased intracranial pressure include headache (the presenting symptom of approximately one-third of the patients with a glioma), nausea, vomiting, diplopia due to palsy the trochlear or abducens nerves and papilledema. The premier sign of increased intracranial pressure is lethargy and obtundation. The headaches are characteristically worst in the morning because of differences in CSF circulation between the supine and upright positions. There is often a regional correlation to the headache, especially with frontal astrocytomas causing frontal headaches and occipital lesions causing occipital or posterior cervical pain. This may be due to local stretching of pain fibers in the dura. There is an urgent need to begin treating patients who present with increased intracranial pressure.

A far better prognostic sign is the presentation with local symptoms, e.g., seizures. Almost half the patients have experienced a seizure at the time of first presentation. The seizure may be the focal Jacksonian type, which aids in localization, or the generalized grand mal type. Often, the first seizure is a momentary loss of alertness and may be ignored by the patient.

Other focal signs observed in patients with supratentorial hemispheric gliomas include personality changes, weakness, sensory loss, visual deficits, hearing loss, anosmia, speech deficits, memory deficits, and other defects in mental functions.

An important characteristic of the symptom complex in the patient with an astrocytoma is the *relentless progression* of the symptoms and signs, which correlates with continued tumor growth.

The evaluation of a patient with a suspected glioma begins with a detailed history and neurological examination. Approximately 50 percent of the patients with a glioma have one of the following findings at the time of presentation: hemiparesis, cranial nerve palsy, mental deterioration, papilledema. It is the *level of consciousness* that determines the urgency of work-up and treatment. The disoriented patient or one with a declining level of consciousness requires immediate evaluation and treatment to lower intracranial pressure. Hyperactive reflexes and a Babinski sign are also indicative of an intracranial lesion.

Adjuncts to the physical examination include visual field testing. This is useful in that the visual fibers can be specifically affected by local lesions in each of the cerebral lobes. Electroencephalography (EEG) is useful in managing patients who have seizures. In general, brain tumors produce a regional slowing of electrical activity. However, a specific epileptogenic focus may produce spikes or spike and wave foci. Examination of the cerebrospinal fluid (CSF) by lumbar puncture carries significant risk and should only be performed when intracranial mass effect or increased intracranial pressure has been definitively ruled out by neurological examination and CT scan. The primary indication for examination of CSF is to rule out meningitis. CSF protein above 40 mg/100 ml is highly suggestive of a tumor, although it can be a consequence of bleeding or infection. Tumors may lower CSF sugar, as do infections or viral encephalitis. CSF Millipore filtration for cytology as well as tissue culture are specifically indicated for the diagnosis of tumors in the CSF. Tumor markers, such as alpha fetoprotein, hCG, polyamines, and angiogenesis factor, are useful for following tumor response to treatment.

Radiographic evaluation of the patient with a suspected astrocytoma may begin with a plain skull film. Approximately 20 percent of astrocytomas have calcifications, which generally are suggestive of slow tumor growth. Chronic increased intracranial pressure is demonstrated by erosion of the clinoid processes of the sella turcica. In children, chronic pressure erosion of the inner table can lead to a "hammered metal" appearance.

Computerized tomography (CT) scanning is the most definitive diagnostic measure for evaluating the patient with a possible glioma. The CT scan demonstrates the configuration of the lesion, its relative vascularity and calcification, and its effects on surrounding structures. The edema and consequent mass effect can also be evaluated. The presence of increased intracranial pressure and hydrocephalus is also apparent.

CT scans can be obtained in axial and coronal directions in order to better localize the tumor for surgical intervention. Dynamic CT scanning, whereby a pulse of contrast dye is injected with rapid sequential scanning, is useful for determining the vasculature of the tumor and for ruling out the presence of vascular lesions mimicking an astrocytoma. A low-grade, well-differentiated astrocytoma occasionally may not be apparent on routine CT scanning. It is therefore necessary to follow some patients with sequential CT scans if their symptoms continue to develop.

Magnetic resonance imaging (MRI) is playing an increasing role in the evaluation of astrocytomas. MRI is frequently more accurate than CT scanning in defining distinct borders of astrocytomas. This has led to an improvement in our ability to surgically resect low-grade astrocytomas. Positron emission tomography (PET) scanning, while still experimental, holds the additional promise of using radioisotope-labeled, metabolically active substances (e.g., glucose or oxygen) to evaluate the functional activity of an astrocytoma.

Cerebral angiography is only occasionally necessary. Its major role is to outline the detailed vascular supply to a tumor as an aid to surgical intervention. Occasionally, a tumor that is not seen on CT scan may be visualized with angiography. For example, with hemorrhage into a tumor, the angiogram may demonstrate the presence of tumor vessels, whereas the CT may not differentiate tumor from clot.

Despite the advances in diagnostic techniques, the definitive diagnosis of an astrocytoma cannot be made without pathologic examination of the tissue. The surgical goals are to remove as much tumor as is safely possible without creating a new neurological deficit. In addition, if the tumor infiltrates through the frontal, temporal, or occipital lobes, a partial lobectomy may be necessary for decompression. Hydrocephalus can be relieved by either ventricular drainage or an internal shunt. For tumors located in a critical area of the brain (e.g., the speech area or motor strip) or for deep-seated lesions, a biopsy may be indicated rather than a resection. Biopsies may be done openly through a small craniotomy and direct observation of the tissue to be examined. A useful adjunct to surgical biopsy is intraoperative ultrasound. With this technique, a cyst or mass can be identified, and the biopsy needle can be observed directly. A further refinement in biopsy technique is the stereotactic CT-guided biopsy. This approach is useful for deep-seated lesions located in critical areas. The techniques are now so refined that a specific area of CT enhancement can be identified for biopsy.

All surgical patients are prophylactically treated with antiseizure medication, usually phenytoin or phenobarbitol, as well as with a corticosteroid, usually dexamethasone, 4 mg every 6 hours. If there is significant mass effect, the dose of steroid is increased. One week after the operation, the steroid doses are slowly tapered and eventually discontinued, whereas the antiseizure medication is continued indefinitely. The operative mortality is less than 1 percent.

The role of postoperative radiation therapy has not been definitively proved. Patients who undergo a subtotal resection generally receive postoperative radiation with apparent benefit. Patients who undergo a gross total resection of a grade I astrocytoma and have no further CT evidence of disease may be followed closely clinically for evidence of recurrence before radiation therapy is given. At present, there is no indication for chemotherapy for the treatment of low-grade astrocytomas.

Ten percent of patients with pathologically proved grade I or II gliomas later present with evidence of a malignant glioma. A variety of explanations have been proposed for this "malignant degeneration". It is possible that the benign astrocytoma represents a time point on the continuum of development of a malignant astrocytoma. In these cases, there would appear to be a steady progression toward malignancy. It is possible that the acquisition of an important biological function, such as the production of tumor angiogenesis factor, may be responsible for allowing a tumor to express its malignant growth potential. It is also possible that cases in which "malignant degeneration" occurs may be misdiagnosed initially owing to sampling errors. For example, a glioblastoma may have sections that appear more benign or a specimen adjacent to the actual tumor nodule may be interpreted as having a low-grade glioma. With the refinement of CT-guided biopsies, this problem should be reduced. Finally, it is conceivable that the radiation therapy itself may contribute to further malignant transformation of tissue that is already defective.

Low-grade astrocytomas are generally looked on favorably when compared to the poorer course of the glioblastoma and because there is such variability in results of treatment. Indeed, a certain percentage of patients are "cured" of a low-grade glioma. However, the overall outlook is still grim, with an average survival of 4 years for all grade I astrocytomas and $2^{1}12$ years for all grade II astrocytomas. Progress needs to be made in a number of areas. Diagnostically, stereotactic CT scan biopsies and MRI scanning techniques need to be further utilized. The role and method of radiation therapy need further investigation. The role of interstitial radiation in the poor-risk group needs to be defined. Finally, newer approaches, such as the development of new chemotherapeutic agents or drugs that could inhibit neovascularization of tumors, need to be developed and tested. With an increased understanding of the fundamental biological characteristics of the astrocytomas, we should be able to improve the outlook for these patients.

SOLITARY INTRACRANIAL METASTASIS

JOSEPH H. GALICICH, M.D.
NARAYAN SUNDARESAN, M.D.
BARRY H. SMITH, M.D., Ph.D.

The brain is a common site of metastasis in systemic cancer. At autopsy, approximately 15 percent of cancer patients have such metastases. Based on projections of 430,000 cancer deaths in 1983, some 60,000 patients were so affected. Beyond the matter of frequency is the important fact that the majority of these metastases become symptomatic and often disabling. Problems range from headaches, seizures, and loss of intellectual and/or cognitive function to ataxia, paralysis, and brain herniation and death.

Tumors of the lung, breast, colon, skin (melanoma), kidney, thyroid gland, and sarcomas frequently metastasize to brain, but virtually all tumors can do so. The incidence of brain metastases seems to be increasing as survival lengthens with improving systemic therapy. Overall, 40 to 45 percent of the parenchymal metastases are solitary, with renal cell carcinomas and lung carcinomas being especially prominent in this group. Roughly 80 percent are located in the cerebrum; 16 percent in the cerebellum; and 3 percent in the brain stem.

Although rational therapy for multiple metastases includes radiation therapy and, perhaps, chemotherapy, as well as supportive measures such as steroids and anticonvulsants as required, the question of optimal therapy for the solitary intracranial metastasis has been controversial. The major issue is whether radiation therapy alone or surgery followed by radiation is the optimal course.

Surgical excision of the tumor offers histologic diagnosis and provides rapid decompression of the brain in patients who are deteriorating rapidly, as well as the removal of the primary cause of the surrounding brain edema. Because parenchymal metastases arise from emboli most often trapped near the surface where there is arterial narrowing and because they grow in a soft matrix, these tumors are frequently superficial and spherical, thus enhancing surgical attack. Advances in brain imaging techniques, including precise CT as well as MRI localization, together with improving anesthesia and new surgical techniques including magnification, the use of ultrasonic aspirating devices, and "no-touch" CO_2 and other lasers, have combined to make surgical mortality acceptably low. Surgery ensures that, for subsequent radiation therapy, the tumor burden is minimal, thus optimizing the therapeutic benefit of this modality. In certain cases, when the brain metastasis is the only site of tumor in the body, there is a small chance that surgical excision can be "curative". For relatively radioresistant metastatic tumors, such as those arising from colon, melanoma, and renal primaries, surgical excision offers the only hope of palliation. A solitary metastasis in a patient who has already had prophylactic brain radiation (e.g., in oat cell carcinoma) may only be approachable surgically since the additional radiation therapy required would not be tolerated.

Radiation therapy, on the other hand, offers several advantages. It is, of course, applicable to virtually all patients with brain metastases, whether they are solitary or multiple. Whereas surgery may be ruled out by the location of the metastasis (such as deep thalamic), radiation is not limited by site considerations. Although radiation therapy, by virtue of dose-fractionation, may be time-consuming, it is compatible with other ongoing therapy, whereas surgery, for example, may require the cessation of bone-marrow toxic chemotherapy. Initial clinical improvement, as reported in most major series to date, is seen in 39 to 92 percent of patients. Eighty percent of those patients responding to radiation therapy are alive at 3 months posttreatment, and 60 percent of those alive at 6 months remain improved with respect to neurological status. Many of these patients can be taken off steroids without recurrence of symptoms or neurological deterioration. CT scan follow-up, furthermore, shows disappearance or significant improvement in over half the cases.

Several factors need to be considered in making a decision as to optimal therapy for a given patient with a solitary brain metastasis. These include overall medical status, neurological status, extent of systemic disease, sensitivity of the primary tumor to radiation and chemotheray, and interval from diagnosis of the primary tumor to that of cerebral metastasis. With regard to medical status, the suitability of the patient for craniotomy must be determined. Coexisting medical conditions including cardiorespiratory abnormalities or evolving hepatic insufficiency, leukopenia, thrombocytopenia, and significant coagulation abnormalities may make surgery too great a risk in relation to expected gains. Patients with minimal or no neurological deficit at the time of consideration for craniotomy seem to do better in terms of median survival. However, even patients with moderate neurological deficits may derive significant palliative benefits from craniotomy, including prolongation of the time to neurological progression or maintenance of neurological improvement until death from systemic disease.

It is not unreasonable to think that the presence of persistent primary tumor or one or two sites of metastatic disease should preclude surgery. However, our data suggest that such disease does not always affect survival after craniotomy. Obviously, no hard and fast rules as to the significance of a given systemic metastasis can be made. Extensive systemic disease or metastasis to a vital organ that is life-threatening makes surgery unattractive. However, if the systemic disease is under control, even if persistent, then surgical excision of the solitary brain metastasis may make sense. Added impetus for a decision for surgery may derive from the fact that the primary tumor is known to be of a radioresistant type. A highly radiosensitive tumor, such as lymphoma or choriocarcinoma, suggests that radiation may be the best initial therapy.

The value of the interval between diagnosis of the primary tumor and appearance of the intracerebral metastasis is a relative one. Evaluating a series of patients who underwent excision of solitary intracranial metastases between 1972 and 1978 at Memorial Hospital, we found that patients who presented with a cerebral metastasis one year or more after the diagnosis of the primary cancer had a significantly longer survival than those in whom the metastasis was detected within one year. This makes biological sense, if one assumes that those in the latter group had more aggressive tumors. However, the matter is not so simple. In another group of patients who underwent surgical resection of non-oat cell lung cancer cerebral metastases between 1978 and 1981, long-term survivors were found in those who presented with both the brain metastasis and the primary tumor at the same time and actually underwent craniotomy prior to thoracotomy. Clearly, one cannot make too simple generalizations about the biology of different tumor types. Although the ideal candidate for surgical excision of an intracerebral mass lesion may be the patient with little or no neurological deficit and no systemic metastases in whom the diagnosis of the primary tumor was made a year or more earlier, much can be done for the patient with more extensive and, perhaps, aggressive disease to achieve palliation.

Aside from the standard medical and preoperative evaluations, the CT scan or the MRI scan is critical, not only for ascertaining that the brain lesion is indeed solitary, but also for the precise localization of the tumor. Precise localization of the tumor, utilizing the techniques now available in tomographic brain imaging, means not only less operative time but less patient morbidity because the brain is disturbed as little as possible. With careful preparation of this sort, even lesions in the dominant hemisphere near the speech or motor control areas can be removed without increasing, and often reducing, the neurological deficit. Steroid preparation for surgery is essential for all patients.

At surgery, complete excision of the metastases is the goal. Because of the fact that a plane between the tumor and the surrounding compressed and edematous brain tissue can be developed, the likelihood of complete removal is enhanced. Removal with magnification helps to ensure this. The metastatic tumors thus differ from the primary central nervous system tumors of glial origin which have a greater tendency to invade and/or infiltrate surrounding brain tissue. With the best anesthetic and surgical techniques, perioperative mortalities can be less than 5 percent and rapid recovery is the rule. Occasionally, in addition, the final pathologic examination reveals a diagnosis different from that expected. Sometimes a second primary is revealed. At other times, benign disease is determined.

For properly selected patients, the surgical removal of a solitary brain metastasis offers substantial benefits that outweigh the risks of surgery. In a series of 75 patients who had this procedure at Memorial Hospital from 1977 to 1980, median survival time was 8.9 months. For patients whose disease was limited to the central nervous system, 75 percent were alive at one year. For those who had disease in the chest or elsewhere, median survival was 4.5 months and less than 10 percent survived for one year. Two-year overall survival was 18/75 or 24 percent. Five patients have survived for 5 years. Thirty-day mortality for the entire series was 9 percent, but 0 percent in the 40 patients who had no evidence of disease outside the CNS. The relapse rate was 11 percent at the operative site, and an additional 10 percent developed other intracranial metastases. Those who did not receive postoperative radiation had more recurrences, emphasizing the value of postoperative radiation. In a recent series of non-oat cell lung cancer patients with solitary brain metastases who underwent surgical excision, median survival was 14 months. With no local or systemic disease at the time of craniotomy median survival was 23 months, and even with the primary tumor present, median survival rose to 18 months with a combination of craniotomy and aggressive primary tumor therapy. These figures are important for patients with this tumor since, at Memorial, approximately 20 percent develop brain metastasis, many within the first year after diagnosis.

Although no one can minimize the seriousness of CNS metastasis, whether solitary or multiple, the fact is that meaningful palliation can be achieved for many patients. For the patient with the solitary brain metastasis, even more can be gained, including, for a few, long-term survival. The use of steroids, radiation therapy, and surgery, either alone or in combination, depending on individual patient circumstances, is indi-cated. Although no rigid rules can be used to determine the optimal therapeutic combination, vigorous clinical efforts can be rewarding for the patient. In this setting, surgery is a viable and valuable option.

PINEAL REGION TUMOR

JEFFREY A. WINFIELD, M.D., Ph.D.

The current recommended management of masses in the pineal region reflects the advances made during the last thirty years in the fields of neuroradiology, endocrinology, neuropathology, neuroanesthesia, and the development of microneurosurgical techniques. Prior to 1960, surgical mortality ranged from 30 to 70 percent, with morbidity in excess of 50 percent. Surgical conservation was therefore advocated, with treatment directed at CSF diversion followed by radiotherapy. This method of treatment carried less than a 5 percent mortality and a 5-year survival of 60 to 75 percent. The previously reported acceptable 5-year survival with shunting and radiotherapy probably reflects the high percentage of germinomas found in this region and this tumor's radiosensitivity.

Owing largely to the efforts of Russel and Rubinstein, pathologists have arrived at the following classification of tumors of the region:

I Tumors of germ-cell origin (teratomas)
   1. Germinomas
   2. Typical teratoma (benign)
   3. Teratoma (malignant)
      a. Teratocarcinoma
      b. Choriocarcinoma
      c. Embryonal carcinoma
      d. Endodermal sinus tumor
      e. Mixed teratoma and germinoma
II Pineal parenchymal cell origin
   1. Pineocytoma
   2. Pineoblastoma
III Other cell origin
   1. Glioma
   2. Meningioma
   3. Hemangiopericytoma
IV Cystic tumors
   1. Epidermoid
   2. Dermoid

In the early 1970s, several surgeons reported excellent surgical success with pineal tumor surgery. The refinements in anesthetic techniques and development of microsurgical instruments and the operative microscope allow for biopsy and/or partial-to-gross total resection of tumors in this deep brain area, with mortality less than 5 percent and minimal morbidity. With the development of high-resolution CT scanning, the neuroradiographic "fingerprints" of tumors in this region could begin to be correlated with the precise histologic types obtainable with safe surgical biopsy. Furthermore, survival could then be assessed, and the biological behavior of these individual tumors determined. Thus, Cushing's dilemma regarding radiation of these tumors as "a therapeutic shot in the dark so long as the tumor's precise histologic type is unknown" has been resolved. Advances in endocrinology have allowed for both hormonal replacement postoperatively, when needed, and the identification of associated secretions of beta human chorionic gonadotropin (hCG) and alpha fetoprotein (AFP) from these tumors. These secretants, when present, provide a valuable tool for assessing tumor response to treatment and for identifying specific tumor types.

The clinical presentation of pineal area tumors is usually a fairly typical one, with symptoms attributed to mass effects which cause obstruction of CSF outflow from the third ventricle, leading to the development of hydrocephalus and mesencephalic brain stem compression. Endocrine disorders, although less common, are usually associated with specific tumor histopathology. The clinical presentations can be categorized as follows: (1) CSF outflow obstruction or hydrocephalus (headache, vomiting, drowsiness, papilledema with decrease in visual acuity), (2) mesencephalic compression or Parinaud's syndrome (upgaze palsy, light/accommodation dissociation, failure of covergence), and (3) endocrine abnormalities (diabetes insipidus in one-third of germinomas, precocious puberty with some teratomas, decreased libido). Endocrine abnormalities are rarely seen with pineal parenchymal tumors. Diagnostic studies following admission should include: (1) endocrine evaluation of serum and CSF (if safe to perform lumbar puncture) including studies for hCG and AFP as well as sex hormone levels if endocrine abnormalities exist, (2) CSF cytology, which is positive in 60 percent of germinomas, and (3) neuroradiological studies such as CT scans with and without contrast, MRI, and, if necessary, angiogram to rule out possible aneurysm).

Although the radiographic features of the tumor noted on CT cannot always predict the histologic type, for the tumors most commonly found in the pineal region (germinomas, teratomas, and pineal parenchymal tumors), CT appearance is fairly typical. Germinomas tend to be hyperdense uniform masses with an increased incidence of premature pineal gland calcification. These tumors enhance homogeneously with IV contrast. Although similar in radiographic appearance, pineal parenchymal tumors are not associated with premature pineal calcification, and the absence of clinical endocrine abnormalities and the presence of normal hCG and AFP levels favor the latter diagnosis. Irregularities, tumor calcification, fat densities within the tumor, and the presence of cysts favor a diagnosis of teratoma, dermoid, or epidermoid. Peritumor edema with intravenous contrast ring enhancement is strongly suggestive of malignant disease.

Correlating age, sex, clinical presentation, endocrine evaluation, CSF cytology and hCG and AFP levels, and CT findings, the following treatment plan is suggested. If a uniformly enhancing lesion is found on CT studies and the patient is a teenage male, the diagnosis is strongly suggestive of a germinoma. A short course of radiotherapy is given, and the known biological behavior of a germinoma is such that tumor shrinkage occurs with 600 to 2000 rads. If a repeat CT shows that the tumor mass has decreased, the diagnosis is germinoma, and radiotherapy can be completed. Although lumbar CSF cytology may not confirm the diagnosis of germinoma, positive lumbar CSF cytology does not correlate with the presence or absence of drop metastases. Failure of treatment for pineal germinomas often is associated with intradural metastasis along the neuroaxis. Craniospinal radiation is advocated.

On repeat CT, if the uniformly enhancing mass has not decreased in size, a pineal parenchymal tumor or, rarely, a meningioma should be suspected, and surgery is required for definitive diagnosis. In the patient whose CT shows calcification, tumor irregularities, cysts, contrast ring enhancement, and/or fat density, surgery should be the initial form of treatment. Twenty-five percent of tumors in the pineal region are benign and therefore not radiosensitive.

In patients with severe hydrocephalus and clinical deterioration, emergent ventriculoperitoneal shunting may be required prior to definitive surgical exploration of the pineal region. Preoperative extracranial ventricular drainage provides an alternative and eliminates the potential for peritoneal seeding from germinomas and pineoblastomas, which have a high incidence of CSF spread.

If available, CT-guided stereotactic biopsy can be performed. Cystic structures can be aspirated or shunted with dramatic clinical improvement.

When direct surgical exploration is required, we prefer the infratentorial supracerebellar approach originally described by Krause in 1926. Other approaches to the pineal region include the posterior transcallosal approach championed by Dandy and the Jamieson right occipital transtentorial approach (modified Poppen approach). Several anatomic relationships make the infratentorial supracerebellar approach preferable because (1) minimal brain retraction is required, (2) transneural tissue dissection is not required, (3) allows early visualization of the brain stem/tumor plane, and (4) permits tumor resection beneath the great draining veins, which are lateral and superior to the tumor mass.

At surgery, following intubation, a right frontal extracranial ventricular drainage catheter is placed. This allows for CSF diversion intraoperatively. CSF specimens should be sent for cytopathologic study. Even if tumor resection is complete, postoperative edema in the mesencephalon usually causes aqueductal stenosis, and temporary CSF diversion may be required. Intracranial pressure monitoring postoperatively will assess the need for permanent shunting procedures. Standard anesthetic techniques are used for surgery in the sitting position. With the head held in the Gardner Wells tongues, the patient is placed in the sitting position with the head flexed forward. The operative table is positioned with the head tilted so that a knee-chest sitting position is established. A midline incision is made 4 cm anterior to the inion and carried inferiorly to C_2. Standard subperiosteal dissection is carried out, exposing the entire suboccipital area. A trapezoid craniotomy is then performed with the apex over the torcular. Both lateral sinuses should be skeletonized. The posterior portion of the foramen magnum does not have to be removed. The dura is opened in one large triangle or three small adjacent triangles with the bases of the triangles on the sinus. The dural flaps are retracted superiorly, exposing the superior surface of the cerebellum. The cisterna magna is then opened, allowing for further decompression of the posterior fossa as well as establishing a CSF pathway for flow of CSF out of the posterior third ventricle, over the cerebellum, and into the cisterna magna following tumor resection. Once the cerebellar surface is covered by cottonoids, self-retaining retractors are placed. Gravity provides the greatest cerebellar retraction, and little downward retraction is required. The anterior cerebellar veins, which may be multiple, are then coagulated and cut, allowing for further cerebellar retraction and exposure of the hiatus of the tentorium. The operative microscope is then brought into the surgical field. A thickened, milky white arachnoid is then encountered, which covers the quadrigeminal plate, tumor, and vascular structures. Care must be taken in opening this arachnoid to prevent damage to vascular structures. Once inside the quadrigeminal cistern, the brain stem is visualized inferiorly and the tumor above and superiorly. Using microbipolar coagulation on the tumor and sharp dissection, a plane of clearance is developed. Working circumferentially, the plane of dissection is developed laterally between the tumor and the ventral basal vein of Rosenthal bilaterally, superiorly between the tumor and the great vein of Galen, and inferiorly between the tumor and the quadrigeminal plate. Once the posterior half of the tumor has been dissected free from these structures, interval tumor debulking can be performed using the micro cup forceps, cavitron, and laser. Specimens are also sent for pathologic study at this time.

The anterior half of the tumor is fixed to the velum interpositum and internal cerebral veins superiorly and the habenular trigeon inferiorly. The tumor's most anterior inferior surface rests against the posterior roof of the third ventricle.

The most critical part of the microdissection now remains. Interruption of the internal cerebral veins would result in venous infarct of the thalamus. Damage to the mesencephalon below the tumor would leave the patient with disabling vertical gaze problems.

Two layers of arachnoid lie between tumor and the internal cerebral veins. Once again, by means of micro-bipolar coagulation and sharp dissection, the anterior superior half of the tumor is removed from the internal cerebral veins with dissection between the two plains of arachnoid. With the dissection now completed superiorly, the tumor can be rolled forward and the dissection completed anterior to the superior colliculi. If the tumor is pineal parenchymal, the stalk of the pineal gland has to be transected and the tumor can be removed. The posterior portion of the third ventricle will have been opened and the entire third ventricular visualized. The dorsal medial thalamic nucleus and posterior medial portions of the pulvinar should be inspected. These surfaces should be "glossy white". Several small thrombin-soaked pieces of gelfoam are applied to the tumor bed and irrigated free after several minutes. Great care should be taken to ensure that no bleeding occurs on the tumor bed and that all blood is irrigated out of the third ventricle. The retractors and cottonoids are then carefully removed.

The dura is then closed in a watertight fashion. Periosteal grafts or commercially available dura can be used to ensure a watertight closure. The muscles are closed in multiple layers. Care should be taken in closing the superior portion of the incision as only galea and scalp layers are present.

Postoperative care is routine with a one-week steroid taper. Ventricular drainage and ICP monitoring are indicated for 24 to 48 hours to assess the need for possible shunting. Parinaud's syndrome may be worse in the initial postoerative period. Although the patient may have difficulty with upward gaze on command, Bells phenomenon can be checked. When the patient is asked to tightly close the eyes, the eyes rotate outward and upward. If this persists, the upward gaze palsy is supranuclear and usually recovers over several weeks.

Further adjuvant therapy depends on the final pathologic diagnosis of the tumor. We do not radiate pineocytomas, whereas patients with pineoblastomas receive craniospinal irradiation. Unless the tumor is a malignant teratoma, no radiation is given to patients with teratomas, epidermoids, or dermoids. Chemotherapy can be given to the patient with choriocarcinoma, and AFP levels must be monitored. If either hCG or AFP levels were initially elevated, they can be periodically monitored. The role of chemotherapy for pineal parenchymal tumors remains speculative. The pineal gland does not have a blood-brain barrier and may therefore be susceptible to intravenous chemotherapy.

CRANIOFACIAL NEOPLASIA

GEORGE W. SYPERT, M.D.

The management of craniofacial neoplasia involves the treatment of extensive malignant tumors originating in the orbit, the paranasal sinuses, and the ear. The most frequent histologic diagnoses include squamous cell carcinoma, basal cell carcinoma, rhabdomyosarcoma, and fibrosarcoma. Severel features of these neoplasms indicate that they, like other head and neck cancers, may be best treated by radical surgery. There is frequently bone invasion at the time of initial diagnosis. This substantially increases the incidence of complications with curative doses of radiation therapy. Although 5-year survival rates of 30 to 40 percent have been reported, the risk of radionecrosis is high. In addition, these neoplasms tend to grow by local invasion and only rarely are associated with distant metastases. They are therefore at least curable by a single therapeutic modality, that is, radical surgical excision.

The clinical experience with piecemeal resection and radiation therapy in the treatment of these lesions repeatedly has yielded dismal survival statisitics for these patients (i.e., less than 8% after 5 years). This eventually led to the adoption of Halsted's traditional principles of en bloc resection in the surgery of neoplastic lesions.

En bloc craniofacial surgery requires an extensive knowledge of both head and neck (facial) surgical and neurosurgical techniques. The potential for complications, including meningitis, exsanguinating hemorrhage, and neurological deficits, is high. Indeed, in some of the early surgical reports, operative mortality rates exceeded the average 5-year survival. It became clear that a team approach, utilizing the skills of both a neurosurgeon and a facial surgeon, would provide the optimal results. During the past two decades, excellent survival rates with minimal morbidity and mortality have been routinely reported, using the combined approach.

Patients afflicted with craniofacial neoplasms are among the most difficult and challenging problems encountered by the neurosurgeon and facial surgeon.

EVALUATION

The en bloc resection of an extensive craniofacial neoplasm is a formidable procedure, even for an experienced neurosurgical-facial surgical team. It must be kept in mind that this type of procedure is only appropriate when there is a reasonable chance of cure. If the tumor has invaded structures that render it incurable, surgical palliation can be achieved through a much easier, and less risky, piecemeal resection. Therefore, the entire aim of the preoperative evaluation should be to assess the extent to which the tumor has invaded contiguous structures.

The preoperative evaluation should include naso-pharyngoscopic examination, skull films, and skull tomography. Skull tomography may be accomplished by polytomographic techniques and/or thin-section computed tomography (CT). Chest roentgenograms, bone scans, and metabolic studies are used to rule out distant metastases. Brain scans, EEG, and CSF analysis have not proved helpful in evaluating the neoplasm. Although some authorities also advocate the use of angiography and venography, I have not found these studies to be routinely necessary. In rare hypervascular neoplasms and certain special cases in which the neoplasm involves major cerebral vascular structures, these latter studies may prove to be invaluable.

If any of the aforementioned studies reveals invasion of the brain, sphenoid sinus, ptyergoid fossa, or cervical vertebrae, or evidence of metastases below the clavicle, the patient is considered to be a poor candidate for en bloc resection. In many cases, the extent of invasion can only be fully assessed at the time of surgery. For example, clouding of the sphenoid sinus may be secondary to either infection or neoplasm. A sphenoid biopsy at the beginning of the surgical procedure can resolve the question. The neurosurgeon must initially assess the extent of intracranial disease to determine whether a potentially curable en bloc procedure is appropriate.

SURGICAL THERAPY

Some general principles are essential to achieving an excellent result, regardless of the specific craniofacial area involved. The prevention of meningitis is obviously of great concern. Because portions of the operation must cross unsterile areas (i.e., the nasopharynx), the use of prophylactic antibiotics is deemed essential. Oxicillin or a cephalosporin, administered from 12 hours prior to surgery through the tenth postoperative day, has proved to be a successful regimen.

Varying degrees of brain retraction are required. Accordingly, spinal CSF drainage and mannitol are routinely used to reduce the amount of force required to obtain adequate exposure. Moreover, continued CSF drainage over the first postoperative day may reduce the incidence of CSF leakage through small undetected dural tears.

Finally, if the neoplasm invades dura, the dura must be widely resected, and a graft must be applied. The neosurgeon must ensure that the dural graft is covered by tissue with an intact vascular supply. It is imperative that such areas be covered with full-thickness pedicle grafts or by a galeal pedicle graft interposed between the dura graft and a split-thickness skin graft.

Orbital Neoplasms

Cranio-orbital resection is an en bloc excision of the orbit and the floor of the anterior cranial fossa. It is an appropriate procedure for extensive and/or recurrent neoplasms of the orbit that have not invaded the paranasal sinuses. A circumorbital incision is made in the soft tissues, exposing the bony margins of the orbit. Multiple small bur holes are connected with a small osteotome. The roof of the orbit is then carefully separated from the dura and pushed downward. The operative exposure is generally excellent, requiring very little brain retraction. Any involved dura is resected en bloc and replaced with a suitable graft. All dural lacerations must be meticulously repaired to avoid CSF leakage and resultant meningitis, and this can best be accomplished after the en bloc specimen is removed. The optic nerve is exposed, coagulated, and divided carefully without damaging the optic chiasm.

Laterally, the resection includes the zygomatic bone and anterior sphenoid bone. Medially, the resection includes the ipsilateral lacrimal bone, ethmoid sinuses, lateral nasal bone and turbinates, and the anterior sphenoid sinus. Inferiorly, the orbital floor and malar bone are taken. Great care is exercised in mobilizing the posterior orbit in order to avoid damage to the middle fossa contents and cavernous sinus.

Adequacy of resection may be assessed by means of biopsies from the surgical margins. The large defect is usually covered with a split-thickness skin graft held firmly in place with a suitably shaped stent. If a dural graft is required, it cannot be supported by a split-thickness skin graft alone because this frequently leads to breakdown of the graft and infection. Definitive cosmetic reconstruction, if desired, is generally undertaken after a 2-year tumor-free period.

Paranasal Sinus Neoplasms

Most of these lesions originate in the maxillary sinuses. At the time of initial diagnosis, however, almost all sinus cancers have invaded the ethmoids and are consequently unresectable via a transfacial approach. Hence, a combined craniofacial approach is required if curative surgery is contemplated.

The first step of the craniofacial procedure is to carefully dissect the dura from the floor of the anterior cranial fossa via a small supraorbital craniectomy in order to inspect the intracranial contents to determine whether an en bloc curative resection is possible. The en bloc resection includes the middle portion of the anterior cranial fossa back to the sphenoid sinus, both medial orbital walls (lateral ethmoid walls), and the walls of the involved maxillary sinus laterally to include the zygomatic arch. If neoplasm is identified within the orbit, an en bloc exenteration is included in the procedure, as described for the orbital tumors. By utilizing the principles previously enumerated, appropriate skin coverage is selected to cover the surgical defect.

Ear Neoplasms

Neoplasms of the external and middle ear, invading the temporal bone, have long been regarded as incurable. This impression originated from the dismal experience associated with piecemeal resection and the high mortality rates that were reported with early attempts at en bloc resection. With modern combined craniofacial surgery, however, some of these malignant tumors can be surgically cured.

The en bloc resection involves a subtotal temporal bone resection. A circular skin incision is made about the external ear. Through a linear neck incision, the soft tissues at the base of the skull are dissected. The sternocleidomastoid muscle is transected and the jugular vein is ligated. Great care must be taken to avoid damage to the carotid artery and to the ninth, tenth, and twelfth cranial nerves. Lymph node biopsies are performed, and if necessary, a radical neck dissection can be undertaken as part of the en bloc procedure. The ascending ramus of the mandible and the zygomatic arch are transected. The squamous portion of the temporal bone is removed. If inspection of the intracranial contents confirms the possibility of en bloc resection for cure, the operation proceeds.

The floor of the middle fossa is transected to the foramen spinosum. A suboccipital bur hole is placed, and the bony removal is carried across the transverse sinus. Occipital bone is removed inferiorly and anteriorly until the jugular foramen is reached. The dura is progressively dissected from the bony groove of the transverse and sigmoid sinuses, with coagulation of any emissary veins. The petrous pyramid is transected in a sagittal plane with an osteotome at the arcuate eminence and the specimen is delivered from the wound en bloc.

The surgical defect is covered with a posteriorly based scalp flap. Split-thickness skin grafts are used to cover the donor site.

RESULTS

The best results are obtained in patients with orbital tumors, in whom 5-year tumor-free survivals are reported to be in excess of 90 percent. This follows because these lesions are generally more localized at the time of surgery than those involving either the paranasal sinuses or the temporal bone. Operative mortality is also quite low in patients with paranasal sinus cancers, and their long-term survival rate is 50 to 75 percent. In cases involving the temporal bone, the operative mortality is higher (15 to 20%), and the long-term survival is generally less than 33 percent.

Meningitis was responsible for the only death in my series and for most of the other reported operative mortalities. This can be directly attributed to CSF leakage from inadequately repaired dural tears and attempts to cover dural graft with split-thickness skin grafts. Free frontal bone flaps are at great risk of late infection. Consequently, an enlarged bur-hole craniectomy has become the preferred technique for anterior fossa exploration and exposure.

Severe hemorrhage was a problem in the early reports. The shift to team surgery, with improved knowledge of the anatomy and control of intracranial vascular structures, has largely eliminated this difficulty. Transient neurological deficits, usually related to frontal lobe retraction, have also been reported. They have been minimized with the routine use of CSF drainage and/or mannitol. Many patients who undergo temporal bone resection experience vertigo for 1 or 2 weeks afterward. In these latter patients, ipsilateral hearing and facial nerve function are sacrificed.

The results of combined craniofacial surgery must be judged in comparison to those obtained with other modes of therapy. For instance, although the long-term tumor-free survival for invasive temporal bone neoplasms treated with radical combined craniofacial resection may at first glance appear not to be worthwhile, a comparable group of such patients treated with radical mastoidectomy and radiation therapy had a 5-year survival of only 8 percent. Most of the patients referred for radical surgery have already undergone standard therapeutic procedures and have recurrent tumors. Many of the long-term survivors of combined craniofacial resection had previously been pronounced "incurable".

DISCUSSION

Dismal results with standard therapeutic modalities in the treatment of orbital, paranasal, and temporal bone cancers have led to the development of combined craniofacial surgery. The potential advantages of this approach are manifold. For example, the intracranial inspection allows the surgical team to assess the feasibility of an operative cure accurately. The brain is well protected. The control of hemorrhage and CSF leaks is facilitated. Orbital exenteration is not mandatory, as with purely transfacial approaches, and most importantly, Halsted's proven principles concerning the en bloc resection of cancer are observed.

Although operative morbidity and mortality were unacceptably high in some early series, great advances have since been made, and further improvement may be expected in the future. This can be attributed to several factors. Improved diagnostic techniques, especially the use of the thin-section CT scan and magnetic resonance imaging, have helped to eliminate inappropriate surgical candidates. Also, because the exact extent of the disease can be better delineated properatively, more precise surgical plans can be formulated in advance. Most important has been the adoption of the team approach, wherein the unique skills of the neurosurgeon and the facial surgeon can be fully utilized. Resultant improvements in operative procedures have included CSF drainage, complete control of intracranial vascular structures, meticulous management of the dura, and well-planned scalp flaps and skin grafts.

Currently, combined craniofacial surgery for craniofacial malignant tumors provides an excellent mode of therapy for heretofore "hopeless" patients.

PEDIATRIC TUMORS

CRANIOPHARYNGIOMA

DEREK A. BRUCE, M.B., Ch.B.

Craniopharyngiomas account for 2 to 3 percent of all brain tumors and 5 to 9 percent of brain tumors in children below the age of 15 years. These tumors are believed to arise from epithelial cell rests in the infundibular stalk of the hypothalamus, and in the sella turcica between the two lobes of the pituitary gland. When the tumors are thin-walled single cysts arising from the intrasellar area, they may be difficult to separate from epidermoid cysts or Rathke's pouch cysts, all of which have epithelial cell origins. It may be that these represent varieties of the same tumor type. Twenty percent of craniopharyngiomas are intrasellar. These are usually single cysts with compressed pituitary tissue in the cyst wall. Eighty percent are suprasellar, arising in the pituitary stalk, hypothalamus, or occasionally truly intraventricular. The location of these tumors places them in intimate contact with the optic chiasm, optic nerves, infundibular stalk, vessels of the circle of Willis, and the third cranial nerve. The posterior boundaries of the tumor are the cerebral peduncles and the basilar artery. Superiorly, the boundaries are the floor of the third ventricle and, still more superiorly, the foramen of Monro. The site of these tumors, then, predicts their presentation, and thus hormonal control to the pituitary gland may be lost as a result of interferences with the infundibular stalk, resulting in diabetes insipidus, short stature, hypothyroidism, hypogonadism, or hypoadrenalism. If the chiasm or optic nerves are affected, visual field defects occur. These are most commonly bitemporal hemianopsia. If the tumor is large, extending up into the third ventricle, interference with CSF drainage from the lateral ventricles will occur, with the production of hydrocephalus and signs of symptoms of increased intracranial pressure.

In children, the first sign of craniopharyngioma is usually poor linear growth. However, this is rarely considered to be significant, and only when puberty is obviously delayed is a physician consulted. Ten to 15 percent of children with craniopharyngiomas present because of short stature and delayed puberty. The single most frequent presentation in children is headache and vomiting (signs of increased intracranial pressure). Papilledema and visual field or acuity defects are the most frequent clinical signs. These may or may not be associated with short status, obesity, or delayed puberty. In adults, the tumors tend to be smaller, the most frequent symptoms are visual, and the most frequent sign is bitemporal hemianopsia.

Except in cases of the largest tumors, endocrine symptoms are usually mild. Indications for further studies are the continuation of headaches, which are frequently nonspecific, and visual complaints, even if no objective abnormalities are found on field examination. Because of the subtlety of the symptoms and the onset of diabetes insipidus, which frequently presents as bedwetting, a psychological reason for the symptoms is a common misdiagnosis, and 30 percent of the children I see have been treated by psychologists or psychiatrists for emotional difficulties.

Routine blood studies are usually normal. The most useful screening test is a plain skull film. This will be positive in approximately 80 percent of children with lesions in this area, showing one of the following: (1) suprasellar calcification, (2) erosion of the posterior clinoid process, (3) ballooning of the sella turcica, or (4) evidence of intracranial hypertension with splitting of the sutures and demineralization of the sellar floor. The conclusive neuroradiographic study is the CT scan, and this should be done with and without contrast injection and in coronal as well as in horizontal plane. Very small lesions may require metrizamide CT scan to be certain that a suprasellar component is present. The MRI scan has proved of enormous benefit in this area and can pick up small lesions with probably greater accuracy than the plain CT scan. Cerebral angiography usually is not necessary, but the indications for it are (1) to rule out any vascular lesions, such as an aneurysm, and (2) to look for evidence of displacement of the anterior cerebral arteries, anterior choroidal arteries, and the basilar vein of Rosenthal. All of these structures are displaced in a different way, depending on the exact locus of the tumor. In children, the tumor is usually large, frequently posterior to the chiasm and rising up into the third ventricle. Under these circumstances, the angiogram is often almost normal. Because of this, if the CT scan is clearly diagnostic of the craniopharyngioma, angiography is often not necessary.

TREATMENT

The treatment alternatives for this tumor are limited to surgery, surgery plus radiation therapy, or radiation therapy alone. Chemotherapy has not proved effective, although there is at least one report of the use of methotrexate in this tumor.

The surgical approach varies, depending on the tumor location. Intrasellar tumors can be operated on via the transsphenoidal approach through the nose. In children less than 10 years old, however, we do not advise this approach because of the limited amount of room and the risk of fracturing the facial bones and nasal structures. Furthermore, it is rare for these tumors in children to be truly intrasellar. The transcranial surgical approach has also varied from the truly subfrontal approach, the bifrontal approach, and, most recently, what is called the pterional approach. I prefer to operate on all of these lesions using the pterional approach. In children, there is no indication for radiation therapy without at least surgical biopsy of these lesions.

These tumors are in the infundibular stalk and grow in the suprasellar and interpeduncular spaces. They are best visualized if approached from an inferolateral direction. The pterional approach permits one to do this best.

An incision is made behind the hairline, stretching from just anterior to the ear to the midline of the forehead. A small bone flap is removed, based on the lateral margin of the lesser wing of the sphenoid bone. The remainder of the lateral 50 percent of the lesser wing of the sphenoid is drilled away, allowing the brain to be approached from an inferolateral direction. This minimizes the amount of traction that is required for normal brain. These tumors are frequently partially cystic, and thus fluid drainage allows better exposure of the area and immediately relieves compression of the optic chiasm. The tumor is covered by two layers of arachnoid. Both of these have to be dissected off the tumor capsule. Otherwise, the small vessels that supply the chiasm and hypothalamus may be damaged.

Even with large tumors, a total surgical resection is possible in 75 to 80 percent of cases. The mortality should be zero. There is some definite morbidity, however. Since the tumor is in the pituitary stalk, the stalk must be divided if the tumor is to be totally resected. Thus, 90 percent or more of patients undergoing total resection of the suprasellar cranipharyngioma are left with postoperative diabetes insipidus. This is usually quite easily controlled with nasal DDAVP taken once or twice per day. However, problems with fluid balance can be seen (1) in cases of damage to the hypothalamic thirst mechanisms, which occurs in 4 to 5 percent of operative cases, or (2) in children under 3 years of age, in whom adequate balance between thirst, fluid intake, and DDAVP dosage can be quite complex. The most frequent complication is postsurgical hyperphagia. Unless the cortical steroids that are used to prepare for surgery are rapidly tapered to minimum replacement dosages quickly and the parents instructed to be strict about the early eating habits, 50 percent of these children will show a marked increase in weight within the first few months. Concomitant with this increase in weight is an increase in linear growth despite the absence of growth hormone. It has been suggested that insulin or insulin-like compounds may function as a secondary growth hormone-like agent. This hyperphagia is usually self-limiting, and although the children tend to remain somewhat overweight with dietary control and minimal replacement steroids, constant weight can be achieved with continued linear growth often in the absence of growth hormone. A less frequent but more serious complication is further deterioration of visual function and/or motor dysfunction (i.e., hemiplegia) due to carotid injury or spasm. These complications are exceedingly rare, but disastrous when they occur. In the immediate 1- to 2-day postoperative period, an unusual syndrome similar to interpenduncular hallucinosis is seen. This is especially true in children with large tumors stretching up into the third ventricle. This syndrome consists of confusion, excitation, usual visual hallucinations, and failure of response to visual stimuli despite normal pupil responses and normal visual evoked responses. My own explanation for this is that there is spasm of the small perforating vessels to the interpeduncular area and to the geniculate bodies. These vessels are all dissected out during the surgical resection. I have never seen this syndrome remain longer than 2 or 3 days, and it has always resolved completely.

In the immediate postoperative period, the first 12 hours, there is usually a period of very little urine output. This is followed by several days of large urine outputs and true diabetes insipidus. There is then a third phase of decreased urine output as residual ADH is released from the pituitary gland. Patients then enter a fairly stable period in which there may or may not be a persistent need for DDAVP. In the first few postoperative days, the diabetes insipidus, if mild, is best treated with fluid replacement. Care must be taken not to give large amounts of dextrose-containing fluids intravenously since this, in combination with steroids, can produce very high serum glucose levels and contribute to osmotic diuresis and electrolyte imbalance. If the patient is awake and alert, the ideal fluid intake is achieved by oral administration of water. It is unusual for this phase to pass without some replacement ADH, given as (1) intramuscular aqueous pitressin in doses of 3 to 5 units, or (2) slow intravenous infusion of aqueous pitressin, or (3) intranasal DDAVP. All of these agents work well. The advantages of aqueous ADH are (1) it has a short effect, and (2) it is less likely to cause problems with electrolyte imbalance. Seizures in the postoperative period are more common in patients with craniopharyngiomas than in those with other tumors in this area and are probably related to the osmotic, fluid and sodium changes. Consequently, routinely prescribe dilantin in the immediate postoperative period to be continued for one month.

Vision was worse postoperatively in 5 percent of the children operated on for craniopharyngiomas in our institution. It improved in 60 percent of the patients, and remained unchanged in the other 35 percent. These figures correlate fairly well with other people's experience. Initial gross total resection of these lesions was felt to be possible in 80 percent of cases. However, 10 to 20 percent of patients in whom a total resection was felt to be achieved can be expected to suffer a recurrence within the first 5 years. In patients who had residual tumor postoperatively, it is usual to advise radiation therapy, except in those very young children in whom radiation is more likely to be detrimental. Our experience, although limited, shows that one-third of the children treated with surgery and radiation have had a recurrence within a 3-year period. Recurrent tumor presents a problem. If the children have not previously been irradiated, I usually suggest reoperation followed by radiation therapy. This therapy has been used in only three patients in our own experience, and as yet no recurrences have been seen during a 5-year follow-up. Of tumors that recurred and were reoperated on without radiation therapy, one in four has recurred.

Intellectual function is generally well preserved in children after surgical removal of craniopharyngioma. Of 13 children who are 5 years old or older, in whom testing is available, 11 have a normal or superior IQ and two have a low normal IQ. Of the five children who received radiation therapy, two are in the normal range and three low normal. This is certainly not an adequate experience to declare that radiation therapy is disadvantageous, but it does serve to confirm in our own minds that radiation is not necessary in every case and, furthermore, that radiation therapy is not a guaranteed cure in every case.

Our current recommendations then for children and adults with craniopharyngiomas is primarily an effort to remove the tumor completely. Radiation therapy is advised only if gross residual tumor remains, either at surgery or repeat CT scan. Careful follow-up with annual CT scans is necessary, but recurrence, when it occurs, appears to recur early in the first 3 years. Annual visual examinations and careful endocrinologic follow-up are most important since most of these children have panhypopituitarism. However, there is no reason that they should not lead full and productive lives. As with all children with brain tumors, intensive support for the family and the child through the few years following surgery is an extremely important aspect of their social, educational, and psychological rehabilitation.

BRAIN STEM GLIOMA

BERNARD L. MARIA, M.D.
BERNARD J. D'SOUZA, M.D.

For purposes of this discussion, the brain stem consists of the thalamus, midbrain, pons, and medulla oblongata. Brain stem tumors, which most often involve the pons and medulla, account for approximately 10 to 20 percent of intracranial tumors in children and adolescents. The peak age of onset is between 5 and 8 years, with 77 percent of patients with brain stem tumors being under the age of 20 years. In most patients, the period from onset of symptoms to diagnosis is less than 6 months and usually under 2 months. Brain biopsy is not often done because of the morbidity associated with this procedure in the region where several vital functions are localized. Anatomic involvement is often difficult to establish on the basis of radiographic appearance since there might be microscopic extension of the tumor. The diagnosis is frequently based on the combination of clinical and radiologic features. The intrinsic nature of the tumor and its location do not allow for a surgical cure, leaving radiotherapy as the principal treatment. Despite treatment, the prognosis for these patients remains extremely poor at a time when the outcome for patients harboring other posterior fossa tumors has improved.

CLINICAL FEATURES

One must suspect a brain stem glioma in a child who has a history and clinical findings of brain stem dysfunction. The typical clinical presentation of a brain stem glioma is manifested by a 2- to 5-month history of cranial nerve dysfunction with diplopia and/or facial weakness and difficulty in walking. Although hydrocephalus is usually a late occurrence, upper brain stem tumors may compress the aqueduct of Sylvius early on and cause headaches and vomiting. Behavioral changes have also been noted and sometimes appear several months before the brain stem glioma is diagnosed. Many unusual presentations have been reported with brain stem glioma; nightmares, night terrors, enuresis, psychiatric disorders, hyperkinetic behavior, and deterioration in school performance. Although these symptoms may be vague, ultimately the child develops major neurological deficits. The most common presenting symptom is ataxia. Unilateral or bilateral lateral rectus weakness develops early and is followed by facial weakness, paralysis of the soft palate, depressed palatal sensation, and sensory involvement of the fifth cranial nerve.

RADIOLOGIC DIAGNOSIS

CT scanning is the noninvasive diagnostic tool of preference. The earliest changes are reflected as distortion, displacement, or obliteration of the prepontine and perimesencephalic cisterns. Most often the tumor is iso-dense with the brain parenchyma on a noncontrasted CT scan. One may also see cystic change or necrosis. If calcifications are present, the CT scan density is high, as in the case of a prominent exophytic component. CT of the brain stem with intrathecal metrizamide is a reliable and sensitive diagnostic technique. It provides better definition and extension of the tumor along with subtle changes in brain stem morphology which can be missed on conventional CT scan. We also use brain stem audi-tory evoked responses (BAER) in patients with brain stem glioma in follow-up since they may accurately reflect changes in brain stem involvement by the tumor. However, it is not clear whether BAER are specific in the diagnosis. In summary, CT scanning with metrizamide appears to be the most sensitive and available way of diagnosing a brain stem glioma radiologically. However, magnetic resonance imaging (MRI) holds a very promis-ing future in diagnosis and follow-up of these patients.

DIFFERENTIAL DIAGNOSIS

A number of entities can mimic the presentation of a brain stem glioma including parasitic cysts, vascular disease, brain stem encephalitis, and tuberculomas. Clin-ical symptomatology in the population at risk, labora-tory data, and CT scans should distinguish parasitic cysts from a brain stem glioma. Neurological symptoms and signs of brain stem vascular malformations are often multiple, episodic, and progressive. Vascular disease can be difficult to distinguish from a brain stem glioma and sequential CT scans may be necessary. A preceding his-tory of viral infection and the presence of severe lethargy should point toward encephalitis rather than a brain stem glioma. One usually finds a CSF pleocytosis sup-porting brain stem encephalitis rather than tumor. Tuberculomas are now a rare pediatric entity. Neverthe-less, signs of infratentorial lesions can mimic those of brain stem gliomas and are more common in children than in adults. Systemic work-up, family history for tuberculosis, the results of skin testing, and CT scan help to establish the diagnosis. Finally, multiple sclerosis should be considered in any young adult with brain stem dysfunction. Visual and brain stem evoked responses and examination of the CSF for myelin basic protein, IgG and oligoclonal bands may be helpful in the diagno-sis of multiple sclerosis.

TREATMENT

Surgery

There is considerable controversy in the literature about the role of surgery in the management of most patients with brain stem gliomas. Histologic grading of the tumors has not been helpful in establishing the prog-nosis. Variations in histologic pattern occur within the same tumor, and sampling errors can easily provide misleading information. Obtaining biopsy material is often difficult in a diffusely swollen brain stem and may carry significant risks. In my opinion, surgery plays an important role when a large exophytic mass has been identified on metrizamide CT scan. At that time, surgery plays a role in removing a significant part of the tumor without impairing neurological function. At the same time, a specimen is obtained for histologic examination before therapy is instituted. In addition, the patient who presents with hemorrhage into a brain stem tumor may benefit from evacuation of the hematoma. Newer micro-surgical techniques now make this procedure feasible. Ependymomas, which sometimes mimic brain stem gli-omas in their presentation, can be removed with greater ease, and when there is reasonable doubt whether the child has a brain stem glioma, surgery should be under-taken. The most common indications for biopsy prior to radiotherapy are on atypical presentations, an atypical CT scan, or both. In patients with hydrocephalus, a ventriculoperitoneal shunt may be required.

In general, the advent of the CT scan removed much of the concern about misdiagnosis. Even so, some lesions may be difficult to differentiate from brain stem gliomas. For instance, children with von Recklinghausen's disease often form meningiomas in the foramen magnum area or neurofibromas of the lowest cranial nerves, and these lesions may present a diagnostic problem. Even with metrizamide cisternography, it may be virtually impos-sible to distinguish an intramedullary tumor from an extramedullary tumor. Exploration can be considered early in such patients because the extramedullary lesions are actually more common than are brain stem tumors and surgical verification may be the only way to differen-tiate between them. Clival tumors situated anterior to the brain stem present the same diagnostic problem, but are usually defined on coronal sections of a metrizamide cisternogram with more certainty than are those that occur at the foramen magnum. Preliminary reports indi-cate that magnetic resonance imaging (MRI) will improve diagnostic accuracy of brain stem lesions and eliminate the need for surgical exploration in some cases.

Radiotherapy

The mainstay of therapy of brain stem gliomas is radiation therapy. Prior to radiation therapy, treatment with Decadron is instituted to minimize the edema that follows radiation. The majority of patients are given a dose of 5000 to 5500 rads (200 rads/day) to the tumor bed. The port should include an area 4 to 5 cm beyond the area of involvement rostrally and extend to C2 cau-dally. In some cases, larger ports encompassing the whole brain are used or craniospinal radiation is given because of the suspicion of a malignant glioblastoma. Temporary remission of signs and symptoms almost always occurs, often after a lag period of several weeks following therapy. However, this encouraging early response does not seem to help the prognosis or survival. Survival rates have not changed significantly in the last 20 years and range from 40 to 50 percent at 3 years to 13 to 15 percent at 5 years. In the few long-term survivors, there is the potential for late complications from radiation therapy. Radiation given in higher doses but more frequent fractions (hyperfractionated radiation) is now being studied in these patients.

Chemotherapy

The use of chemotherapeutic agents has not been encouraging. In a few patients, stabilization may occur with cisplatin, vincristine, or the nitrosoureas (BCNU, CCNU). Few long-term survivors have been reported, and chemotherapy is used at first recurrence following radiation therapy.

POSTERIOR FOSSA EPENDYMOMA

ROBERT L. McLAURIN, M.D.

Posterior fossa tumors are more commonly seen in the pediatric age group than in adults. Various reported series have recorded the incidence of infratentorial tumors in children to be between 50 and 65 percent. In the adult population, the percentage is considerably less and the histologic types vary from those seen in childhood. Because of the greater experience and higher incidence of cerebellar tumors in the younger age groups, the following discussion will focus principally on that aspect of the problem.

The tumors occurring in the pediatric age group include, in order of frequency, cerebellar astrocytoma, medulloblastoma, and ependymoma. Each of these tumors has been reported to occur in adults, but the incidence is extremely low. Instead, tumors occurring in the cerebellum in the adult population are most often hemangioblastomas or metastatic tumors.

CLINICAL DIAGNOSIS

The clinical presentation of posterior fossa tumors, especially in children, is essentially the same, regardless of the type of lesion. The symptoms and findings on examination are the result of two pathophysiologic events. The most prominent of these is intracranial hypertension resulting from obstruction of cerebrospinal fluid circulation. Depending on the exact position of the tumor in the cerebellum, this obstruction may occur at the level of the aqueduct or in the fourth ventricle. The second pathophysiologic phenomenon involves the neurological deficit resulting from focal invasion or compression of neurological structures. Since the tumors are usually confined to the substance of the cerebellum, the neurological deficit is most likely to reflect cerebellar dysfunction. Certain types of cerebellar tumors, however, may extend into the lateral recesses of the posterior

fossa and produce deficit of one or more cranial nerves. Generally speaking, it is rare for cerebellar tumors to directly invade the brain stem and cause symptoms arising from that portion of the central nervous system.

As previously stated, the symptoms and findings on examination in children with posterior fossa tumors fall into two basic categories: those due to increased intracranial pressure and those due to altered local neurological function. Since these are stereotyped in most cases, the diagnosis usually is not difficult and can be made on clinical grounds in most cases.

The findings that are due to obstructive hydrocephalus and intracranial hypertension include increased head size, headache, vomiting, and certain visual and oculomotor signs. Although posterior fossa tumors are rare in infancy, they occur often enough to require inclusion in the differential diagnosis of macrocrania. There is nothing characteristic regarding the cranial configuration, although there have been occasional instances of asymmetric bulging of the posterior fossa on palpation which seems to correspond with an underlying expanding mass. Historically, it should be noted that the head was normal in size at the time of birth and the progressive macrocrania occurred thereafter; this obviously does not exclude other causes of macrocrania, but if the macrocrania was present at birth, the possibility of a posterior fossa tumor is remote.

Since most children with posterior fossa tumors are between 4 and 10 years of age, macrocrania is a rare finding, but the other symptoms of intracranial hypertension are extremely common. Headache is almost invariably present and has a rather characteristic pattern. The headache is generally present in the morning on first awakening and may be relieved after the child arises or after vomiting has occurred. The headaches begin insidiously and progressively increase in frequency and severity, presumably related to the rapidity of tumor growth. The headaches are usually felt in the frontotemporal areas and are therefore considered to be the consequence of hydrocephalus rather than the direct irritation of contiguous structures by the subtentorial mass.

Vomiting is probably the second most frequent symptom and, like the headache, has a characteristic pattern. It also occurs in the morning after the child arises, and after vomiting the youngster usually feels relief of headache and nausea. The basic pathophysiology responsible for the occurrence of morning headache and vomiting has not been documented. It is presumed that one possible factor may be the increased intracranial venous pressure associated with recumbency during the night. Another possible contributory factor may be mild hypercarbia due to hypoventilation while asleep. It is postulated that when the child arises, intracranial venous pressure begins to subside, and the hyperventilation that may occur associated with vomiting further reduces intracranial pressure and the consequent symptoms.

Oculomotor weakness is seen in approximately one-third of patients with cerebellar tumors. The most common form of extraocular weakness is that involving one or both abducens nerves. This is of no localizing value in relation to the tumor, but simply is a reflection of the downward displacement of the brain stem due to hydrocephalus. Much more common than esotropia is the presence of papilledema on funduscopic evaluation. Unfortunately, papilledema may be recognized only late in the course of the illness, and permanent damage to the optic nerve may have occurred. In rare instances, the visual loss resulting from papilledema may progress significantly, even after removal of the posterior fossa tumor.

Although plain radiographs of the skull are much less commonly done at present than they were several years ago, chronic intracranial hypertension is frequently manifested by widening of the incompletely fused cranial sutures during this period of childhood and also by increased digital markings, giving the "beaten silver" appearance of the skull. The latter radiologic finding is increasingly rare at present because of the fact that it represents long-standing intracranial hypertension, and the present methods of diagnosis are such that neglected increased pressure is uncommon.

Objective signs of altered neurologic function are usually later in occurrence. It is noteworthy that a head tilt or some degree of nuchal rigidity may be found on examination. Indeed, the head tilt may be part of the initial observations noted by the child's parents. This phenomenon and the signs of meningismus that may be present are presumably the result of herniation of the cerebellar tonsils through the foramen magnum. Although this observation is not truly a neurological deficit it is the result of local displacement of the neural tissue at the craniocervical junction.

The true neurological signs are principally those relating to cerebellar dysfunction. Tumor occurring in the midline cerebellum leads to truncal and gait ataxia. The child is unsteady in a sitting or walking posture, with instability of the trunk and sometimes inability to maintain an upright posture of the trunk. There may be no cerebellar disturbance involving the extremities in midline tumors. Ataxic gait, however, with a wide base and lack of ability to perform tandem walking, is generally part of the truncal ataxia. If the tumor involves the cerebellar hemispheres, the ataxic incoordination is more likely to involve the extremities. This results in dysmetria of the upper extremities with dysdiadocho-

kinesia as well as ataxia of the lower extremities.

Nystagmus may also be noted in youngsters with cerebellar tumors. There is still considerable uncertainty whether this results from cerebellar involvement or from secondary dysfunction of the brain stem due to extrinsic pressure. It is possible, therefore, that this finding is nonspecific in relation to the location of the tumor.

As noted previously, certain tumors that originate in the fourth ventricle and cerebellum may become exophytic into the lateral gutter on one side or the other. This is particularly characteristic of ependymomas. When the tumor does, in fact, extend into the lateral gutter and cerebellopontine angle, it may involve one or more of the cranial nerves. The most common nerves involved by such a process include the facial, glossopharyngeal, and vagal nerves. Rarely does such a tumor cause facial weakness, and even more rarely does it extend cephalad sufficiently to involve the trigeminal outflow.

In the latter stages of tumor symptomatology and CSF obstruction, the child may experience episodes of extensor posturing, including opisthotonus and extension of the extremities. Bradycardia and apnea may accompany these "cerebellar fits". These are of ominous significance as they probably represent transient episodic ischemia of the brain stem. These episodic occurrences do not respond to anticonvulsant therapy, but only to decompressive measures.

COMPUTED TOMOGRAPHIC DIAGNOSIS

At present, CT scans represent the most precise noninvasive method of preoperative diagnosis. The correlation between CT diagnosis and histology is remarkably good.

Astrocytomas, because they do not characteristically grow directly into the fourth ventricle, do not have halos around the tumor mass, it is frequently seen with medulloblastomas and ependymomas. The fourth ventricle is more likely to be displaced and deformed rather than filled by the tumor mass. The tumors may have a characteristic cystic appearance or may be solid and are usually seen as round or oval, sometimes lobulated, and usually well-defined lesions. A mural nodule can usually be identified within a cystic tumor, and the cyst is characteristically unilocular. The cyst wall is not enhanced with contrast material. The mural nodule and the solid astrocytomas usually do show distinct enhancement. Calcification may be present in approximately one-fourth of astrocytomas.

The medulloblastoma is usually accompanied by a halo because of its growth characteristics within the fourth ventricle. These tumors become densely enhanced and appear to be solid tumors rather than cystic. They are usually seen as fairly large tumors and, in most instances, are central in location. Enhancing lesions seen elsewhere over the surface of the cerebral hemispheres strongly suggests that the tumor is a medulloblastoma.

The ependymoma may be difficult to distinguish by

CT scan from the medulloblastoma. It is invariably an intraventricular tumor and therefore usually has a halo around the tumor mass. In contrast to medulloblastomas, which are characteristically solid in appearance, the, ependymoma may have small cystic lucencies, although these are not invariably present. As with the previously described tumors, contrast enhancement invariably occurs.

Extension into the cerebellopontine angle from the region of the fourth ventricle is more commonly seen with ependymomas than with the other tumor types.

It may be concluded from the preceding description of CT appearance that the cystic astrocytoma can usually be distinguished unequivocally. The solid astrocytoma, the ependymoma, and the medulloblastoma can usually be distinguished, but not invariably so. All other diagnostic methods have far less precision.

TREATMENT

Treatment of all posterior fossa tumors in children include surgical exploration and partial or complete removal of the lesion. Surgery is necessary regardless of the histology of the tumor because of its mechanical effect in blockage of the cerebrospinal fluid pathways. Therefore, regardless of whether a complete removal can be achieved and regardless of the potential effectiveness of radiation and chemotherapy, it is necessary that the mass of the tumor be removed to relieve the effects of ventricular obstruction.

Since there is generally some delay between the initial recognition of the existence of a posterior fossa tumor and its definitive treatment, certain specific measures are available to relieve the symptoms and prevent intracranial decompensation from the obstructive process. In most instances, corticosteroid therapy produces sufficient temporary shrinkage of the tumor mass to relieve headache and vomiting and to promote a transient subsidence of the obstructive and the neurological effects of the tumor mass. Dexamethasone is the pharmaceutical agent most frequently used, and after a loading dose of 10 mg, it should be continued in doses of 2 to 4 mg every 6 hours, depending on the size of the patient and the severity of symptoms. The exact mechanism by which corticosteroids reduce the tumor size and symptoms is not known.

A second method of controlling intracranial hypertension prior to definitive surgery is the use of ventricular shunting. The value of placement of a ventricular shunt prior to definitive surgery was first recognized in 1963. Since that time there has been considerable controversy regarding the advantages and disadvantages of using this procedure on a routine basis. Proponents of ventricular shunting justify its use on the grounds that it relieves all sense of urgency about definitive surgical intervention and allows stabilization of the nutritional and metabolic state of the patient prior to a major surgical undertaking. Although this argument had some merit prior to the development of the present means of rapid and accurate

noninterventional diagnosis, the CT scan has altered this situation by providing easy and fairly precise diagnosis.

The opponents of routine preoperative ventricular shunting indicate that corticosteroids, in most instances, provide adequate relief of obstructive symptoms, and that the complications of shunting are significant. The complications are twofold: (1) upward herniation of the brain stem through the incisura due to the expanding subtentorial mass, and (2) the potential for dissemination of the neoplasm through the shunting device into the peritoneal cavity or the vascular system. Although this latter complication is admittedly rare, and perhaps can be minimized or eliminated by the use of a filter in the shunt system, it has nevertheless been reported with disturbing frequency.

Another satisfactory way of temporizing with problems of intracranial hypertension is placement of an external ventricular drainage system. This can be used if the corticosteroids have not effectively reduced the symptoms of pressure. A plea is made for the placement of a one-way valve in the external ventricular system and complete avoidance of violation of the drainage system between the patient and the one-way valve. If this method of drainage is used, the incidence of secondary infection is extremely low.

Regardless of the elected method of control and management it should be reemphasized that priority must be given to relief of those aspects of the clinical picture resulting from ventricular obstruction since this aspect of the pathophysiology may be rather abruptly fatal.

The definite operative procedure is a posterior fossa craniotomy with the objective being to remove, either partially or completely, the cerebellar tumor. Details of the operative technique will not be defined here, but the procedure may be carried out with the patient in a prone or sitting position. There are recognized advantages and disadvantages to each posture, and ultimately the decision is made on the basis of the surgeon's personal preference. Our practice has been to use the sitting position in nearly all youngsters over 3 years of age. It is perhaps unnecessary to note that neuroanesthetic competence and experience contribute considerably to the success of the surgical undertaking.

What may be accomplished in the individual case depends entirely on the location, size, and character of the tumor. In many instances, as will be noted below, the tumor can be completely excised. In other situations, debulking of the tumor is the most that can be achieved, and further radiation or chemotherapy is necessary. Although histologic diagnosis can be predicted with a reasonable degree of accuracy on the basis of the CT scan and the gross appearance at surgery, it is nevertheless often necessary to define the histologic nature of the tumor at surgery by frozen section for purposes of establishing surgical objectives.

As stated earlier, the three principal tumor types occurring in the cerebellum during childhood include astrocytoma, medulloblastoma, and ependymoma, in that order of frequency. Since certain details of operative and postoperative management, as well as prognosis, depend on the tumor type, the remainder of this discussion will focus on the characteristics of the ependymoma.

The least frequent of the principal cerebellar tumors is the ependymoma, which arises from the ependymal lining of the fourth ventricle. As with the medulloblastoma, the tumor tends to fill the fourth ventricle and may spill out into the lateral recesses or through the foramen of Magendie into the upper cervical canal. However, the tumor much more frequently involves the floor of the fourth ventricle as it may, in fact, arise from that location. It is usually not possible to be certain that complete removal is achieved when the floor of the fourth ventricle is invaded. Nevertheless, as complete a removal as possible relieves the CSF obstruction and provides the optimal conditions for postoperative management.

Ependymal tumors may appear histologically benign (ependymomas) or malignant (ependymoblas-tomas). Postoperative radiation treatment does not distinguish between these histologic gradings. Although ependymomas arising in the posterior fossa are less likely to extend throughout the subarachnoid system, the tumor does so with sufficient frequency to make the entire central nervous system suspect. Therefore, as with medulloblastomas, myelography should be done to determine whether any implants in the spinal axis can be identified. In general, the recommended dosages of radiation therapy to the craniospinal axis are similar to those that were described for medulloblastoma.

Chemotherapy is reserved only for ependymoblastomas. There appears to be a definite beneficial effect of chemotherapy, which again employs prednisone, CCNU, vincristine, and procarbazine. Despite all present methods of treating ependymal tumors, the prognosis remains rather dismal. The 5-year survival rate is approximately 15 to 20 percent.

MEDULLOBLASTOMA

LARRY K. PAGE, M.D.

Medulloblastoma is a malignant tumor of the cerebellum that accounts for 20 percent of all the intracranial neoplasms of childhood and for 40 percent of tumors occurring in the posterior cranial fossa of infants and children. It is found much less commonly in adolescents and young adults and is extremely rare in those over 50 years of age. This tumor routinely arises within the cerebellar vermis, expands ventrally into the fourth ventricle to cause obstructive hydrocephalus, and has a propensity to seed metastases throughout the cerebrospinal fluid (CSF) pathways. Secondary deposits may become clinically evident preoperatively, but are found much more frequently after operation in the latter stages of the disease, when they may grow within the basal cisterns, over the cerebellar convexities, within the lateral or third ventricles, or anywhere along the spinal cord, especially at lumbosacral levels. Metastases outside the central nervous system to bone and viscera have been reported in as many as 9 percent of cases.

Medulloblastoma occurs at least twice as frequently in males as in females. The majority of cases become clinically evident in patients younger than 8 years of age. In those cases that do present in the third, fourth, and fifth decades, the tumor is usually located laterally within one cerebellar hemisphere rather than within the vermis.

Typically, the patient experiences vomiting on arising in the morning. This may initially occur only one day per week or less often, but becomes progressively more frequent. It is often of a projectile type, the patient then becoming completely asymptomatic for the rest of the day. Later, headache, unsteadiness of gait, and diplopia develop, with enlargement of the head in the infant and papilledema in the child or adult. Neurological examination of the patient with a midline medulloblastoma reveals truncal ataxia and a broad-based gait. The infant will have regressed in his ability to sit, stand, or walk. Paralysis of one or both sixth nerves and nystagmus may be found. The older patient with a laterally located tumor shows unilateral ataxia and a slow, coarse nystagmus when gazing toward the side of the tumor. Symptoms may occur more acutely following a relatively minor traumatic event and can first become manifest after spontaneous hemorrhage has occurred within the tumor. The latter presentation has been reported to occur in 5.6 percent of cases. Rarely, a metastatic supratentorial tumor, or one in the spinal canal, produces symptoms before the primary cerebellular tumor does so.

Medulloblastoma can be localized by air or contrast pneumography, angiography, ultrasound, or radioisotope scanning. Computed tomography (CT) is currently the most frequent technique used to locate this tumor. The typical appearance is that of an isodense mass that enhances markedly after contrast. Areas of hypodensity and hyperdensity and even small calcific deposits may be present. I have recently been impressed with the superior results obtained by the magnetic resonance imaging (MRI) of these lesions. MRI circumvents the problems of allergy to contrast agent and bone artifact in the posterior fossa and provides better sagittal views. MRI may ultimately replace CT as the best imaging technique for lesions of the posterior fossa.

Patients with medulloblastoma usually present with a shorter history, less than 3 months in the great majority, and appear to be more incapacitated than do patients with other types of tumor within the posterior fossa. With the widespread use of CT, I have seen several relatively smaller medulloblastomas, even prior to the development of hydrocephalus in two cases. However, most patients are admitted to the hospital with marked symptoms of increased intracranial pressure (ICP) due to obstructive hydrocephalus. Dexamethasone (0.4 mg/kg up to a total dose of 16 mg per 24 hours) should be given promptly to these patients. This often results in reduction of the peritumoral edema, relief of hydrocephalus, and amelioration of all symptoms of increased ICP. Surgical excision of the tumor can then be carried out more safely and effectively.

I do not recommend the placement of a ventriculo-peritoneal shunt prior to posterior fossa craniectomy for a number of reasons. First, even if rapid CSF drainage is avoided at the time of shunt placement, only one valve—e.g., high, medium, or low— can be selected. CSF then is decompressed to the selected pressure level over a relatively short, but unknown and uncontrollable period of time. This exposes the patient to the risk of subdural hemorrhage, epidural hemorrhage, and upward herniation of posterior fossa contents through the tentorial incisura. Second, patients with medulloblastoma who have been shunted are more likely to develop systemic metastases than those who have not. Once these occur, the average survival time is reduced to seven months. Millipore filters have been used in conjunction with shunting devices to prevent the passage of tumor cells, but systemic metastases have occurred despite this precaution. In addition, millipore filters add an increased resistance to the flow of CSF through the shunt that often results in continuing symptoms of increased ICP. Last, the surgical goal of gross total removal of tumor, or at least of tumor resection sufficient to allow free passage of CSF through the fourth ventricle, should be routinely accomplished. Postoperative shunting can then be avoided in all but about 20 percent of patients.

In the few cases in which dexamethasone does not relieve the symptoms of increased ICP, external drainage is established via twist drill hole placement of a catheter within the frontal horn of the right lateral ventricle. This bedside procedure, instead of shunting, avoids the necessity for another general anesthesia as well as the increased possibility of systemic spread of tumor. Furthermore, it allows for the constant monitoring of ICP and for its gradual reduction. Intracranial hemorrhage and/or upward herniation can follow external ventricular drainage as well as permanent shunt implantation, unless careful attention is paid to this gradual reduction in pressure. Intracranial pressure should not be lowered initially more than half the opening pressure, and under no circumstances should it be allowed to drop below 100 mm of H_2O. The patient should be kept in an Intensive Care Unit with the head elevated 30° and restrained if necessary. When the initial ICP is 300 mm of H_2O or higher, it is gradually reduced over 2 to 3 days only to the extent necessary to relieve vomiting, headache, somnolence, and bradycardia.

This level of ICP is maintained throughout the induction of anesthesia and suboccipital craniectomy. It is then lowered further, as needed, while the dura matter is being opened.

Posterior fossa surgery is carried out with the patient in the prone position or in the sitting position. The prone position should be used in the rare case in which massive hydrocephalus is present or in the neonate or infant with very thin skull bones. The head is flexed forward and toward the shoulder opposite the side on which the surgeon and assistant will stand. The back of the operating table is elevated about 30° so that the posterior fossa is higher than the shoulders and the vertex of the skull. The sitting position, with bone fixation of the head, is used in most other situations. It provides the best opportunity for gross total removal of a medulloblastoma, but certain precautions are mandatory when it is used. A central venous line and a Doppler monitor, as well as a good peripheral venous line, are used to detect and treat air embolism and to provide for the rapid and accurate replacement of blood. The U-bar that connects with the head holder must be fixed to the back of the table so that this can be quickly lowered without loosening the head holder, if hypotension secondary to air embolism or blood loss occurs. An arterial line for pressure and EAS monitoring must be available and is referenced to the level of the head rather than the heart. The legs are elevated and wrapped with ace bandages. An indwelling urinary catheter is inserted. Hypothermia must not be allowed to develop in neonates.

A paramedian incision is used if the lesion is limited to one cerebellar hemisphere, as is usual in adults. Otherwise, a midline incision is made from well above the inion to the C2 spinous process. Twenty percent mannitol, 0.5 g/kg, is given just prior to the removal of the occipital squama. The craniectomy extends from the transverse sinuses down through the foramen magnum and out toward the mastoid processes. If tumor and/or cerebellar tonsils have nerniated through the foramen magnum, laminectomy of C1 and perhaps C2 is necessary. The dura is opened with a Y-shaped incision beginning inferiorly and extending bilaterally upward toward the lateral extent of the transverse sinuses. The occipital sinus is not discretely developed in some young infants. Instead, there is a large lake of blood between the two leaves of the dura that may extend over most of the exposure. Then the dural incision must be lined with metal clips prior to its incremental extension. The intradural portion of the procedure is carried out under the surgical microscope.

This gray-purple tumor may be seen immediately beneath the pia of the cerebellar vermis, or it may extend posteriorly through the foramen of Magendie into the cisterna magna and even down into the upper cervical spinal canal. One or more satellite seedings may have spread to the pia of a cerebellar hemisphere or to the meninges in the cisterna magna. Even if no tumor is visible after the dura is opened, it can routinely be seen through the foramen of Magendie, filling the fourth ventricle. A narrow cottonoid strip pledget is placed between the floor of the ventricle and the anterior surface of the tumor to identify this plane when it is approached later in the dissection from other angles. It is usually necessary to incise the vermis well upward toward its superior extent, since the epicenter of this tumor is often at the anterior medullary velum. Each cerebellar hemisphere must be retracted laterally during lateral tumor dissection, but the weight of the lesion when the patient is in the sitting position makes the rostral and superior aspects of dissection rather easy. It is necessary for the surgeon to sit on a low stool and to direct the microscope well above its horizontal axis while this is being accomplished, particularly if the tumor extends into the aqueduct of Sylvius. A gush of CSF signals the relief of obstructive hydrocephalus.

Though occasionally quite vascular, medulloblastoma has a soft and "suckable" consistency that, when viewed with the near-perfect lighting and magnification provided by the operating microscope, allows it to be removed cleanly from adjacent cerebellar white matter. Gross total removal is the goal. It is quite unusual for this tumor, as seen at the initial operation, to invade the brain stem itself, although small metastases on the surface of the floor of the fourth ventricle may occur where the ventral surface of the primary tumor has rested on it. The wound is closed meticulously in layers. It is particularly important to close the dura, although this may be tedious and exasperating. To do so significantly minimizes the risk of pseudomeningocele and effectively prevents postoperative aseptic meningitis.

Daily lumbar punctures are made after operation to monitor CSF pressure, to lower it as necessary, and to remove bloody CSF. These taps are continued until the CSF is clear and the opening pressures remain within normal limits. If an external drain was used prior to and during surgery, it is left in place for the first 2 to 3 postoperative days for ICP monitoring, but not ordinarily for CSF drainage, unless significantly high pressures occur in spite of the daily lumbar punctures. Dexamethasone is tapered rapidly after the fifth postoperative day and is discontinued at the end of the seventh day. A CT scan is obtained at least by the end of the first week. If elevated CSF pressures and ventriculomegaly continue unabated after the second week, a CSF shunt is implanted, usually from a lateral ventricle to the greater peritoneal cavity. This is necessary in about 20 percent of cases.

Surgical mortality should be less than 0.5 percent. Wound hematoma and infection occur at a rate of 3 percent each. The former can be differentiated from edema or pneumocephalus by emergent CT scanning. Wound infection and/or meningitis may not become manifest clinically until dexamethasone has been discontinued. Fourth or sixth cranial nerve paralysis or medial-longitudinal fasciculus injury is uncommon. Paralysis of a seventh or lower cranial nerve is rare. The syndrome of inappropriate antidiuretic hormone may occasionally develop and is treated by simple water restriction and/or demeclocycline.

Medulloblastoma is composed microscopically of a dense collection of small round to oval nuclei with scant and indistinct cytoplasm. The cells occur in no specific pattern, but a slight tendency toward rosette or pseudo-rosette formation is occasionally seen. This neoplasm has been classified in recent years as a primitive neuroectodermal tumor and is the most frequently occurring example of this pathologic grouping. Staining with glial fibrillary acidic protein may reveal varying amounts of glial cell differentiation within the medulloblastoma. Neurofilament protein staining may show cells of neuronal differentiation. Ependymal cell differentiation can be discerned with the electron microscope in some of these tumors. It has recently been suggested that the prognosis is best when these multipotential cells do *not* differentiate. Apparently, as more cell lines occur within a particular medulloblastoma, the prognosis becomes progressively worse.

Patients treated only by surgical removal of a medulloblastoma routinely die of recurrence within 1 to 2 years. Patients who receive radiotherapy to the entire craniospinal axis can expect a 40 to 80 percent chance for 5-year survival. In addition to the lack of histologic differentiation mentioned above, higher survival rates are significantly related to the older age groups, to gross total removal of the primary tumor, and to a lack of demonstrable metastases within the central nervous system or systemically. Presence of the latter is a particularly ominous prognostic indicator.

The standard initial radiation dose is 3500 to 4000 rads to the craniospinal axis and an additional 1000 to 1500 rads to the posterior fossa. If and when recurrence at the primary site or metastatic deposits become evident, additional radiotherapy is often given along with chemotherapy. The currently most popular drug combination for recurrence is chloroethyl-cyclohexyl-nitrosoureal (CCNU), prednisone, procarbazine, and vincristine. Despite a general tendency among therapists to lower slightly the dose of radiation that is given to infants and young children, there is a high incidence of low I.Q., poor short-term memory, learning disabilities, and short stature, as well as the occasional occurrence of frank radiation necrosis. Because of these very likely and significant complications, trials of initial postoperative treatment for the very young patients are currently under way in which significantly reduced total dose craniospinal axis radiation is combined with adjunct combinations of chemotherapeutic agents.

CEREBELLAR ASTROCYTOMA

JOHN SHILLITO Jr., M.D.

A benign cerebellar astrocytoma in childhood usually is consistent with an excellent prognosis. It may be possible to achieve a total excision, and experience has shown that the possibility of a cure is likely. Occasional extension into the brain stem may modify the excellent outlook.

SYMPTOMS AND SIGNS

A tumor may originate in one cerebellar hemisphere. As it grows it produces awkwardness of the limbs on the same side. If a right-handed child has a left cerebellar tumor, it may go unnoticed longer than if it were on the dominant side. Ultimately, hand motions become awkward, and the child may stumble into things on the side of the tumor because one leg is uncoordinated. Later, as the tumor grows, it pushes into the fourth ventricle and begins to obstruct it; symptoms of pressure then begin some time after the neurological signs develop. Frequently, it is the pressure symptoms that prompt the parents to bring the child for medical attention.

If a tumor grows in the midline of the cerebellum, it may grow little into brain tissue, but rather extrude itself into the fourth ventricle right away; there may be no neurological deficit. When it has reached adequate size, obstruction of the fourth ventricle causes symptoms of pressure.

When a midline tumor originates more deeply in the vermis and causes neurological deficit, it does not interfere with the extremities but rather with balance of the trunk. A child is uncomfortable while sitting unless propped up in a chair. If seated on a bed or examining table, he puts his hands behind him for support, somewhat resembling a tripod. When standing he tries to hold onto someone or something. The feet are placed widely apart. He walks like a sailor on a rolling ship. He turns in several careful motions lest he tip over. His Romberg sign is positive,and he is unable to tandem walk.

Wherever it starts, the tumor usually has produced fourth ventricular obstruction and hydrocephalus before the child's parents seek medical attention. Obstruction produces headache. The first headaches are usually in the morning and become less prominent as the child gets up and becomes active. We have equated this phenomenon with the likelihood that the tumor mass is producing a near-total obstruction past which spinal fluid can be driven by the Valsalva maneuver or by normal daily activities. When the child is quietly sleeping at night, the pressure may gradually build up to the point of producing symptoms, which are relieved by activity and particularly by the vomiting that frequently accompanies the headache. As some CSF is blown past the partial obstruction, the pressure is relieved and the symptoms disappear. We have often heard the story of a child who awakens vomiting and complaining of headache, is kept home from school, and is then fine the rest of the day. After a few such occurrences he is considered to be a malingerer!

With enough pressure for a long enough time in a child of any age up to about 10 years, the cranial sutures may split. This releases the rigidity of the skull enough to ease the pressure, and for weeks afterward no symptoms may be noted; this may further confound the diagnosis, particularly when this coincides with a school vacation!

Longstanding increased pressure from hydrocephalus may shift the brain stem downward toward the foramen magnum, as the ventricles above enlarge. The sixth cranial nerve, which runs upward and forward beneath the brain stem, is vulnerable as it pierces the dura. As it is stretched, one or both eyes may fail to abduct properly. This sign may lead the child to an ophthalmologist who may be the first to note papilledema.

As the cerebellar tumor pushes the tonsils or itself grows down into the foramen magnum, extra tissue is jammed against the dura or even the upper cervical sensory roots, and this produces pain. The child guards motion of the neck and may tilt the head to one side to relieve the pain.

The child is examined for head tilt, strabismus, and difficulty in walking and standing and sitting, particularly with the eyes closed. The finger-to-nose test demonstrates ataxia of the upper extremeities, and the ability to stand or to hop on one foot may show the earliest asymmetry in coordination of the lower extremities. There may be nystagmus on lateral gaze. Percussion of the skull may reveal a cracked-pot note, Macewen's sign indicating split sutures. There may be tenderness in the suboccipital region where firm pressure is transmitted against the herniated tonsils and surrounding pain-sensitive structures. Deep tendon reflexes are characteristically hypoactive with an intracerebellar tumor. Unless there is compression of or extension into the brain stem, there are no Babinski signs. All of these signs vary with the location of the tumor, and the rapidity of its growth; sutures may not have time to split. The duration of symptoms, as pieced together retrospectively, may suggest the histologic diagnosis.

DIFFERENTIAL DIAGNOSIS

The CT scanner has made most of our diagnostic tests obsolete except in certain problem cases. Skull films may show asymmetry of the occipital bone, indicating a longstanding change beneath it, which offers a reassuring prognosis if present. Films are also helpful to the surgeon in planning his incision with relation to the transverse sinus and the location of a supratentorial bur hole with reference to the lambdoid suture.

Histologic diagnosis by the CT scan is at times reliable. A cystic astrocytoma with the so-called mural nodule of solid tumor is usually interpreted correctly. The density of the cyst fluid as measured by the scanner is usually denser than spinal fluid, and our astute radiologist may jokingly predict quite accurately the color of the fluid! We have learned by bitter experience that the CT scanner cannot reliably differentiate between high-protein fluid and low-density solid tumor tissue; occasional "cysts" have proved to be very firm solid tissue or very juicy gelatinous tumor material. The cerebellar astrocytoma usually enhances and shows crisp margins; there may be little or no edema around it. The solid astrocytoma enhances and is delineated in much the same way as the mural nodule of a cystic astrocytoma. The location within a cerebellar hemisphere or the vermis is further supportive evidence of the diagnosis.

Tumors that hang into the fourth ventricle from the vermis or project into it from one wall present a greater variety of possibilities, for both medulloblastomas and ependymomas can do this. A tumor projecting inward from the midline of the roof of the fourth ventricle adds the additional diagnostic possibility of a choroid plexus papilloma. Malignant astrocytoma is another possibility. Almost any of these tumors can produce cysts of some size, but usually only the low-grade astrocytoma can produce an immense cyst from a small nodule of tissue. Tumors occasionally may be mixed astrocytomas and oligodendrogliomas.

PREOPERATIVE TREATMENT

What should be done prior to surgery depends in large part on the severity and the nature of the symptoms with which the child presents. Usually headache, nausea, and vomiting respond to dexamethasone started intravenously in loading doses comparable to 10 mg for a person of adult weight, scaled down roughly in proportion to the child's weight. Maintenance dosages comparable to the adult dose of 4 mg *q6h* IV or PO are thereafter usually adequate. Some protection for the gastrointestinal tract should be used; cimetadine, Riopan, Maalox, or just milk. If the child responds to this treatment well, it is advisable to wait a day or two to allow oral rehydration and several good meals.

If the symptoms do not subside promptly, it may be necessary to relieve the hydrocephalus. Some advocate shunting. I have avoided this for three reasons: (1) it may be an unnecessary extra operation; the dexamethasone usually does the job quite readily; (2) with the histologic diagnosis of a tumor not absolutely certain in many cases, it is inadvisable to shunt spinal fluid that may contain tumor cells elsewhere in the body; dysgerminomas, medulloblastomas, and malignant astrocytomas have been implanted in the abdominal cavity by ventriculoperitoneal shunting; (3) the patient may be made shunt-dependent, even after a few months, in situations in which the shunt could have been avoided.

If relief of increased intracranial pressure is urgent, the use of external ventricular drainage can provide prompt relief and the shunting of tumor cells elsewhere in the body can be avoided. I have done this by several methods. In a young child or one with split sutures, a rapidly deteriorating situation can be checked by simply tapping percutaneously through the coronal suture with an 18-gauge spinal needle; this relieves extreme pressure immediately. If this is not possible, a small scalp incision may be made just in front of the coronal suture at a distance (from the midline) equal to that of the ipsilateral pupil, and a twist drill hole placed through which either a long intravenous catheter may be inserted or a plastic catheter passed through an open-ended Cone needle. If one suspects that the posterior fossa tumor may be one that requires radiation therapy, such as a dysgerminoma or medulloblastoma, and particularly a tumor that may not be ideally suited for excision, one may take the child to the operating room and, through a small incision and bur hole, place a ventricular catheter and reservoir, then close the scalp incision. By means of a small butterfly needle like that frequently used for scalp vein intravenous infusions in children, external ventricular drainage can be established with less risk of infection than when percutaneous catheters are passed directly into the ventricle.

Some posterior fossa tumors are so large that they may exert dangerous pressure on the brain stem, in which case the signs may not be relieved by decompressing the ventricles above. Not only may the signs of brain stem dysfunction persist, but the ventricular drainage may permit an upward herniation of the posterior fossa contents and cause worsening of the signs. This situation demands immediate posterior fossa craniectomy and at least debulking of the tumor mass. Only in such situations has it been necessary to use mannitol while preparing for the operation itself. In the more chronic situations, dexamethasone usually is adequate.

MUST EVERY POSTERIOR FOSSA TUMOR BE IDENTIFIED BY BIOPSY?

Biopsy is not necessary in every case. Examples are the aforementioned dysgerminoma and certain other tumors which at the time of discovery show evidence of spread elsewhere in the spinal fluid compartments. In these cases, radiation therapy or chemotherapy may be the most effective means of controlling the tumor and its seeds, and a posterior fossa craniectomy may be not only inadequate but unnecessary. These are important exceptions to the rule that exact diagnosis by radiological studies is not totally reliable, and histologic identification of a cerebellar tumor should ordinarily be made.

THE OPERATION ITSELF

In children over a few years of age, the sitting position has the advantages of permitting optimum flexion of the head and neck, good visibility, and removal of blood by gravity; it also facilitates excision of the tumor.

Precautions Concerning the Sitting Position. An intravenous line placed directly into the right atrium permits aspiration of any significant accumulation of air that may result from opening venous channels above the heart; monitoring techniques such as end-tidal CO_2 determination and Doppler auscultation of the heart, as well as EKG and continuous blood pressure readings, permit the early diagnosis of air in the heart even before serious changes or embolization can occur. The child must be secured in such a way that his trunk will not slide down the operating table and put traction on the cervical spine; a small seat belt across the padded iliac crests will suffice. The head may be held in a pinpoint head rest for good security without the danger of pressure sores on the skin. The use of the Greenberg retractor apparatus facilities working deep within the cerebellum without allowing it to sag and tear. Whether or not I use it, I have always placed a bur hole supratentorially so that the ventricle can be tapped if necessary to relieve pressure before opening the posterior fossa dura, and also to provide access to the ventricle postoperatively should there be bleeding in the tumor bed with sudden obstruction of the fourth ventricle. The dura of the bur hole need not be opened if the dura of the posterior fossa is not tense or if a cystic portion of the tumor can be tapped to relieve the pressure below. It is best not to violate the supratentorial subdural space with the child in a sitting position, for supratentorial subdurals are one complication of this position, particularly when the ventricles have reached a large size.

Technique. Details of surgical technique can be reviewed elsewhere. In general, if the dura is opened in a way that will permit closure, bone regenerates rapidly in the posterior fossa of a child, providing as good protection as was present preoperatively. In a small child, removal of the arch of C1 and C2 may permit the development of a marked kyphosis, which may itself need treatment later in life. In general, the arch of C1 should be exposed, but if it is possible to leave it there, the aforementioned problem may be avoided.

Removing some fluid from a cystic astrocytoma provides room for easier dissection of the mural nodule. It is not usually necessary to remove the entire cyst wall; the limits of the tumor may be detected grossly. If the cyst wall is thicker and not actually transparent, it may be advisable to take biopsies here and there to determine the true extent of tumor tissue and act accordingly.

If the tumor hangs down into the fourth ventricle, it is advisable to elevate the cerebellar tonsils and gently place a long cotton strip on the floor of the fourth ventricle. Then, as dissection continues around the tumor to the fourth ventricle, one can avoid suddenly traumatizing its floor. During dissection it is advisable to work from above downward, but to look periodically beneath the tumor up into the fourth ventricle so that one can better appreciate the proximity of the tumor to the walls of the fourth ventricle. Thus, dissection is not carried too far anteriorly and traction from a sagging tumor is not transmitted continuously to the brain stem.

The sagging cerebellum is quite a sight after a large tumor has been removed. There may be many bridging veins or just little arachnoid adhesions suspending it from the tentorium. If large veins are part of this, they may be coagulated but not divided. Thus, they provide support, but should the structure break, hemorrhage will not result.

Lower portions of the dura are closed first and thus support is provided for the cerebellum. As the closure is completed, irrigations are carried out to remove as much air as possible and to fill the posterior fossa to check for leaks in the suture line. A watertight muscle closure should also be completed in case there are inevitable small leaks. If preoperative ventricular drainage has been utilized, it is well to continue it postoperatively until the wound has had time to heal, and then test the adequacy of the CSF circulation by gradually raising the drainage bottle.

FOCAL EPILEPSY

FOCAL EPILEPSY

JOHN M. VAN BUREN, M.D., Ph. D.

The question of surgical intervention in focal epilepsy is never an easy one. Thus it is important that those considering surgical therapy in epilepsy become part of a team of specialists.

The neurologist who oversees the medical epileptic clinic must remain alert to identify patients with focal cerebral seizures and determine their drug resistance. He must remain particularly alert to changes in seizure patterns, especially around puberty when the focal nature of temporal lobe seizures may become clear. The electroencephalographer should be experienced in the diagnosis of focal seizures since the recording cannot be done in a "routine" fashion and special runs and procedures are needed. The patient's reaction to the restraints placed on him by his disease and the psychological difficulties attending temporal lobe epilepsy require the attention of a psychologist and a psychiatrist. A social worker is needed to evaluate the socioeconomic impact of the patient's seizures and to guide rehabilatation. It is important to summarize the efforts of this group at a formal conference in which the diagnosis and the therapeutic plan can be carefully evaluated.

The surgical treatment of focal cerebral seizures is still regarded by some as an experimental procedure with questionable rationale. This is somewhat surprising since a systematic approach to seizure surgery appeared nearly half a century ago.

CRITERIA FOR CASE SELECTION

Clinical Criteria

The need for care in history-taking cannot be overemphasized. Patients with focal seizures often have a past history of obstetrical difficulty, neonatal distress, early febrile fits, and later trauma or infection of the central nervous system. The characteristic complex partial seizures (psychomotor attacks or automatisms) often are not seen before adolescence. When multiple patterns of attacks are found, they should be carefully separated. Usually the lesser attacks have the greatest localizing value, although they are often ignored by the patient and his family (Table 1).

Dysphasia, particularly anomia, prior to or following a complex partial seizure provides strong evidence of a focus in the dominant temporal lobe, whereas understandable speech during an automatism suggests a focus on the other side. An intracarotid injection of Amytal (Wada test) may be needed to identify the dominant hemisphere and to assist in planning surgery.

Fearing that they will be considered "crazy", patients may not volunteer accounts of hallucinations and illusionary phenomena. Features useful in distinguishing epileptic from psychotic hallucination are the stereotyped nature of the epileptic phenomena and the lack of emotional significance to the patient. Like the "broken record" character of epileptic auditory hallucinations, the visual aurae are "TV replays".

Partial seizures without an aura, although frequently associated with a primary (nonfocal) disorder, are compatible with a focal onset in either the temporal or the frontal lobe.

Complex partial seizures (automatisms, psychomotor attacks) frequently accompany temporal lobe seizures and are characterized by loss of eye contact (staring), followed by handling or plucking at clothing and autonomic phenomena. Involvement of the anterior

TABLE 1   Aura and Ictal Patterns in 124 Patients* with Temporal Lobe Epilepsy

	N	%
Aura		
Epigastric—abdominal	54	43.5
Oropharyngeal	19	15.3
Cephalic	24	19.4
Feelings of fear	20	16.1
Deja vu — jamais vu	13	10.5
Visual†	21	16.9
Auditory†	17	13.7
Olfactory–taste	17	13.7
Vestibular	21	16.9
None	12	9.7
Ictal pattern		
Akinetic with loss of posture	24	19.4
Akinetic without loss of posture	34	27.4
Automatisms (with chewing, swallowing, etc.)	51	41.1
Automatisms (gestural, etc.)	42	33.9
No automatism	34	27.4
Only automatism	30	24.2
Automatism + tonic posture(s)	11	8.9
Head and eyes adverse	10	8.1
Clonic motor phenomena, unilateral	11	8.9
No generalized convulsions (regardless of medication)	62	50.0

*More than one type of aura and/or ictal pattern may coexist in some patients.

†Includes crude, elementary sensations as well as illusions and/or more complex hallucinations.

insula and adjacent opercular cortex may lead to chewing, smacking movements, swallowing, or drooling. The patient may walk about, and it is useful to inquire whether after an attack he has found himself in a strange place.

It is important to separate the epileptic automatism from psychotic fugue states and outright malingering. Epileptic automatism usually lasts no more than a few minutes. Although a patient in an automatism may struggle in a confused fashion if forceably restrained by misguided attendants, I have never observed complex, goal-oriented antisocial acts during this state. This may be claimed as defense by those accused of criminal acts. Complex planned activity would seem incompatible with the "psychoparesis" that appears to be the concomitant of temporal lobe discharge.

Ictal automatisms should be separated from postictal psychosis as care is different and urgent. Usually after a flurry of small seizures, the psychosis has a gradual onset with alteration in emotional response, usually with a paranoid character. The patient refuses medication and may leave the hospital in pajamas. Since the state may last several days, it is trying on the open ward. Early use of adequate doses of chloropromazine and antiepileptic drugs must be instituted before the patient becomes inaccessible to medication without physical restraint.

Physical examination is usually unrewarding except in those instances in which a tumor or destructive lesion produces focal signs or increased intracranial pressure. On interview, the patient may show mental changes that are somewhat difficult to define. The patient is easily frustrated and may overreact in such situations. There may be a tendency to concreteness of thought, difficulty in abstraction, lack of humor, and a poor self-image.

Radiologic Criteria

Plain films of the skull may suggest atrophy of the cerebral hemisphere (flattening or thickening of the cranial convexity, elevation of the petrous ridge, or asymmetric enlargement of the accessory nasal sinuses). The CT scan permits the discovery of low-grade neoplasms or atrophic scars. It is important to use an adequate dose of iodinated contrast material and to allow sufficient time for diffusion into lesions with only a minor inadequacy of the blood-brain barrier. Angiography may be useful if there is a hint of a vascular malformation.

Electroencephalographic Criteria

Electroencephalographic evidence is crucial in the diagnosis of focal cerebral seizures, but only a few points are considered here.

Twenty-one electrode arrays, arranged in the standard 10–20 inernational system, usually with nasopharyngeal or sphenoidal electrodes, are basic for evaluation. It is important to distinguish true epileptic "spikes" with a short-rising phase and a longer falling curve,

which often overshoots the baseline, from summed sinusoidal activity, which may appear as a sharply pointed wave. Phase reversal of spikes, particularly if observed in both the transverse and sagittal linkages, are important signs of focality. Repeated examination, both with and without medication, probably is required. Electrographic observation of the onset of a seizure is particularly important, and telemetering methods make prolonged periods of observation more tolerable for the patient.

Perhaps the most difficult evaluation is that of determining the surgical indication in patients displaying more widespread discharges or discharges arising independently from both sides. This is particularly frequent in focal temporal seizures (Table 2). We have abandoned activating drugs (e.g., Metrazol) because of the frequency with which they provoked nonspecific generalized seizures and the occasional vertebral compression fractures that ensued.

Since there is a definite, although small, risk of intracranial hemorrhage with implanted electrodes (epidural, subdural, or stereotactically implanted depth electrodes), they are reserved for the purpose of resolving conflicting scalp electrographic findings when therapy is seriously needed. In the final analysis of cases showing a complex electrographic pattern and no overt structural lesion on x-ray studies, the decision in favor of surgery must rest on a predominance of interictal epileptiform activity from one area, and this is particularly compelling if an electrographically demonstrated seizure can be seen to arise from this site. These findings should be compatible with the clinical seizure pattern. As the focal features of the clinical, x-ray, and electroencephalographic examinations become increasingly blurred, the good results of cerebral excision markedly diminish.

TABLE 2   EEG Localization of Epileptiform Discharges in Temporal Lobe Epilepsy

	N	%
Temporal unilateral	78	62.9
Temporal bilateral	46	37.1
Left, or predominantly left temporal	48	38.7
Right, or predominantly right temporal	76	61.3
Temporal, also suprasylvian	45	36.3
Only temporofrontal	20	16.1
Temporo-extrafrontal	10	8.1
Also posterior temporal	36	29.0
Maximum midposterior temporal	18	14.5
Maximum ant-inferior-mesial temporal	72	63.2
No involvement of inferior-mesial temporal	28	24.6
Temporal unilateral, maximum ant-inf-mesial, no posterotemporal, no suprasylvian	35	30.7
Temporal unilateral, no posterotemporal	61	49.2
Temporal unilateral, also posterotemporal	17	13.7
Temporal bilateral, also suprasylvian	15	12.1
Temporal bilateral, also posterotemporal	19	15.3
Temporal bilateral, no posterotemporal, no suprasylvian	15	12.1

EVIDENCE FOR DRUG RESISTANCE

Although generalized convulsive seizures respond relatively well to antiepileptic medication, the partial complex seizures of temporal lobe epilepsy frequently prove refractory. With the large variety of antiepileptic drugs currently available, medical therapy on varied drugs and in various combinations can be continued indefinitely. On the other hand, if seizure control is not achieved and there is reasonable evidence of a focal onset, continued medical therapy may not be in the patient's best interest.

Although medical treatment can usually be handled on an outpatient basis, close supervision and family cooperation are essential. The patient who is considered a candidate for surgery is one who has been maintained on three of the major drugs (diphenylhydantoin, phenobarbital, primidone, carbamazepine), with adequate blood levels or evidence of toxicity and poor seizure control, for 2 years. The inability of the patient to follow adequate drug therapy is a rare but occasionally compelling reason to consider surgical therapy.

SOCIOECONOMIC FACTORS

The disability associated with epilepsy usually bears little relationship to the actual duration and even the frequency of the attacks. The stigma of epilepsy among co-workers, employers, and their insurers too often dooms an otherwise capable individual to joblessness or loss of educational opportunities. Too often an epileptic child is carried thoughtlessly on medication despite emerging features of surgically treatable focal seizures while the golden years, when he could be receiving useful training, are lost.

Postoperative relief of seizures does not guarantee immediate reintegration into society. The sudden relief of chronic invalidism may suddenly present the patient with normal social demands and precipitate acute feelings of inadequacy and anxiety. A self-image characterized by failure in job and social competition may continue to dog the patient and interfere with his efforts to rehabilitate himself.

Supportive care by the social worker and psychiatrist must continue after surgery, and particular efforts are needed in the first postoperative year. Continued contact is urgently needed, if seizure suppression is less than complete, to encourage the patient to make the best use of his capabilities. Frequently the family requires counseling as overprotection and unwise to frankly neurotic manipulation of the patient may seriously impair his potential.

TECHNIQUE OF CORTICAL RESECTION

I have continued to perform the cortical resection with local anesthesia following Penfield's technique. Since this permits more useful electrocorticography and cortical mapping of the actual position of sensorimotor and speech representations, the procedure can be tailored to the particular patient's focus without increased risk of postoperative neurological deficits. Many surgeons perform a "standard" temporal lobectomy under general anesthesia, taking no more than the anterior 5 cm of the dominant temporal lobe and usually conserving the first temporal gyrus for fear of producing dysphasia. In my view, however, if temporal lobe seizures followed a routine clinical or electrographic pattern, routine surgery seems reasonable. Unfortunately, the pathologic and electrographic foci are quite individual and require individual consideration.

As with any procedure performed under local anesthesia, the surgeon must spend time with the patient describing the procedure and answering questions. The patient must be aware that his role is not passive, but that he is an important and active member of the surgical team since his responses are essential for effective mapping of vital cortical areas. To allay anxiety without significantly altering cortical electrical activity, I have used chlorpromazine, 100 to 200 mg IM, 1 hour prior to surgery for many years. More recently, droperidol and fentanyl, given in small doses during the procedure, have been used with better results.

Following exposure of the brain, electrocorticography is used to outline the epileptic focus. Then the sensorimotor region and speech representation are mapped by means of gentle electrical stimulation. Using the cortical mapping as a guide to areas which must be conserved, a line of resection is established which best removes the epileptic tissue. After resection, electrocortigography is especially useful in detecting residual regions of electrically unstable cortex, which then may be removed to complete the ablation of the epileptic focus. Using this technique, we have gradually resorted to more radical removals, especially in removal of the mesial temporal structures (uncus, amygdala, and hippocampus) with a significant increase in the patients cured and markedly improved (see Table 3).

RISKS AND PROGNOSIS

Owing to the relative frequency of temporal focal seizures, the most extensive statistics are in this group. Over a period of 25 years I have performed 200 temporal lobectomies for epilepsy with two deaths (one postoper-

TABLE 3 Temporal Lobe Excision: Postoperative Results

Results	All resections		"Total" resections		"Partial" resections	
	N	%	N	%	N	%
Seizure-free	26	21	24	31.6	2	4
Very rare seizures	17	14	14	18.4	3	6
Rare seizures	24	19	16	21.1	8	17
Moderate improvement	16	13	7	9.2	9	19
No improvement	41	33	15	19.7	26	54
	(124)		(76)		(48)	

tive hemorrhage; one fatal transfusion reaction). About one-third of patients who underwent removal of the dominant temporal lobe had dysphasia during the period of postoperative cerebral swelling. All of these cleared as the edema subsided. Two cases of contralateral hemiparesis occurred without evident cause, although spasm of the middle cerebral arterial branches exposed during temporal removal was hypothecated. Fortunately, in both instances the hemiparesis cleared slowly but completely. A small homonymous upper quadrantanopia usually occurs, but is unnoticed by the patient. When a major posterior temporal removal is planned, however, a complete hemianopia, often macula-splitting, may ensue, and the patient should be warned of this. Since such removals can only be done on the right (nondominant) side, the defect does not interfere with reading.

Review of our material 3 to 15 years following temporal lobectomy gave the following results in otherwise intractable epileptics: one-third seizure-free and off medication; somewhat more than one-third markedly improved, but still requiring medication; and somewhat less than one-third on medication and without significant benefit (Table 3). Thus, the salvage in lives seriously blighted by epilepsy has been significant and most encouraging. Our present interest is in the earlier detection of resectable foci in medically intractable young epileptics so that their education and life styles can develop in a normal fashion.

PITUITARY TUMORS

PROLACTIN-SECRETING PITUITARY ADENOMA

IVAN CIRIC, M.D.

CLASSIFICATION

Prolactin-secreting pituitary adenomas are the most common pituitary lesions. In a series of 281 pituitary adenomas treated surgically since 1968, 114 (31.3%) were classified as prolactin-secreting. There were 95 (83.3%) females and 19 (16.7%) males.

In 60 (52.6%) patients, the adenoma was less than 10 mm in size and was situated within a normal-size sella (microadenoma, grade I). An enlarged but otherwise intact sella (grade II) was presented in 37 (32.5%) patients. In the remaining 17 (14.9%) patients, the adenoma was invasive into the surrounding structures (grades III and IV).

CLINICAL PRESENTATION

Female patients presented with endocrine symptoms such as amenorrhea, galactorrhea, and infertility. The most frequent endocrine symptom in males was impotence. Patients with large adenomas (macroadenomas) often presented with fatigue owing to an anterior pituitary insufficiency. Headaches in some form were present in over 80 percent of patients with macroadenomas. A visual abnormality was present in 16 (14%) patients.

DIAGNOSIS

The diagnosis of a prolactin-secreting adenoma is based on the presence of an elevated serum prolactin level (greater than 20 to 25 ng/ml in females and 15 ng/ml in males), on a blunted serum prolactin response to TRH stimulation, and on a radiologic demonstration of the lesion. Until the introduction of high-resolution CT scanners, the radiologic diagnosis of a pituitary microadenoma was made on sella polytomograms. The presence of a slanting sella floor or of focal erosion was the most common abnormal finding. Pituitary macroadenomas were studied further by means of cerebral angiography, pneumoencephalotomography, and CT scans. Today, however, the radiologic diagnosis

of pituitary micro- and macroadenomas depends on their demonstration by high-resolution CT scans. Recently, MRI scans are obtained in selected cases of microadenoma and in all patients with macroadenoma. Preliminary experience has shown that this study can be useful in demonstrating the presence of a constrictive diaphragma sellae and in revealing the exact relationship of the suprasellar tumor extension to the third ventricle. In addition, the MRI scan is capable of distinguishing between a vascular lesion, such as an aneurysm, and an adenoma, obviating thereby the need for invasive cerebrovascular studies.

TREATMENT

The therapeutic goals in the management of a prolactin-secreting pituitary adenoma are (1) eradication of the mass lesion (if present), (2) cure of the endocrine abnormality with preservation of the normal anterior and posterior pituitary functions, and (3) prevention of a recurrence. In addition, the treatment should be relatively simple, safe, and cost-effective. All of these goals are best achieved by surgical removal of the lesion utilizing the transsphenoidal approach. Relief of pressure and endocrine symptoms can also be accomplished with medical management using dopamine agents, specifically, bromocriptine (Parlodel).

RESULTS

Eradication of the Mass Lesion

The most serious mass effect of a pituitary macroadenoma is visual impairment secondary to compression of the optic nerves and chiasm. In a series of 108 patients with adenomas larger than 2 cm, 59 (63.7%) had visual symptoms. All were treated with transsphenoidal decompression. A visual improvement occurred in 90 percent of patients. When the adenoma extends in a lateral direction, it can endanger the oculomotor nerves in the cavernous sinuses. A sudden visual or oculomotor abnormality due to a hemorrhage into the tumor occurred in 4.5 percent of patients in this series. This was preceded by a period of severe headaches. The apoplectiform onset of visual or oculomotor symptoms constitutes an absolute indication for emergency surgical decompression.

In the same series of 108 patients with macroadenomas, there were three patients (3.2%) who presented with hydrocephalus secondary to a marked suprasellar adenoma extension, which caused an obstruction of the foramen of Monro. In two of these patients, the hydrocephalus was symptomatic preoperatively. They were treated with dexamethasone and improved. In the third patient, the preoperative borderline hydrocephalus became acutely symptomatic postoperatively, requiring emergency bilateral ventriculoperitoneal shunts.

Bromocriptine was used to reduce the size of the tumor preoperatively in four patients with invasive tumors. An appreciable reduction in the tumor size occurred in three patients. Three of these patients were operated on within 6 weeks of initiation of bromocriptine therapy. At operation, the tumor was rather fibrous and difficult to remove in two patients. Bromocriptine was administered postoperatively to six additional patients with incompletely removed tumors and effected an appreciable reduction in the tumor size in five patients.

Endocrine Cure

The incidence of endocrine cures following transsphenoidal surgery was the function of the tumor size and the preoperative secretory potency of the tumor. The highest incidence of cures (89%) was achieved when the prolactin-secreting microadenoma did not exceed 10 mm in size and the preoperative serum prolactin level was 100 ng/ml or less. The overall endocrine cure in patients with prolactin-secreting macroadenomas was 27 percent.

Bromocriptine can provide a relatively fast and safe endocrine palliation in most patients with prolactin-secreting adenomas. The beneficial endocrine effect of bromocriptine, however, ceases with the discontinuation of therapy. Thus, endocrine cures following administration of bromocriptine in patients with prolactin-secreting adenomas are rare or uncertain at best.

Preservation of Normal Pituitary Function

In two (1.2%) patients with prolactin-secreting pituitary microadenomas, diabetes insipidus occurred postoperatively and lasted longer than 3 months. In only one of these patients (0.6%) was there evidence of postoperative anterior pituitary insufficiency. The presence of postoperative anterior insufficiency in patients with macroadenomas was directly related to the patient's preoperative endocrine status and to the completeness of tumor removal. If pituitary insufficiency was present preoperatively, it was likely to persist postoperatively. The more extensive the tumor removal, the greater was the chance of postoperative pituitary insufficiency. Nevertheless, even the small amount of residual normal anterior pituitary tissue that usually adheres to the undersurface of the diaphragma sellae at the completion of the procedure is sufficient to maintain normal pituitary function after surgery.

Recurrences

A gross total tumor removal, with no demonstrable evidence of a residual tumor tissue on the postoperative CT scan, was accomplished in 41 percent of the 108 patients with pituitary macroadenomas. If radiation therapy was withheld from these patients, a recurrence rate of 20 percent was observed over a follow-up period of up to 15 years. In contrast, when there was evidence of some residual tumor tissue on the postoperative CT scan and the patients received postoperative radiation therapy, the incidence of recurrences was only 10 percent. This indicates that postoperative radiation therapy is probably more important in prevention of recurrences than the completeness of tumor removal. Radiation treatment has no place in the therapy of prolactin-secreting pituitary microadenomas.

Morbidity and Mortality

There were no operative mortalities in this series. No patient developed a permanent postoperative neurological deficit. One patient with a macroadenoma developed a temporary postoperative sixth nerve paresis. The patient with acute postoperative hydrocephalus had a transient recent memory defect lasting for 2 weeks. He subsequently made a full recovery. A cerebrospinal fluid rhinorrhea requiring reoperation occurred in two patients (1.2%). In one of these patients, the rhinorrhea occurred 18 months following transsphenoidal resection of a recurrent and invasive adenoma and after a year of treatment with bromocriptine. In this patient, the rhinorrhea was associated with meningitis (0.6%). Rhinorrhagia requiring operative hemostasis occurred in two patients. One patient had deep vein thrombosis and pulmonary embolism.

The usual hospital stay averaged 7 days. When radiation therapy was necessary, it was administered on an outpatient basis usually 3 to 4 weeks after surgery.

The natural course of a prolactin-secreting pituitary adenoma is not well understood. There is evidence in the literature that approximately 10 percent of microadenomas enlarge significantly without treatment over a period of 5 years. Given an unequivocal diagnosis of a prolactin-secreting microadenoma, the preferred treatment should be surgical in younger patients, especially in those of childbearing age. The administration of bromocriptine is an accepted therapeutic alternative, although prolonged treatment over a period of months or years will probably be necessary. In patients with prolactin-secreting macroadenomas, a direct surgical decompression utilizing a transsphenoidal route is the preferred treatment when the adenoma is confined to the sella or has a straight suprasellar extension. In patients with a constrictive diaphragma sellae or an asymmetric suprasellar tumor growth, and in those with invasive adenomas, preoperative administration of bromocriptine for a period of 6 to 12 weeks is advisable. Bromocriptine has also proved useful as an adjuvant therapy in patients with incompletely removed macroadenomas. Postoperative radiation therapy, however, appears to be the single most important factor in the prevention of recurrences in patients with macroadenomas.

GROWTH HORMONE-SECRETING PITUITARY TUMOR

EDWARD R. LAWS, Jr., M.D.

The revival of the transsphenoidal approach to the pituitary gland has revolutionized the current management of patients with acromegaly. Along with improvements in surgical technique, advances in endocrinology and neuroradiology have allowed much more accurate preoperative diagnosis of such patients and have influenced the entire spectrum of pituitary disease. The diagnosis of acromegaly is now being made more frequently when the disease is in its early stages. The proportion of patients having large tumors with accompanying visual field defects is smaller than in the past, and it is already evident that early surgical intervention when tumors are small results in much more satisfactory long-term management. At this time, 95 percent of all pituitary tumors beeing treated surgically at our institution are approached transsphenoidally rather than by craniotomy.

This chapter describes a personal experience with 100 consecutive patients with acromegaly treated by transsphenoidal microsurgery. Accurate follow-up information, including basal growth hormone levels and visual field examinations, were available in virtually every case and have been analyzed.

MATERIALS AND METHODS

The case records of 100 consecutive patients with acromegaly who were operated on by the same surgeon were reviewed with regard to presenting symptoms and signs, preoperative endocrine evaluation, findings at surgery, postoperative endocrine evaluation, and overall results of neurosurgical management. In addition, pre- and postoperative visual field examinations were performed on all patients with visual complaints and on a majority of those who had no disturbance of vision. Human growth hormone (hGH) levels in serum were determined by quantitative radioimmunoassay. Because the normal basal value for serum hGH in females in our laboratory is less than or equal to 10 ng/ml, and because this level is commonly utilized in reports of the results of treatment of acromegaly, it was used as the "normal" postoperative hGH value. More precise assessment requires the use of dynamic endocrine testing, and results of glucose or insulin tolerance tests were not available in all the patients.

The study group consisted of 59 men and 41 women whose ages ranged from 16 to 75 years with an average of 42 years. Complete follow-up review, including growth hormone determinations, was available in 98 of the 100 cases. In one patient, tumor removal (diffuse adenoma) was not completed because of hemorrhage; one patient (microadenoma) lives abroad and has not returned for follow-up examination. At the time of analysis, the follow-up period ranged from 2 to 74 months following surgery with a mean of 24 months. Previous therapy had been given in 22 of the 100 cases: radiation therapy in 19, radiofrequency (RF) thermocoagulation in two, and craniotomy and two courses of radiotherapy in one case of gigantism and acromegaly. Two of the patients had been treated unsuccessfully with heavy particle radiation therapy via the proton beam.

Tumors were classified on the basis of radiologic findings and appearance at surgery. *Microadenomas* were those tumors less than, or equal to, 10 mm in diameter that could be demarcated from normal pituitary gland. *Diffuse adenomas* were those tumors that filled the sella, but remained confined by the dura, though some of these had suprasellar extension. *Invasive adenomas* were those tumors that had invaded dura or both dura and bone and some of these also had suprasellar extension.

CLINICAL PRESENTATION

All the patients had hormonally active acromegaaly and presented with a wide spectrum of symptoms and signs characteristic of this disease. Four of the patients had gigantism, and one teenage girl had gigantism and active acromegaly. Associated visual complaints were present in seven of the 100 patients, all of whom had bitemporal visual field defects when examined. Headache, osteoarthritis, and arthralgia were common complaints. Diabetes mellitus was present in approximately 50 percent of the cases, and many patients had histories of thyroid disease or menstrual irregularity. Four patients had multiple endocrine neoplasia syndromes.

Two of the patients who had undergone prior therapy (one RF thermocoagulation, one craniotomy) presented with associated cerebrospinal fluid rhinorrhea.

LABORATORY STUDIES

Preoperative basal hGH values ranged widely. Among patients with active acromegaly, there were some who had "normal" baseline values as well as those who had markedly elevated levels. By tumor category, there were 24 cases of microadenoma with a mean basal preoperative hGH of 25.4 ng/ml, 52 cases of diffuse adenoma with a mean preoperative hGH of 52.4 ng/ml, and 24 cases of invasive adenoma with a mean of 69.7 ng/ml. Preoperative prolactin values were elevated in 12 of the 60 patients in whom it was measured.

The presence of a pituitary adenoma was confirmed by appropriate radiologic studies in each case.

SURGICAL CONSIDERATIONS

All patients were operated on by a standard transseptal transsphenoidal route. Enlargement of the facial features and bony structures made the surgical approach difficult in some cases, with the depth of the sella occasionally being 11 cm or more. Abandonment of the procedure was thought advisable in one case when excessive hemorrhage occurred from a large intracavernous sinus.

RESULTS

Transsphenoidal surgery produced improvement in the signs and symptoms of acromegaly in all but eight of the 100 patients. No significant postoperative change occurred in any of the four acromegalic giants, in the patient whose operation was abandoned because of excessive bleeding, in one patient whose persistent postoperative hGH elevation was eventually cured by craniotomy, in one patient who developed a recurrent tumor, and finally in the single patient who is not alive at this time. He died of an adenocarcinoma of the colon, and his growth hormone was higher than when determined preoperatively.

All seven patients who presented with visual field defects had improvement in vision both subjectively and objectively following surgery. No patient had vision worsened by the surgical procedure.

On the basis of findings at surgery, 24 tumors were characterized as microadenomas ($\leq$ 10 mm in diameter), 52 as diffuse adenomas (including 13 with suprasellr extension) and 24 as invasive adenomas (including 4 with suprasellar extension). "Total" removal of the tumor with preservation of normal gland was the goal in most cases. Total hypophysectomy was purposely performed in two patients, one of whom was an acromegalic giant with diabetic retinopathy.

Follow-up basal hGH values were available in 98 of the 100 cases and are presented in Table 1 along wih the results of postoperative assessment of remaining anterior pituitary function. Radiation therapy has been given or recommended to 37 of the 81 patients who had not received it previously, the recommendation usually being based on the invasiveness or extent of the tumor and/or the postoperative hGH value.

There was no operative mortality in this series. Surgical complications consisted of one case with transient cerebrospinal fluid rhinorrhea, four cases of partial anterior pituitary insufficiency, and 14 cases of complete anterior pituitary insufficiency. Permanent diabetes insipidus occurred in one case and transient diabetes insipidus, which lasted more than one month, occurred in two other patients. Perforation of the nasal septum developed in one patient. One patient suffered subdural hemorrhage and decrease of vision as a complication of her postoperative radiation therapy 3 months following surgery.

Four patients underwent more than one operation. One man initially thought to have a microadenoma had a diffuse adenoma as the cause of his persistently elevated hGH. Another patient, whose tumor activity remained uncontrolled after RF thermocoagulation and a transsphenoidal operation, was ultimately normalized by craniotomy and removal of an extrasellar tumor nodule. One of the patients with gigantism and acromegaly had a postoperative hGH level of 22 and was reexplored transsphenoidally one year after the initial procedure. Additional tumor tissue in the wall of the left cavernous sinus was removed, but the hGH values continued to be abnormal. One patient required reexploration for repair of postoperative CSF rhinorrhea. There has been one recurrence of an intrasellar diffuse adenoma in a patient whose hGH values initially fell and then progressively rose during an 18-month period of observation. She has been referred for proton beam therapy. The ultimate true recurrence rate is not known,

TABLE 1   Results of Transsphenoidal Surgery in 100 Patients With Acromegaly

		Postop hGH			Postop pituitary function		Suprasellar extension	Visual field defect	Elevated prolactin†	MEN syndrome
	N	$\leq$ 10	>	?	unimpaired	impaired				
Microadenoma										
TS surgery only*	20	19(95%)	1	0	20	0			1	1
Prior Rx	1	0	1	0	1	0			0	0
Surgery and radiotherapy	3	1	1	1	2	1			1	1
Total microadenoma	24	20	3	1	23	1	0	0	2	2
Diffuse adenoma										
TS surgery only	27	22(81%)	4	1	25	2	6	2	4	2
Prior Rx	8	7	1	0	5	3	1	0	1	
Surgery and radiotherapy	17	8	9	0	15	2	6	3	1	
Total diffuse adenoma	52	37	14	1	45	7	13	5	6	2
Invasive adenoma										
TS surgery only	7	4	3	0	5	2	2	0	1	
Prior Rx	4	1	3	0	0	4	0	0	0	
Surgery and radiotherapy	13	8	5	0	9	4	3	2	3	
Total invasive adenoma	24	13(54%)	11	0	14	10	5	2	4	0
Total acromegalics	100	70	28	2	82	18	19	7	12/60	4

*Includes 2 invasive microadenomas
†Preoperative Prolactin levels available in a total of 60 patients

but is probably 8 to 12 percent.

Five of the seven young women with amenorrhea have resumed menstruating, and three of the five have become pregnant. Postoperative prolactin values are normal in all the patients whose values were abnormal preoperatively, and galactorrhea has not persisted in any of the patients who had this symptom preoperatively.

DISCUSSION

Because the follow-up period is relatively short, the effects of successful surgery on the natural history of the disease cannot be evaluated fully. It is anticipated, however, that long-term control will be better and that the recurrence rate will be lower than those resulting from other forms of therapy.

Classification of tumors into categories of microadenoma, diffuse adenoma, and invasive adenoma appears to be validated by the postoperative hGH values. Clearly, the most favorable results occur in those patients with microadenoma, in concurrence with most recent reports. That persistent fraction of uncured

patients in every series of acromegalics is probably best accounted for by tumors that involve the sellar dura or parasellar structures and therefore cannot be resected totally. It is important to note that our overall plan of management does include radiation therapy postoperatively for a significant number of patients, and the results of postoperative endocrine evaluation are the most accurate means of determining the success of the surgery and the possible need for follow-up radiation therapy. Bromocriptine therapy is occasionally utilized, but has not proved effective for most patients as large doses are generally required. The results in terms of preservation of normal anterior pituitary function have been most encouraging and represent a significant advance over previous systems of therapy for acromegaly.

Transsphenoidal microsurgery currently has an excellent potential for achieving ideal results—the removal of the pituitary adenoma with preservation of normal pituitary function. Every effort should be made to treat acromegalics at the earliest possible phase of the disease, when the selective removal of a small microadenoma is most readily accomplished.

PITUITARY CHROMOPHOBE ADENOMA

JOHN C. VanGILDER, M.D.

Pituitary tumors are divided into those that produce an excessive amount of one or more pituitary hormones and those that are nonsecreting, affecting pituitary hormone production by destruction or compression of the pituitary gland. The latter, or chromophobe adenomas, were originally so named because of their lack of affinity for vital stains.

In the older literature, chromophobe adenomas comprised approximately 80 percent of pituitary tumors; this percentage is comparable to the percentage of chromophobe cells in the normal pituitary gland. Subsequent histochemical scrutiny and the development of pituitry hormone assay techniques have resulted in a more precise classification of pituitary tumors. Thirty to 40 percent of all pituitary tumors are now diagnosed as chromophobe adenomas.

Symptomatic pituitry adenomas account for approximately 10 to 20 percent of all intracranial tumors. The true incidence cannot be accurately stated because autopsy studies have shown that the adult pituitary gland commonly contains one or more circumscribed foci of adenomatous proliferation on microscopic examination.

Minimal changes may be interpreted as foci of hyperplasia, and there are many gradations between hyperplasia and the encapsulated tumor nodule enlarging the pituitary gland.

Paralleling the development of assays to measure pituitary hormones in serum or cerebrospinal fluid and more precise neuroradiographic diagnostic studies, the incidence of diagnosed pituitary tumors has increased. Hormone-secreting tumors are commonly diagnosed when small and are successfully managed with both medical and surgical treatment. In contrast, nonhormone-secreting tumors, chromophobe adenomas, when symptomatic, are usually larger in size and are frequently associated with neurological symptoms secondary to compression of parasellar neural structures or medical symptoms related to pituitary hormone deficiency. The management of symptomatic chromophobe adenomas consists of surgical removal and/or radiation therapy. Experience with over 250 such pituitary chromophobe adenomas over the past 8 years at the University of Iowa is the basis for this chapter.

TUMOR CHARACTERISTICS

Symptomatic chromophobe adenomas occur predominantly between the ages of 30 and 50 years. The mean age in this series was 44 years. Less than 2 percent of patients were below 10 years of age and 3 percent were 80 years old or older. There is no significant sex difference.

For practical purposes, the tumor arises from the anterior pituitary lobe in the sella turcica, although other potential sites exist along the embryonic migration tract ventral to the sella. With growth, the tumor expands the sella turcica and rises above the diaphragm sella to encroach on the brain. This process is one of invagination, the neural tissue being pushed ahead of the tumor and separated from it by a capsule of leptomeninges. Expansion is usually upward in the midline. When lateral extension occurs, the tumor may escape from its leptomeningeal capsule and extend between bone and dura often as far as the gasserian ganglion or invade the mucosa of the sphenoid sinus. Chromophobe adenomas are usually soft, solid and vary in color according to their vascularity. Secondary changes due to degeneration or hemorrhage may result in the tumor being largely cystic, and calcium is present in less than 3 percent of tumors. Malignant changes are extremely rare, and when reported, they are usually associated with tumor penetration of the dura with nodules on the inner dural surface.

SYMPTOMS AND SIGNS

The most common symptoms of pituitary chromophobe adenomas are headache, visual loss, and pituitary hormone deficiency. Headache is characteristically bifrontal or bitemporal in location, corresponding to the distribution of the first division of the trigeminal nerve, which innervates the dura in the sella turcica. Because of binocular vision, visual field loss may be severe before the patient is aware of this deficit. Visual acuity is usually decreased later than visual field loss because of central retinal fiber preservation. Endocrine symptoms are usually those of hypothyroidism, impotence, decrease in sexual drive, and alteration of menses. Hypoadrenalism is a less common endocrine symptom. Sudden loss of vision is usually associated with hemorrhage into the tumor or a rapidly developing cystic component.

The most frequent neurological deficit is visual field loss, and this was found in 80 percent of patients. The characteristic ocular deficit is a bitemporal hemianopsia, although many field irregularities may be present. Optic atrophy is usually evident and is more severe when symptoms are of longer duration. Eighteen or 5 percent of patients had diplopia secondary to oculomotor, trochlear, or abducens nerve palsies. Extraocular palsy is most often associated with larger tumors invading the cavernous sinus. Other cranial nerves are rarely involved, the most common of these being the first division of the trigeminal nerve.

Eleven patients had pituitary apoplexy associated with altered level of consciousness. Five of these had subarachnoid hemorrhage, and extraocular nerve palsies were present in nine cases. Three patients, or less than 1 percent, had papilledema coincident with increased intracranial pressure secondary to obstruction of the foramen of Monro from suprasellar tumor growth.

There are remote effects from glandular insufficiency. The skin is pale from defective pigmentation and is often smooth and of fine texture. The hair is frequently fine with scant distribution over the pubes and axilla. In males, the testes may be small.

DIAGNOSTIC STUDIES

Endocrine Evaluation. It is important to assess both thyroid and pituitary-adrenal axis function. If either hypothyroidism or hypoadrenalism is present, there is an associated increased operative risk unless corrected. These tests include measurement of serum thyroxine and thyroid-stimulating hormone for the former, and compound S (before and after metapyrone) in the latter.

Additional hormone assays should include serum prolactin, luteinizing hormone, follicle-stimulating hormone, and growth hormone. To be meaningful, growth hormone measurements should evaluate the response to insulin stimulation and glucose suppression. Other chemistries of value are serum electrolytes, testosterone in the male, and cholesterol. Approximately 63 percent of patients were found to have insufficiency of one or more pituitary hormones prior to treatment.

Neuroradiologic Studies. Plain skull roentgenograms in patients with pituitary adenomas characteristically demonstrate altered configuration and enlargement of the sella turcica. The initial bone change is usually expansion of the sella beneath the anterior clinoid process; this is followed by enlargement of the sella turcica, whose maximum dimensions should not exceed 17 × 13 mm on the lateral view. Thinning and erosion of the sella cortical bone accompany these expansile changes.

Lateral and anteroposterior polytomograms are helpful to further define the bony anatomy of both the sella turcica and the sphenoid sinus. This latter is important to identify anatomic landmarks in patients who subsequently undergo surgery by the transseptal sphenoidal approach.

The most important radiographic study is computerized tomography, with and without contrast enhancement. Chromophobe adenomas usually are enhanced, and the tumor can be precisely outlined with its relationship to the adjacent neural structures. Both sagittal and coronal reconstruction, as well as transaxial planes with sections 3 mm in thickness, are obtained. Solid and cystic tumor components can be identified by computerized tomography. Early experience with nuclear magnetic scanning has been helpful to further clarify tumor and brain anatomy outlined by computerized tomography scanning.

Air and/or contrast (metrizamide) encephalography has not been useful in providing additional information. Similarly, contrast angiography has been replaced by digital venous angiography if the CT scan raises suspicion of a diagnosis of giant aneurysm.

The differential diagnosis of intrasellar and parasellar lesions from pituitary adenomas includes giant aneurysms originating from the carotid or basilar artery.

Other suprasellar tumors such as optic nerve and hypothalamic gliomas, craniopharyngioma, chordoma, meningioma, and bone and metastatic tumors, as well as granulomas and abscesses, may mimic the symptoms and signs of pituitary adenomas. A precise diagnosis can usually be established by clear neuroradiographic studies prior to treatment.

TREATMENT

The treatment of chromophobe adenomas is surgery and/or irradiation. The preferred operative approach for excision of the tumor is the extracranial transseptal sphenoidal approach to the sella turcica. Giordano, in 1897, first proposed a transnasal approach, which was subsequently modified and perfected by Eiselsberg, Kocher, Halstad, and Cushing in the early 1900s. With better anesthesia and the introduction of the operating microscope, the latter resulting in improved illumination and magnification, this surgical operation has been the procedure of choice for the past 15 years. Its advantages, as it is compared to the transcranial approach, include direct visualization of the tumor and pituitary gland in the sella turcica, less manipulation of neural tissue, an extracranial procedure that does not violate the subarachnoid space, and decreased morbidity and mortality. Large as well as small pituitary adenomas can be resected, usually with identification of normal pituitary gland and preservation of pituitary function. Pituitary adenomas with suprasellar extension, which have an hourglass configuration with the waist at the diaphragma sellae, cannot be removed by the transsphenoidal operation. Similarly, tumors with extensive growth lateral to the sella require transfrontal craniotomy for removal or decompression of neural structures.

Surgical treatment of pituitary adenomas is preferred to radiation therapy because a definite tissue diagnosis is obtained, the tumor may be removed completely, and compromised neural structures can be decompressed. Radiation therapy, which consists of 5500 rads delivered through two lateral ports over $5\frac{1}{2}$ weeks, is indicated for patients with medical contraindications to surgery and is effective in controlling progressive tumor mass effect. However, in the latter case, it may be several months following treatment before reduction of tumor size occurs.

Irradiation is most effective when used as a supplement to subtotal tumor removal by surgery. Complications of irradiation include development of panhypopituitarism or optic nerve atrophy in a small percentage of patients, the symptoms usually appearing several months after completion of treatment. Sarcomatous degeneration has rarely been reported to develop in the irradiated field.

Other methods of treatment, such as stereotaxic surgery, interstitial irradiation, and proton-beam irradiation, have been described, but seem to have no advantage over the more conventional methods except in selected cases.

RESULTS

In patients who had visual field deficits preoperatively, 78 percent showed improvement following transseptal sphenoidal removal of chromophobe adenomas. An analysis of these improved patients demonstrated that 60 percent returned to normal, 21 percent had greater than 50 percent improvement of visual fields, and 19 percent had less than 50 percent improvement of visual fields. Eighteen percent of patients had no change in their visual field deficit postoperatively. Four percent had an increased visual field deficit subsequent to surgery. All patients with preoperative extraocular nerve palsies had subsequent complete resolution; however this is slow and may require several weeks to occur.

Endocrine evaluation is done at 3 months, 6 months, and thereafter at yearly intervals. Forty-one percent of the patients had thyroid deficiency preoperatively; postoperatively, 19 percent returned to the euthyroid state. Among patients who had normal thyroid function preoperatively, 10 percent were hypothyroid following surgery. In contrast, 18 percent of the patients demonstrated pituitary-adrenal axis insufficiency preoperatively. Subsequent to surgery, this number increased to 27 percent of patients. No patient who had pituitary-adrenal axis insufficiency prior to surgery had improvement of this function.

Surgical morbidity and mortality are low with the transseptal sphenoidal removal of pituitary adenomas. Five patients developed signs of meningitis, two of whom had positive bacteria culture. All cases with clinical meningitis recovered without neurological deficit. Four patients had transient diplopia, and one required re-exploration of the tumor bed for a postoperative hematoma. Cerebrospinal fluid rhinorrhea occurred in 6 percent of patients; however this was usually transient, responding to bed rest with head elevation. One patient required reoperation for repair of rhinorrhea 2 months after surgery.

The most common complication is diabetes insipidus, which was present in 22 percent of patients. This is usually of a transient nature, is easily controlled with pitressin nasal insufflation, and resolves in less than 2 months. In approximately 5 percent of cases, diabetes insipidus persisted beyond 2 months, but all eventually recovered.

Mortality is less than 1 percent. In this series there were two deaths: one from pulmonary embolism and the other from infarction of the hypothalamus.

RECURRENCE

Although pituitary chromophobe adenomas are benign, the incidence of recurrence is not insignificant. There are differences of opinion among physicians regarding supplemental irradiation after surgery. It is my practice to remove mass effect of the chromophobe adenoma with surgery. If residual tumor is present, as evidenced by subtotal tumor removal at surgery or on evaluation of the postoperative computerized tomography scan, irradiation to a total dosage of 5500 rads is administered to the tumor bed. If the tumor was believed to be completely removed, based on surgical observation and confirmed by computerized tomography scan, I do not administer radiation therapy.

In our 5- to 8-year follow-up of 167 patients with chromophobe adenoma, 28, or 17 percent of cases, have been irradiated subsequent to surgery. Two have demonstrated recurrence during this period, an incidence of 7 percent. One hundred and thirty-nine patients have not received irradiation, and 15 patients, or 11 percent, have had recurrence. Of these 15 patients, four were symptomatic with signs secondary to compression of parasellar structures and underwent reoperation prior to irradiation. The other 11 patients had evidence of tumor recurrence by computerized tomography scan and were treated with irradiation 1 to 8 years after surgery.

ACTH TUMORS AND NELSON'S SYNDROME

NICHOLAS T. ZERVAS, M.D.
PETER McL. BLACK, M.D.

In his book, *The Pituitary Body and Its Disorders*, Harvey Cushing described a patient, Minni G, Case #XLV, with "polyglandular syndrome". The photograph of Minnie G shows a young woman with severe asthenia, abdominal swelling and abdominal striae. Two decades later, Cushing had acquired almost a dozen similar cases, a few from his own clinic and the rest from colleagues around the world. He studied the autopsy material and concluded that the patients had a small tumor of the pituitary gland (in some cases almost microscopic in size) which was the basophilic adenoma that Cushing deduced was the cause of this devastating illness.

Since then, several etiologies of Cushing's original description have been discovered. The term, *Cushing's syndrome*, is used today to group these entities, and it encompasses ACTH-producing pituitary adenomas, ectopic ACTH-producing tumors such as carcinoid tumors or malignant lesions (especially from the lung), and adrenal lesions such as hyperplasia, adenoma, or carcinoma. The term *Cushing's disease* is reserved strictly for pituitary adenoma or pituitary hyperplasia. The manifestations are fundamentally the same. The key features pointing to a malignant etiology are rapidity of onset and severity of symptoms. In addition, a number of several nontumorous etiologies have to be considered, especially alcoholism, obesity, and depression.

Cushing's syndrome causes a variety of clinical abnormalities, some minor and some especially striking or potentially fatal. Diabetes mellitus and hypertension are significant features in longstanding cases. Hirsutism, abdominal striae, easy bruisability, excessive weight, and proximal muscle weakness are common. Indeed, muscle weakness from myopathy occurs frequently, and osteoporosis with compression fractures can be a disabling complication. When examined, the patients may easily be recognized because of the roundness and fullness of the face ("moon facies") and reddening of the cheeks. In addition to the hirsutism, acne is prominent, especially around the lower face and jaw. A fatty accumulation in the posterior lower cervical area is termed "buffalo hump".

Many patients complain of depression and lassitude or irritability. In fact, these may be the most prominent symptoms and may subside fully following successful treatment so that patients return to their former state of well-being. The emotional symptoms should not be underestimated since they may be the most severe disability reported by the patient.

On physical examination, the key findings should include rounding of the face, an excessive mass of fat at the low cervical area, evidence of bruisability such as ecchymoses, muscle wasting, and abdominal obesity due to fatty deposition in the mesenteric bed. Hypertension may or may not be present.

General laboratory findings frequently are not helpful, although the eosinophil count may be low and neutrophils may be slightly raised. In more advanced stages, serum potassium and chloride may be diminished. Some patients demonstrate low urinary specific gravities and have a history of polyuria and polydipsia. Glycosuria is often present, and frank diabetes mellitus on a glucose tolerance test is found in approximately 25 percent of patients.

Radiographic examination often demonstrates both osteoporosis and vertebral compression fractures, or rib fractures, especially in longstanding cases.

X-ray films of the skull are most frequently normal, although larger tumors enlarge the sella turcica, making the diagnosis much more certain. The very best computed tomographic scanning today may show small adenomas, but in the majority of cases, the adenoma, though present, cannot be seen with certainty. Tumors greater than 6 to 7 mm, however, may show some mottled density of the intrasellar contents on a contrast-enhanced scan, as well as asymmetry of the floor of the sella turcica and thinning of the surrounding bony confines. CT scanning of the adrenals usually demonstrates a symmetric enlargement in patients with pituitary tumors. CT examination is important for ruling out unilateral adrenal adenoma or carcinoma. Iodine-131 tagged 19-Iodo cholesterol and ultrasonic scanning of the adrenals may also help to detect unilateral adrenal mass, thus excluding pituitary adenoma.

A diagnosis of a pituitary-based cause of Cushing's disease depends on demonstrating either excessive ACTH production by the pituitary or hypercortisolemia attributable to the pituitary. Since one definition of Cushing's disease is hypersecretion of cortisol, the first step is to prove that hypercortisolemia exists. The normal secretion of ACTH by the pituitary gland is dependent on corticotropin-releasing factor (CRF) emanating from neurons in the anterior median eminence of the hypothalamus. ACTH secretion has a circadian rhythm, with the lowest levels found in the late evening or early morning and the highest levels at the time of awakening from sleep in the morning. Although there are occasional spikes in the afternoon, the basic pattern is high in the morning and low in the evening. Because of this rhythmic secretion, the diagnosis cannot be made on a single value of serum cortisol, but on the basis of a number of samples taken during the 24-hour period, with the mean value being high (>25 μg/ml). Since it is difficult to obtain many plasma levels for cortisol, a better test of basal function is the 24-hour collection of urine to measure 17-OH corticosteroids and free cortisol. Cushing's syndrome or disease is probably present if the free cortisol level for 24 hours is greater than 100 μg. Also, the same is true if 17-OH corticosteroids are greater than 12 mg over a 24-hour period.

Dynamic tests of adrenal function, however, are relied on heavily to differentiate a pituitary tumor from other lesions. Under normal circumstances, glucocorticoids inhibit the hypothalamic stimulation of ACTH production by the pituitary gland. This negative feedback system is one of the major controlling mechanisms of ACTH secretion by the pituitary gland. Consequently, in normal individuals, the administration of dexamethasone late in the evening will reduce plasma cortisol or urinary excretion of free cortisol or 17-hydroxysteroids by at least 50 percent. However, in patients with Cushing's disease, the hypothalamus is relatively insensitive to glucocorticoid feedback and the threshold is raised, requiring greater doses of glucocorticoids to suppress ACTH secretion. The classic test used today is the low-dose, high-dose dexamethasone test. In patients with Cushing's disease, it is found that the administration of small doses of dexamethasone (i.e., 1 mg) fails to suppress hypercortisolemia, whereas the administration of higher doses (8 mg) does suppress hypercortisolemia. This observation is perhaps the best determinant for the presence of a pituitary adenoma or, more rarely, pituitary hyperplasia. There are two variations of the test, a quick overnight test or a longer and more accurate 2-day test. In either event, patients with Cushing's disease fail to suppress with low-dose dexamethasone and do suppress cortisol production by 50 percent with higher doses. Conversely, ectopic ACTH-producing tumors or primary adrenal lesions are not affected, i.e., they do not show suppression of cortisol with either low or high doses of dexamethasone.

Measurements of ACTH are not as useful since the radioimmunoassay can be unreliable. In Cushing's disease, ACTH levels are slightly raised or normal, and it is difficult in many cases to detect a slight rise in ACTH. It is hoped that better antibodies for ACTH will be found in the future. Also, beta-lipotropin synthesis from pro-opiomelanocortin (the precursor molecule for ACTH) is equimolar to that of ACTH, and it is hoped that a good assay for beta-lipotropin may help in the diagnosis of Cushing's disease.

Hypercortisolemia from other causes must be ruled out in studying Cushing's syndrome. Some depressed patients may appear to have some of the stigmata of Cushing's disease and may, in fact, fail to demonstrate suppression of cortisol following the administration of small doses of dexamethasone. However, stress is a major stimulus for the production of cortisol in normal patients. Insulin-induced hypoglycemia (a severe stress) causes a rise in cortisol in normal individuals. This does not occur in patients with Cushing's disease. On the other hand, depressed patients are able to produce cortisol following insulin-induced hypoglycemia. This has proved to be a satisfactory dynamic study to exclude emotional instability as a cause of Cushing's syndrome. A number of tumors, benign and malignant, such as pancreatic carcinoma, carcinoid tumors, thyroid tumors, and oat cell carcinoma, secrete ACTH. However, the levels of ACTH in these patients are much higher than in patients with Cushing's disease, and there is failure to suppress either ACTH or cortisol with extremely high doses of dexamethasone. Furthermore, CT body scanning can detect unsuspected tumors of the organs involved. The principal clinical features in malignant tumors are the rapidity of onset and the debilitated state of the patients.

The accuracy of endocrine diagnosis of a pituitary cause for Cushing's syndrome by the tests just described is in the range of 90 to 95 percent. Other procedures to improve diagnostic endocrine testing have proved unsuccessful so far. Attempts have been made to measure ACTH levels in both jugular veins. Differential levels would indicate a unilateral tumor and also possibly disclose the side of the tumor. However, the test is difficult and is confounded by the asymmetry in the drainage from the cavernous sinuses. Consequently, this test has not found wide popularity.

TREATMENT

Until recently, bilateral adrenalectomy was the surgical treatment for Cushing's disease. Today, exploratory surgery of the sella turcica is the primary procedure of choice of many endocrinologists. First described by Hardy on the basis of Cushing's prediction, exploratory surgery has quickly been adopted by neurosurgeons, and the results have been encouraging. In a recent survey of surgeons familiar with this operation, it was reported that approximately 15 percent of cases had macroadenomas, and the remainder had microadenomas or hyperplasia. When the endocrine diagnosis of microadenoma had been made preoperatively, the surgeon actually found the tumor in 82 percent of patients. If the microadenoma actually was found at operation, full remission was achieved in 91 percent of those patients. In the 18 percent of patients in whom a microadenoma was not found, approximately 50 percent were brought into a state of full remission by partial or total hypophysectomy. With present diagnostic methodology and the current state of precision and technical mastery in surgery, 86 percent of patients thought to have a microadenoma before operation probably will achieve remission following operation. Data are not available, at least to our knowledge, to determine what the recurrence rate will be 5 to 10 years following operation.

If operation is unsuccessful, extensive postoperative testing should be carried out to make sure that the preoperative diagnosis was correct. The laboratory studies should be repeated, and if they are equivocal both before and after operation, the diagnosis of a pituitary tumor should be strongly doubted, and an extensive search should be made for another source. This includes re-examination of other organs using ultrasound and CT and MRI scanning. If the diagnosis still points to a pituitary source which apparently was missed at the time of operation, it is appropriate to discuss with the patient a second operation for total removal of the pituitary gland, assuming a tumor is not identified at the time of the second procedure. However, there may be reluctance on the part of the patient or the endocrinologist to follow this tactic. Other options are photon therapy or heavy-particle radiation (such as alpha- or proton-beam therapy.

Various forms of medical therapy have been proposed. Medical adrenalectomy using metyrapone, aminoglutethimide, or o,p'DDD has been evaluated, but none of these drugs seems to have a long-term satisfactory effect on Cushing's disease or syndrome. Treatment with serotonin-blocking agents has been suggested since a serotonergic innervation of the pars intermedia has been verified. Cyproheptadine, however, has not been truly effective in bringing about satisfactory clinical response in the great majority of patients, although 30 to 50 percent of reported cases have had some benefit.

Following successful pituitary operations, patients are almost immediately relieved of most of the stigmata of this disease. The most promising finding within the first week is the dramatic cessation of emotional disturbances such as depression and irritability. This is almost a certain indicator of a substantial remission. In addition, the mild hypertension that is present begins to subside within a week or two, and after several months, the cutaneous stigmata resolve.

Treatment of patients in the postoperative period requires the administration of replacement doses of glucocorticoids, most commonly prednisone, 5 to 7.5 mg per day. This is necessary because the adrenal glands are unresponsive to the normal or low levels of ACTH now being secreted by the normal pituitary gland. Many months (4 to 6) may elapse before the adrenal response is satisfactory, at which time the administration of prednisone is no longer necessary. It is a mistake to attempt to reduce prednisone dosage too early in the patient's course.

An early indicator that remission is under way is the measurement of serum cortisol 3 to 4 mornings following operation, after the patient has received 1 mg of dexamethasone the evening before. If the cortisol level is $4 \mu g/ml$ or less, a remission is probably in process. Higher levels may be found which eventually subside, but if the level is $>10 \mu g/ml$, it is necessary to consider that the operation was unsatisfactory or incomplete and to take steps to re-evaluate the pituitary adrenal axis.

In children, the same set of standards apply. It should be noted that children are likely candidates for surgical removal, and the results can be as rewarding as those seen in adults. We have found that the operation is no more difficult, despite the smaller surgical field, and if the diagnosis is correct, the success rate is virtually the same. Radiation therapy was once thought to be a satisfactory modality for treating these youngsters, but operation is now preferred as the first procedure.

NELSON'S SYNDROME

One of the major complications of adrenalectomy for Cushing's syndrome in the past has been the stimulation of pituitary adenomas, some of which go on to malignant transformation. This is called Nelson's syndrome. Several factors are believed to be at work in the development of Nelson's syndrome. The principal mechanism is thought to be the chronic absence of the negative feedback of cortisol on the hypothalamus following adrenalectomy for Cushing's syndrome. In this situation, chronic CRF overstimulation of the pituitary gland (and/or an already present pituitry adenoma) is thought to stimulate an existing adenoma or to initiate a neoplastic process. The patients have excessive secretion of both ACTH and MSH and demonstrate local symptoms such as oculomotor palsies, diabetes insipidus, and visual disturbances, as well as classic hyperpigmentation of the skin. Nelson's syndrome occurs in approximately 10 percent of patients who undergo adrenalectomy, and of these, perhaps 10 percent undergo malignant changes that resist any form of therapy. The treatment is removal by either the transsphenoidal or the transcranial route, followed by radiotherapy. However, these are difficult tumors to control, and in some cases death cannot be prevented. The diagnosis depends on CT scanning, hyperpigmentation of the skin, and high levels of MSH and ACTH in the blood.

VASCULAR DISEASES

TRANSIENT ISCHEMIC ATTACKS AND STROKE FROM CAROTID ARTERY DISEASE

JAMES I. AUSMAN, M.D., Ph.D.
FERNANDO G. DIAZ, M.D., Ph.D.
JEFFREY PEARCE, M.D.

Transient ischemic attacks of the anterior circulation are episodes of focal cerebral dysfunction with rapid onset, variable duration, and rapid resolution. TIAs most frequently last for 2 to 15 minutes; however, by definition they may extend to 24 hours. Anterior circulation TIAs are characterized by the following symptoms, alone or in combination: (1) motor deficits—unilateral motor impairment ranging from mild clumsiness to dense paresis, (2) sensory deficit—unilateral numbness with loss of sensation or paresthesias, (3) aphasia—language disturbance which can involve expression, comprehension, reading, writing, or calculation, (4) complete or partial loss of vision in one eye only, (5) homonymous hemianopsia or dysarthria alone may be a manifestation of either anterior or posterior circulation ischemia.

Patients with actively changing neurological deficits in the anterior circulation demonstrate a change in their severity or recruitment of new deficits (listed above) while under observation. This is frequently referred to as stroke in evolution or progressing stroke. Many authors include patients who present with carotid distribution deficits of less than 24-hour duration in this category.

Completed stroke includes deficits that are relatively stable for more than 24 hours. This category is further subdivided into reversible ischemic neurological deficits (RIND)—deficits of 24-hour to 3-week duration—and completed stroke of greater than 3-week duration.

TRANSIENT ISCHEMIC ATTACKS

Numerous studies have followed the natural history of TIA patients. Milliken has recently reviewed these studies and found the incidence of cerebral infarction to vary between 20 and 40 percent over 5 years. The results of the Mayo Clinic study are frequently quoted. They found a TIA incidence of 31 per 100,000 population with subsequent infarction in 36 percent. Of those developing infarction, 21 percent occurred within one month and 52 percent within one year.

The first priority in managing patients with the stroke syndrome should be to establish a firm diagnosis. Although myriad systemic and vascular pathologies have been linked to stroke, a reasonably comprehensive evaluation can generally be carried out rapidly with little morbidity. An accurate and complete history and neurovascular examination are the single most important features in the evaluation of this syndrome. They determine the direction and extent of proposed invasive and noninvasive studies and should be used in considering the significance of any abnormality uncovered.

All patients presenting with the stroke syndrome deserve a screening laboratory examination of cardiovascular, renal, and metabolic activity. This should include a baseline chest roentgenogram, EKG, urinalysis, complete blood count with differential, electrolytes, BUN, creatinine, prothrombin time and partial thromboplastin time, platelet count, sedimentation rate, and fasting glucose. Further testing must be tailored to specific findings and clinical judgement.

Therapeutic objectives in the management of cerebral ischemia vary with the patient's clinical presentation. For those with TIAs prevention of cerebral infarction is the first priority, followed by treatment of associated disease states and the amelioration of risk factors. The patient with a progressing stroke presents the most complex and challenging problem. Goals include prevention of infarct progression, reversal of relative ischemia in the boundary zone, and prevention of secondary complications which can lead to increased injury. Patients with completed stroke require a risk assessment and treatment plan for prevention of recurrent infarction, alteration of risk factors, and rehabilitation.

As previously noted, patients with TIAs are at high risk for developing cerebral infarction early in their course. Almost all TIA patients without major contraindications to surgery will need eventual cerebral angiography. Since angriography is the most informative test and to a large extent determines the course of subsequent therapy, it should be performed early in the course of evaluation rather than as a last resort. In our opinion, patients who have had recurrent TIAs within the past 2 months or a recent increase in frequency should undergo immediate CT scanning followed by cerebral angiography. If any delay in their evaluation is anticipated, anticoagulation with intravenous heparin is instituted.

In patients who have well-defined but more chronic TIAs and are acceptable surgical risks, we believe that noninvasive screening is unnecessary. Significant surgical pathology can be mised even when the best noninvasive methods are used, making angiography necessary in TIA patients with negative studies. If noninvasive testing does suggest significant disease, angiography is needed for evaluation of surgical accessibility, intracranial pathology, tandem lesions, and collateral circulation. Digital intravenous angiography can be a useful screening procedure in some patients. However, significant disease can be missed with current technology.

The complication rate for angiography in patients with cerebral vascular disease varies widely in different series. The joint study reported a serious complication rate of 1.2 percent. This study failed to find an increased risk in patients with recent or severe deficits.

Medical Management of TIA

A significant number of patients with classic TIA symptoms have definite contraindications to surgery or lack an appropriate surgical lesion on angiography.

Cardiac emboli from myocardial infarction, valvular disease, and prosthetic valves are a frequent cause of cerebral ischemia. Unfortunately, these patients usually present with acute infarction without antecedent TIAs. Rheumatic heart disease, especially with atrial fibrillation or mitral valvular disease, is a frequent source of embolism. There is a recurrent stroke rate of 50 percent in the first year, which is significantly reduced with anticoagulation.

Cardiac dysrhythmia is rarely related to focal transient cerebral ischemia without underlying atherosclerotic flow-limiting lesions. Because of the low incidence of TIA in patients with cardiac dysrhythmia or embolization and the high incidence of atherosclerosis in this patient population, angiography probably is indicated in the majority of older patients with transient focal cerebral ischemic events, despite cardiovascular disease, unless a definite source of embolization is documented.

Transient ischemic symptoms have been attributed to polycythemia, anemia, hypolycemia, and a variety of other causes. Once again, atheromatous disease should be ruled out in patients with systemic disease but focal symptoms. A sound diagnosis of migraine variants or hypertensive crises with focal ischemia can sometimes be established by history and examination. Mass lesions and focal seizures may be difficult to identify on a clinical basis; however, CT scanning and EEG are now widely employed in the management of this disorder. The medical management of patients who are not surgical candidates include anticoagulants, antiplatelet agents, control of hypertension, and manipulation of other risk factors.

Anticoagulant Therapy of TIA

Several authors have recently reviewed antiplatelet and anticoagulant therapy. The number of patients reported in most series of anticoagulant treatment have been quite small. In general, all studies failed to demonstrate differences in mortality between treated and untreated groups; randomized studies failed to show significant benefits; and nonrandomized studies tended to favor anticoagulant therapy. Because of the small number of patients and methodologic problems, no indisputable evidence exists favoring anticoagulants. However, more recent reassessment of patients with TIAs does demonstrate decreases in stroke rate over the first 6 months which were then maintained over the following 5 years. This reduction was statistically significant only in patients with vertebrobasilar symptoms. The group studied was relatively small and lesions were not defined by angiography. Little additional benefit was accrued after 6 months, and the risk of complications from the anticoagulants greatly increased after one year of treatment.

Larger series have been completed on the use of antiplatelet agents for TIA. They have shown statistically signifiant efficacy for aspirin, but at a marginal level. The primary benefit was seen in males, in patients with multiple TIAs and an approrpiate lesion, or in carotid distribution TIAs. Recent work has demonstrated antagonistic effects of aspirin on platelets and the endothelial cell which are dose-dependent. Combinations of aspirin and dipyridimole are also frequently employed, and a marked dose and dose-interval dependency has been shown for combinations. The optimal dosing schedules and trial with these agents have not yet been documented.

In summary, anticoagulant therapy has documented efficacy in cases of embolization from a central source. It may be of value in nonsurgical candidates with TIAs early in the course of their disease. Antiplatelet therapy does have documented efficacy in at least some patients with TIAs, but the effects are not dramatic.

Carotid Endarterectomy for TIA

The role of carotid endarterectomy in the management of patients with TIAs and significant angiographic carotid lesions is well established, but its therapeutic efficacy remains poorly documented. Both medical and surgical series of various treatment modalities have failed to find significant improvement in mortality over untreated patients. This is not unexpected since the majority of patients with untreated TIAs die of a cardiac cause rather than cerebral infarction.

Many large series have recorded morbidity and mortality statistics for carotid endarterectomy. Risk assessment is based on neurological status and on medically and angiographically determined risk factors. Patients with stable neurological status and no major medical complicating factors have less than 2 percent total morbidity and mortality. Patients with significant medical risks have a higher (1%) incidence of serious morbidity and mortality.

Long-term follow-up of TIA patients who have successfully undergone endarterectomy generally shows decreased morbidity and mortality. The joint study group of TIA patients demonstrated initial hospitalization morbidity and mortality figures of 11.2 percent in surgically treated patients versus 12.4 percent in medically treated patients. However, in those successfully treated surgically, there were significantly more asymptomatic patients and fewer completed infarctions after the acute period. Overall significant infarct or mortality at 42 months in the two groups was about equal; 26.6 percent in those treated surgically and 25.9 percent in those managed medically. A stroke complication rate less than 2.9 percent is necessary to evidence significant superiority in surgically over medically managed patients. Finally, it also appears that postoperative treatment with aspirin in patients undergoing carotid endarterectomy is of value in decreasing postoperative mortality and stroke.

Recent statistics indicate that carotid endarterectomy can lower the rate in patients experiencing TIAs if they are moderate medical risks and have appropriate bifurcation lesions. Most authors would agree that a 50 percent stenoses and/or significant ulceration would constitute an operative lesion in a symptomatic patient. There is a greater risk of infarction in highly stenotic lesions. Surgical therapy may still be considered on an individual basis in patients with heightened medical risks if they demonstrate severe stenoses.

Superficial Temporal Artery to Middle Cerebral Artery Anastomses for TIA

Patients with a stroke syndrome demonstrate lone intracranial lesions in 6.1 percent of cases and combined cervical and intracranial lesions in 33.3 percent. This includes 6.6 percent stenoses and 8.5 percent occlusion of the internal carotid artery intracranially, together with 4 percent stenosis and 2 percent occlusion of the middle cerebral artery.

Surgical treatment of carotid bifurcation disease is generally aimed at removing a thromboembolic focus, whereas bypass surgery is most often performed to increase perfusion in areas of marginal supply. Lesions in the carotid artery begin to limit flow when there is a 60 percent reduction in diameter or when the cross-sectional area of the vessel is less than 90 percent.

The role of hemodynamic factors in the genesis of TIA is not so well documented as that of microemboli. Hypotension and arrhythmia are rarely associated with focal cerebral symptoms. Indirect evidence provided by changes in the EEG and regional cerebral blood flow have been demonstrated in patients with TIAs.

Because of hemodynamic effects, cerebral perfusion in patients with cerebral ischemia may vary with the patient's position. In general, the distal territory of supply of an artery is more sensitive to hemodynamic factors. The watershed zone in man over the motor strip occurs in the region controlling the arm. The retina should also be sensitive to hemodynamic factors since the intraocular pressure is normally 16 ml Hg, more than twice that of intracranial pressure.

ACUTE CAROTID OCCLUSION AND RELATED PROGRESSIVE STROKE SYNDROMES

FERNANDO G. DIAZ, M.D., Ph.D.
JAMES I. AUSMAN, M.D., Ph.D.
JEFFREY PEARCE, M.D.

Medical and surgical management of the stroke syndrome remains a controversial issue despite voluminous clinical and basic science research. Medical therapy has been described in a number of excellent recent articles. We have attempted to outline current therapy of carotid distribution ischemia from a surgical viewpoint. Medical adjuncts to therapy and areas of active current investigation are also addressed.

BASIC PHYSIOPATHOLOGY

Under physiologic conditions, blood flow to the gray matter is 75 ml/100 g/min, white matter 25 ml/100 g/min, and brain as a whole on an average 55 ml/100 g/min. Experiments in animals and observations in humans undergoing carotid endarterectomy would indicate that blood flow between 15 and 20 ml/100 g/min results in decreased cortical evoked potentials and EEG changes; responses generally being abolished below 15 ml/100 g/min. Sodium potassium pump failure does not occur until flow values have decreased to a level below 10 ml/100 g/min. This suggests that for at least a limited period of time the cerebral blood flow may drop below the levels necessary for neuronal function, but will remain above the level needed to maintain viability. The minimum cerebral blood flow compatible with cell survival and the duration of relative ischemia which can be tolerated have been investigated, but are yet to be rigorously defined.

Each carotid artery supplies 200 to 400 cc/min and the vertebral arteries together approximately 250 cc/min to the circle of Willis. From this point, the distribution pool of arteries extends to the level of the penetrating arterioles. Both the arteriolar bed, with a diameter of 70 microns at the cortical surface and 50 microns at the base of the brain, and the capillary bed are the primary source of cerebral vascular resistance and control of cerebral blood flow.

General autopsy studies demonstrate an anatomically normal circle of Willis in only 50 percent of specimens; however, less than 25 percent have one or more posterior communicating arteries less than 1 mm in diameter. Collateral supply may arise from a number of sources and is conveniently grouped by territories. This would include external to internal, right carotid to left carotid, or vertebral basilar to carotid collateral channels. An angiographic study has demonstrated an average of 5.9 sources of collateral filling in patients with unilateral carotid occlusion and 11 in those with bilateral carotid occlusions.

A number of factors, both local and systemic, can alter blood flow and metabolism in the region of an acute infarction. Autoregulation is lost, and local cerebral blood flow becomes dependent on perfusion pressure. Microcirculatory impairment secondary to intravascular sludging, together with endothelial and perivascular swelling, can add further injury. Intracellular calcium uptake secondary to ischemia of the arterioles may precipitate smooth muscle contraction and further increase cerebrovascular resistance. Cerebral edema may cause significant mass effect and herniation with large infarcts, but also probably plays a role in the development of microcirculatory changes.

In addition to a progressive loss of perfusion after an ischemic insult, cellular metabolic damage appears to be an ongoing process process. The role of Ca^{++} flux across membranes in relation to cytotoxicity is just beginning to be appreciated. The intracellular build-up of Ca^{++} following anoxia has been implicated in energy failure due to blockade of ATP synthesis in the mitochondria. Ca^{++} is also instrumental in generating cytoplasmic free fatty acids initiating the synthesis of a number of toxins including: thromboxanes, leukotrienes, and endoperoxides.

CLINICAL PROBLEM

Transient ischemic attacks (TIA) of the anterior circulation are episodes of focal cerebral dysfunction with rapid onset, variable duration, and rapid resolution. TIAs usually last for 2 to 15 minutes; however, by definition, they may extend to 24 hours.

Patients with actively changing neurological deficits in the anterior circulation demonstrate a change in the severity or recruitment of new deficits. This is frequently referred to as stroke in evolution or progressing stroke. Many authors include patients who present with carotid distribution deficits of less than 24-hour duration in this category.

Completed stroke includes deficits that are relatively stable for more than 24 hours. This category is further subdivided innto reversible ischemic neurological deficits (RIND)—deficits of 24-hour to 3-week duration and completed stroke of longer than 3-week duration.

The first priority in managing patients with the stroke syndrome should be establishing a firm diagnosis. Although a myriad of systemic and vascular pathologies have been linked to stroke, a reasonably comprehensive evaluation can generally be carried out rapidly with little morbidity. An accurate and complete history and neurovascular examination are the single most important measures in the evaluation of this syndrome. They determine the direction and extent of proposed invasive and noninvasive studies and should be used in considering the significance of any abnormality uncovered.

All patients presenting with the stroke syndrome deserve a screening laboratory examination of cardiovascular, renal, and metabolic activity. This should include a baseline chest roentgenogram, EKG, urinalysis, complete blood count with differential, electrolytes, BUN, creatinine, prothrombin time and partial thromboplastin time, platelet count, sedimentation rate, and fasting glucose. Further testing must be tailored to specific findings and clinical judgment.

Almost all TIA patients without major contraindications to surgery will need eventual cerebral angiography. Since angiography is the most informative test and, to a large extent, determines the course of subsequent therapy, it should be performed early in the course of evaluation rather than as a last resort. In our opinion, patients symptomatic within the previous 2 months or with a recent increase in symptom frequency should undergo immediate CT scanning followed by cerebral angiography.

Occlusion of the carotid artery may develop secondary to obstruction at either the bifurcation or the intracranial segment of the carotid artery. Acute occlusion due to disease at the bifurcation generally shows occlusion of the entire internal carotid artery on angiography, whereas occlusion intracranially usually is associated with a significant stump remaining at the origin of the internal carotid artery.

Therapeutic objectives in the management of cerebral ischemia vary with the patient's clinical presentation. For those with TIAs, prevention of cerebral infarction is the first priority, followed by treatment of associated disease states and the amelioration of risk factors. The patients with a progressing stroke present the most complex and challenging problem. Goals include prevention of infarct progression, reversal of relative ischemia in the boundary zone, and prevention of secondary complications which can lead to increased injury. Patients with completed stroke require a risk assessment and treatment plan for prevention of recurrent infarction, alteration of risk factors, and rehabilitation.

Patients in the category of stroke in evolution present with the highest potential for salvage and disaster. These patients present with an acute increase in the severity of recruitment of additional symptoms and signs of focal cerebral ischemia. The natural history of these patients is quite variable and less well defined than that of patients with TIA. It has been reported that after 2 weeks, 74 percent developed moderate or severe deficits, 14 percent died, and 12 percent improved.

GENERAL MEASURES

The patient in the early phase of an acute or progressive infarct is in a precarious position. Cerebral infarction is frequently a progressive process when secondary to a major vessel occlusion. The degree of ischemia seen with occlusion of a major vessel varies with collateral supply and is almost never complete. This is attested to by the variable course following carotid or middle cerebral occlusion in man.

Attention should be directed toward maintenance of normal homeostasis in acute stroke patients. Rapid correction of congestive heart failure or arrhythmias which compromise cardiac output is necessary. Pulmonary function must be watched closely to provide adequate oxygenation, ventilation, and prevention of secondary infectious complications. Normal renal function and fluid states must be established to maintain acid base balance and prevent electrolyte abnormalities which can aggravate cerebral ischemia and edema. In addition, adequate nutritional support can be initiated once the acute insult has stabilized. Optimization of the patient's general organ function through strict attention to standard medical therapy can minimize secondary insults to the ischemic brain.

MEDICAL MANAGEMENT OF ACUTE AND PROGRESSIVE STROKE

Anticoagulants

The use of anticoagulants in acute or progressive stroke has both theoretic and experimental support. Elevated concentrations of fibrinogen complexes which can be identified chromatographically are indicative of increased fibrinogen-to-fibrin conversion. In the clinical setting, this is most frequently seen with intravascular thrombus formation. Significant elevation of circulating fibrinogen complexes has been documented for several days following acute cerebral infarction. The same study also demonstrated increased levels of fibrinogen complexes in patients at high risk for stroke.

Several literature reviews supporting anticoagulant therapy in progressing strokes have been recently reported. Factors such as decreased cardiac perfusion, cerebral edema, hypoxia, or metabolic insults must also be identified as they can lead to progressive neurological deficit and would not be responsive to anticoagulant therapy. Lacunar infarcts in hypertensives frequently present as a slowly progressive lesion. They can sometimes be identified clinically by the specific focal nature of the deficit and should not be anticoagulated. Finally, patients with severe deficits have near-maximal ischemia and are unlikely to benefit from anticoagulation.

Antiplatelet Agents

No studies have been completed to date on the efficacy of aspirin or dipyridamole for acute or progressive cerebral infarction. Low-molecular-weight dextran decreases platelet adhesiveness and blood viscosity. Animal studies of dextran have suggested that it may prolong the interval of ischemia that can be tolerated prior to revascularization. Clinical trials, however, have been disappointing.

Osmotic Diuretics

Glycerol tends to delay or prevent acute herniation in massive infarcts, but has no efficacy in preventing severe deficits in patient with major infarctions. A significant or uncontestably beneficial effect of glycerol has not been documented to date, although the therapy appears to have some promise.

Several clinical studies have concluded that mannitol has not been effective in cases of acute ischemia. More recent work has reported beneficial effects when mannitol was used alone and in combination with perfluorochemicals as adjuncts for revascularization.

Massive brain edema with herniation accounts for approximately 30 percent of mortalities in the acute phase after cerebral infarction, frequently in young patients. With some simplification it can be considered to be primarily cytotoxic, but aggravated by late vasogenic changes which can become dominant. The mean survival in cases of herniation was 3.7 days.

Steroids

Conflicting results have obscured the evaluation of steroid therapy in acute or progressing stroke. Five controlled studies inthe 1970s failed to show significant benefit in steroid-treated patients.

Barbiturates

Interest in barbiturate therapy for focal cerebral ischemia has grown as protective effects in animal models became increasingly well documented. Protection in global ischemia is not so well supported.

The mechanism of barbiturate protection has not been conclusively demonstrated. Reduction of cerebral metabolic rate, decreased intracranial pressure, Ca^{++} channel blocking, inverse steal phenomenon, suppression of catechol-mediated hypermetabolism and free radical scavenging have all been offered as possible contributing factors.

Barbiturates cannot be expected to offer any protective effect in cerebral ischemia if local blood flow remains below that necessary for tissue survival. Possible benefits of therapy can only accrue if barbiturates either improve secondary local factors aggravating the ischemic process, thereby limiting infarct size, or provide a period of protection for ischemic tissues during which spontaneous hemodynamic changes or surgical intervention augment cerebral blood flow.

High-dose barbiturate therapy does entail significant risk and cannot be recommended routinely for the patient with an acute focal ischemic insult until indications for, and efficacy of, treatment are better established. Their use does appear to be justified in selected patients at present.

CAROTID ENDARTERECTOMY

In the past, carotid endarterectomy has played a very limited role in the management of stroke in evolution. Early attempts at revascularization were generally unsuccessful. The joint study reported a 42 percent mortality rate with surgical treatment and favored medical therapy. Hemorrhagic infarction has been a significant problem following thromboendarterectomy for acute occlusion.

Several recent studies have reported excellent results in patients demonstrating acute deficits treated surgically. Almost all patients who responded well to surgery demonstrated a fluctuating course with mild to moderate neurological deficit. In patients with crescendo TIAs, stroke in evolution, sudden partial deficits, sudden severe deficits, or postangiographic deficits, 63 percent showed marked improvement and 19 percent some improvement, with a mortality rate of 4 percent after acute carotid surgery. Those with sudden severe deficits, however, had a 44 percent mortality rate, and only one patient demonstrated marked improvement following surgery.

These results are clearly at odds with those reported in the earlier studies. Patients with severe deficits were not operated on in the later surgical series. Although there are scattered case reports of dramatic recovery following surgery for acute severe neurological deficits, the majority of these patients to date have done poorly with acute revascularization. Experimental evidence would indicate that without adjunctive therapy to inhibit progressive cytotoxic and ischemic insults, revascularization following severe ischemia is deleterious after 2 to 4 hours. Until a method of selection based on cerebral blood flow, metabolic parameters, or as yet unspecified criteria can be established, or an effective adjunct to prolong ischemic variability is documented, patients with severe deficits are best managed conservatively.

Hypertension is also clearly linked to the development of hemorrhagic infarction, intracerebral hematoma, and complications following revascularization. Diapedesis of red cells into an area of severe ichemia following revascularization with the formation of a hemorrhagic infarct is seen clinically and experimentally. Loss of autoregulation in ischemic areas is well documented in animal models and humans. After reperfusion, even moderate levels of hypertension would be uncompensated, increasing the propensity to hemorrhagic infarction and hematoma formation. All studies reporting good results following acute revascularization included strict control of blood pressure in their postoperative protocol. It would appear that acute endarterectomy can be of value in selected patients with stroke in progress. Results should improve as more explicit criteria for patient selection are developed.

SUPERFICIAL TEMPORAL ARTERY TO MIDDLE CEREBRAL ARTERY BYPASS

Some atients with stroke in evolution have an established carotid or middle cerebral occlusion. A number of animal models have been devised to evaluate reperfusion after various intervals of ischemia. These studies on the middle cerebral artery revascularization suggest that a short but definite period of time exists between the onset of an ischemic event and irreversible injury. The natural duration of this interval and means of extending it are currently under study.

Early attempts at STA-MCA anastomosis for progressing ischemia were disappointing. Several factors no doubt contributed to these results. Initial mean flow rates through STA-MCA anastomosis have been reported as 28 ml/min which may be inadequate to compensate for a major vessel occlusion with minimal collateral. It is probably more important, however, that bypass operations were generally completed after a significant delay. This was presumably after cytotoxic and vascular injury had been irreversibly initiated.

Recent reports suggest that acute revascularization can be performed with relative safety in selected cases if medical adjuncts known to retard cytotoxic and vascular damage are employed. The patient population that can benefit from these procedures and the most efficacious medical adjuncts have yet to be determined.

INTRACEREBRAL HEMORRHAGE

NICHOLAS T. ZERVAS, M.D.

Hemorrhage within the parenchyma of the brain is a major catastrophe. Medical or surgical management can be lifesaving, but the patient may sustain a major motor, sensory, or cognitive deficit that precludes return to the preictal level of function. Brain hemorrhage is somewhat less disastrous than infarction in that far less tissue may be destroyed. Unless the hemorrhage increases intracranial pressure and impairs cerebral perfusion enough to cause a secondary infarction, recovery can be complete. The hemorrhage usually is reabsorbed gradually over a period of several months. Thus little is gained by the removal of small volumes of parenchymal hemorrhage, even if they temporarily interfere with local brain function. Occasionally the mass effect from a large hemorrhage is such that surgical intervention is necessary to save the patient's life.

GENERAL CONSIDERATIONS

Special considerations in the management of patients with brain hemorrhage include the necessity of both understanding and ruling out various etiologies such as hypertension, vascular lesions or coagulopathies. Anticoagulants and drugs that impair platelet function or cause thrombocytopenia have been frequently implicated in cerebral hemorrhage. These complications must be rectified using vitamin K, fresh frozen plasma, or platelets and cryoprecipitate. It is usually possible to carry out operation if the necessary clotting factors are restored to the blood under the direction of a competent hematologic consultant.

At the time of operation it is also necessary for the surgeon to biopsy the wall of any hemorrhagic lesion to try to ascertain the cause of bleeding. Currently the diagnosis of amyloid angiopathy is being made with increasing frequency. This disorder is especially important to recognize, as these hemorrhages are difficult to treat surgically because the tissue is so friable, and because recurrent hemorrhage is so often the rule.

Most experienced practitioners believe that cerebral hemorrhage has a far better prognosis than cerebral infarction. The restorative processes generally remove the lesion within six months to a year. Operation is indicated primarily when intracranial pressure is high or the patient's condition is deteriorating. Surgery is more successful when the lesion is superficial in the cerebrum, or in the cerebellum. Special procedures for the drainage of angiomatous lesions in the brain stem or elsewhere are often successful, but these lesions are rare. Stereotaxic drainage of deep hemorrhages is in the experimental stage, and its role must await further reporting.

THE ROLE OF SURGERY

Surgical treatment must be directed toward excising the mass, if it is life-threatening, and removing the cause, if it can be found. Many so-called spontaneous cerebral hemorrhages are the result of anatomical lesions such as arteriovenous malformations or tumors. Whenever possible, these lesions should be removed to prevent rebleeding. Failure to demonstrate the cause of the hemorrhage in the acute stage is common. It is necessary to repeat angiography and computed tomography (CT) scanning several weeks or a month or two after the ictus to rule out occult arteriovenous malformation or, possibly, a vascular tumor such as a hemangioblastoma.

The principal natural phenomenon aiding the physician is the knowledge that the hematoma will diminish in size over many months and eventually will become a small cavity, perhaps no larger than a 1 cm ellipse or slit by the end of a year. Surgery cannot improve on this process of repair.

The approach to a cerebral hemorrhage is dictated by its location, although the locus might not be obvious when the patient is admitted to the hospital. The best test to localize the lesion is CT scanning. Lumbar puncture plays no role and may be dangerous in patients with suspected intracerebral hemorrhage.

MEDICAL MANAGEMENT

General tactics that must be employed in acutely ill patients in whom cerebral hemorrhage is suspected include maintenance of the patient's airway, with an endotracheal tube if necessary, control of hypertension, and measures to reduce intracranial pressure such as administration of steroids and mannitol. At the same time, the patient's coagulation studies must be analyzed and any deficiencies rectified. Fluid and electrolyte problems must be corrected promptly.

Since in so many cases intracranial pressure rises sharply with the onset of stupor or coma, it is preferable to intubate a comatose patient and institute hyperventilation. At the same time, we administer 32 mg of dexamethasone (Decadron) and 100 g of mannitol IV. In less urgent cases steroids alone may be sufficient. When the lesion is thought to be in the cerebrum, anticonvulsants should be given. Once a CT scan has been obtained and the location of the hemorrhage is clear, one must exercise judgment regarding therapy for the various types of hemorrhage.

MANAGEMENT OF SPECIFIC HEMORRHAGES

Superficial Supratentorial Hemorrhages

Hemorrhage in the frontal, temporal, or occipital lobes may or may not require evacuation. When the etiology of these lesions is unknown and they are not causing severe intracranial pressure, they can be managed conservatively and will gradually clear up in a majority of cases. Many are due to hypertension, which must be controlled. Tumors, arteriovenous malformations, and hemorrhagic diatheses account for some of the remaining cases, but many are of unknown etiology.

That the hemorrhage caused a neurological deficit such as homonymous hemianopia, speech deficit, or motor or sensory loss is not an indication for operation; rather, the level of consciousness should be the primary determinant. When the patient is alert despite a large lesion, I prefer to allow the hematoma to resorb on its own. An argument can be made for early evacuation, to allow the neurological deficit to clear up sooner. That decision, however, can incur lasting neurological impairment if the operation is complicated by further bleeding, either intra- or postoperatively. Operation should be approached with great circumspection, especially in hypertensive patients.

Thalamus and Putamen Hemorrhages

Deeper hemorrhages involving the putamen and thalamus are more complicated. If they are small, I usually allow them to resolve on their own. Surgery in these deep areas is likely to induce a greater deficit than the original ictus. A great deal of controversy surrounds operation for thalamus and putamen hemorrhages. The outcome is almost always poor for patients with large hemorrhages. Surgical removal of larger lesions is seldom rewarding, although it can be lifesaving.

Patients with small lesions who show progressive deterioration are the best candidates for operation. Those who are already comatose with large hemorrhages seldom, if ever, survive, and surgery in these cases is not good practice, in my opinion. When the lesion is large and the patient is fairly alert, recovery is still associated with major deficits, and surgery again should be reserved for those whose condition deteriorates. The large thalamic hemorrhages, as well as hypothalamus and putamen hemorrhages, have a high death rate regardless of treatment. I am not convinced that operation on them is warranted, unless the patient is awake and the lesion is in the nondominant hemisphere.

Pontine Hemorrhage

Pontine hemorrhage is easily diagnosed because of the classic clinical presentation with rapid coma, pinpoint pupils, and quadriparesis. In general recovery is rare, but patients with hemorrhages from small angiomas of the pons and mesencephalon often do recover. Treatment in most cases includes careful observation and maintenance of vital functions. Surgery may be required in rare patients with large hematomas who are sufficiently alert, retain brain stem function, and appear salvageable. Pontine angiomas usually are located centrally and probably arise from the floor of the fourth ventricle. Removal of the angioma is hazardous; removal of the hematoma alone may allow the patient to recover. Rebleeding is always possible. Direct attack on the lesion is usually less than satisfactory.

Cerebellar Hemorrhage

Cerebellar hemorrhage is a challenge for the neurosurgeon because early decompression of the hemorrhage can allow full recovery. These patients are simple to diagnose: They are generally known hypertensives who develop severe headaches, ataxic gait, and other brain stem disturbances such as paralysis of ipsilateral gaze. The most common mistake is failure to obtain a low enough CT scan, i.e., one that encompasses the posterior fossa. When the lesion is greater than 2 or 3 cm, early surgery is mandatory, because these patients often deteriorate rapidly. Much has been written about not operating on comatose patients with cerebellar hemorrhage. We have seen a few patients make good recoveries so that, even in these cases, we seriously consider operation.

One should be careful during these procedures to obtain biopsies of the lesion wall, especially in patients who are atypical or who are not hypertensive, because an occult arteriovenous malformation, hemangioblastoma, or tumor may be the cause of the bleeding. It may be satisfactory to observe patients with very small lesions, but any evidence of deterioration mandates immediate surgery without further tests.

Intraventricular Hemorrhage

Intraventricular hemorrhage is rather common. In my practice, it is generally the result of a ruptured intracranial aneurysm. In these cases, intraventricular hemorrhage is a serious complication and indicates that the aneurysmal hemorrhage was more severe than usual. Immediate drainage of the ventricles is usually necessary to reduce high intracranial pressure. Spontaneous intraventricular hemorrhage can be caused by an arteriovenous malformation or numerous other factors associated with brain hemorrhage, such as hypertension. When intraventricular hemorrhage is caused by a parenchymal hemorrhage directly into the ventricles, the prognosis is much worse. In these cases, drainage of the ventricles is not a rewarding tactic, both because it is difficult to maintain drainage and because the original lesion usually has had a much more destructive effect upon the brain. However, when a small arteriovenous malformation or benign tumor within the ventricle is the cause, removal of the lesion can be a very rewarding enterprise.

Hemorrhage from Vascular Lesions

Hemorrhages from vascular lesions such as aneurysms and arteriovenous malformations often must be treated before the removal of the offending lesion, if that is possible. We prefer to attack the lesion and the hemorrhage during the same operation, but in life-threatening, high intracranial pressure situations, the hemorrhage alone may be removed and the causative lesion excised later.

CEREBELLAR HEMORRHAGE

DONALD L. ERICKSON, M.D.

The clinical presentation of cerebellar hemorrhage can be varied. In some patients headache and unsteadiness of gait may be the only symptoms; in others there is a rapid onset of coma and multiple cranial nerve deficits. Prior to the advent of CT scanning, the diagnosis of cerebellar hemorrhage required a high index of suspicion and sharp clinical acumen. Delay in diagnosis often resulted in lack of preparation for potential emergency surgical intervention. If the physician is lulled into complacency by the mild presenting symptoms, the course can then be complicated by a crescendo of rapidly appearing brain stem findings, culminating in cardiorespiratory arrest. If appropriate treatment is delayed, cerebellar hemorrhage is perhaps rivaled only by traumatic epidural hematoma for the rapidity with which a completely resolvable situation deteriorates into a neurological disaster. Fortunately, with the wide availability of CT scanning, only the high index of suspicion is necessary to establish the presence of a cerebellar hemorrhage, which then allows institution of the appropriate surgical intervention. This is not to say that all cerebellar hemorrhages need surgical treatment, but the nurses and physicians who are observing the patient must be prepared for very rapid surgical intervention should any of the signs of early brain stem compromise become manifest.

NATURAL HISTORY

The most common cause of isolated cerebellar hemorrhage is hypertension. Cerebellar hemorrhages may occur with trauma, but are likely to be associated with other evidence of intracranial hemorrhage as well. Cerebellar tumors can be a source of hemorrhage, and one must always entertain that possibility, particularly in patients who do not have known hypertension. Posterior fossa arteriovenous malformations (AVM) are uncommon, but when they bleed they are likely to produce intraparenchymal cerebellar hemorrhage. Aneurysms, which are more common, are much less likely to rupture into the parenchymal cerebellum because the major sites of basilar-vertebral aneurysms are more superficially located. Bleeding disorder etiologies, such as hemophilia and, more commonly, iatrogenic anticoagulation, can be established by the history.

The initial onset is most commonly that of abrupt headache with or without brief unconsciousness, unsteadiness of gait, and often some mild brain stem findings such as sixth nerve paresis. If the hemorrhage is large, causing direct brain stem compression, or if the hemorrhage extends into the brain stem along one of the cerebellar brachia, immediate and persistent coma with multiple brain stem findings can ensure. With this latter presentation, prognosis is hopeless, often from the inception of the hemorrhage. It is the mild presentation that presents the most diagnostic challenge, the pathophyisology of which must be understood. A hemorrhage initially causes headaches if some of the blood enters the spinal fluid, while the mass effect of the blood causes compression of the cerebellar hemisphere, producing ataxia or dysmetria. Subsequent progression occurs when edema develops around the hemorrhage, thereby producing brain stem compression. At this stage, one begins to see cranial nerve dysfunction and perhaps some change in state of consciousness. Compression of the fourth ventricle or aqueduct of Sylvius, with subsequent rapidly progressing hydrocephalus, also can occur. It is this lethal combination of posterior fossa mass and hydrocephalus that culminates in the ultimate crescendo of neurological deficits and finally, downward herniation of the brain stem with cardiorespiratory disruption. Direct brain stem pressure from cerebellar hemorrhage, even in the absence of hydrocephalus, can produce a progressive brain stem dysfunction, but it is usually of a much more indolent nature and therefore much more amenable to timely surgical intervention.

DIAGNOSIS

The constellation of historical symptoms and neurological findings, as already outlined, should suggest to the clinician a diagnosis of cerebellar hemorrhage. However, with the easy availability of CT scanners, the diagnosis of this entity often is established before it has been entertained clinically. Nevertheless, familiarity with the symptoms is necessary so that CT scanning can be used wisely and economically. The history of immediate onset of severe headache suggests only one diagnosis, which is blood in the subarachnoid space. The severe headache of encephalitis, migraine, or other etiologies does not rival that of subarachnoid hemorrhage for rapidity of onset. If complaints of unsteadiness of gait, diplopia, or incoordination of one extremity are also present, one can strongly entertain the diagnosis of cerebellar hemorrhage. It is possible, of course, to have little or no headache associated with cerebellar hemorrhage if the blood is entirely contained within the parenchyma of the cerebellum. In that situation, the aforementioned posterior fossa findings are necessary to alert one to the diagnosis. For the patient who presents in coma with multiple cranial nerve findings, one is unlikely to obtain a history of headache, and therefore, distinguishing hemorrhage from brain stem infarction is often impossible. One must therefore depend on CT scanning for the differentiation.

If hemorrhage is suspected, the initial CT scan should be performed without enhancement. If the hemorrhage is visualized, but there is some reason to suspect a lesion in addition to the hemorrhage, enhanced scanning should be added. Only rarely is intracerebral hemorrhage missed on CT scan. Severe anemia or some admixture of blood and tissue fluid could render the lesion isodense. In addition to identifying the size and location of the cerebellar hemorrhage, CT scan defines ventricular size, which can prove important in determining the course of treatment.

Once the diagnosis of cerebellar hemorrhage is established, determining the etiology is not so important as rapid treatment. However, the etiology does affect the course of definitive care, and if the patient is stable, one should attempt to establish the cause of the hemorrhage. If there is reason to suspect something other than hypertensive hemorrhage, an unenhanced and enhanced CT scan might give additional information regarding such lesions as tumor or arteriovenous malformations. If the patient has a mild clinical syndrome with no evidence of progression, angiography prior to hematoma evacuation could at times be very helpful. For the neurologically unstable patient, one must be careful not to allow diagnostic measures to consume that crucial 30 to 45 minutes which often separates an excellent result from death or permanent neurological deficit. Angiographic delineation of aneurysms or AVMs preoperatively might allow definitive treatment at one operation, but can also be performed following hematoma evacuation, if time is of the essence preoperatively. It is also important to assess competency of clotting on an urgent basis.

THERAPY

Therapy can be divided into three general categories, the first of which is medical-expectant. I would prefer not to use the word conservative to describe medical therapy, because it may prove to be the most radical course, if prolonged, in some patients. Along with careful observation, the medical course should in most instances include the institution of steroids, such as dexamethasone or Medrol, for their antiedema effect. Osmotic agents such as mannitol should probably be used primarily as a prelude to surgical intervention, because the beneficial effect is likely to be temporary and could ultimately aggravate the progressive deterioration. If, with medical therapy, the patient returns to a

normal state of consciousness, without any progression of neurological findings, continuation of nonsurgical treatment is appropriate, awaiting ultimate spontaneous clot resorption.

The second general category of treatment is ventricular drainage, which should be instituted in patients with evidence of acute hydrocephalus. Occasionally ventricular drainage might be the definitive treatment, particularly if the cause of hydrocephalus is direct obstruction of the aqueduct of Sylvius or fourth ventricle with clotted blood. Some patients may develop chronic hydrocephalus secondary to the subarachnoid bleeding, necessitating permanent ventricular shunting. However, if the cause of obstruction is a large cerebellar hemorrhage, the ventricular drainage is only an interim step, and one must be prepared to proceed with the third category of treatment, namely, evacuation of the cerebellar hematoma.

Surgical evacuation of intracerebral and intracerebellar hematomas is often a simple uncomplicated procedure, particularly if there is a lapse of severel days between the time of hemorrhage and the surgical procedure. On the other hand, attempting emergency evacuation of acute intraparenchymal hematomas can be a frustrating experience complicated by excessive bleeding and fulminating brain edema. The surgical procedure and ultimate result are also complicated if delay has resulted in a marked increase in intracranial pressure, loss of autoregulation with vasogenic edema, and brain stem herniation. The ideal course, therefore, is to delay surgery only until it becomes evident that there is some neurological progression or lack of improvement, and then proceed with surgical evacuation of the hematoma.

Evacuation of cerebellar hematomas is slightly more difficult than that of intracerebral hematomas, primarily because the suboccipital area is less accessible and the confines of the posterior fossa more limited. Positioning of the patient is important if one is to avoid working in a compromised space with inadequate visualization. Positioning is enhanced by skeletal fixation, which allows adequate flexion of the cranial cervical junction. One can elect a prone, lateral decubitus, or sitting position for exploration of the posterior fossa. Both the sitting position and the lateral decubitus position have the advantage of a clear operative field because the bleeding is gravitationally drained away from the working area. The prone position, like the sitting position, offers easy access to the midline posterior fossa, whereas the lateral decubitus position is extremely convenient for a more lateral approach to the cerebellum. Cardiovascular stability must be considered in selecting the position as well, and older patients with unstable blood pressure or evidence of cerebrovascular ischemic disease are not good candidates for a sitting position. The sitting position has the additional risk of air embolism.

When the position has been established, a small craniectomy is usually sufficient to deal adequately with an uncomplicated intracerebellar hematoma. The operating microscope or surgical head light should allow adequate visualization to control bleeding within the hematoma cavity, and agents such as Gelfoam, Surgicel, or Avitene are particularly helpful when there is small vessel oozing in the edematous brain tissue, which may prove difficult to control with cautery.

If the etiology is other than spontaneous hematoma, lesions such as aneurysm, AVM, or neoplasm may be present, requiring definitive surgery at the time of hematoma evacuation or at a second stage. The need for a two-stage procedure may be determined by several factors, some of which are not under the surgeon's control. If emergency intervention is necessary, the presence of a second lesion may not be known. Vasospasm may be present in patients with aneurysm rupture, making definitive surgery unwise. Surgical resection of complex AVMs should rarely be done at the time of hematoma evacuation, but small focal AVMs can be safely handled at that stage. Benign tumors such as meningiomas or acoustic neurinomas may bleed, and removal of these neoplasms should be attempted, preferably in an ideal setting provided by a second-stage procedure.

The likelihood of early serious rebleeding from any of these lesions apart from aneurysm is small, and therefore a second-stage, definitive procedure may be the prudent course in any but the most ideal situation.

Postoperative management can be complicated by rebleeding into the hematoma cavity or development of marked cerebellar edema acting as a mass and thereby producing recurrent brain stem compression and compromise of CSF pathways. For these reasons, patients with preoperative evidence of hydrocephalus are best managed with a ventricular catheter, which allows both continuous monitoring of intracranial pressure and evacuation of CSF if hydrocephalus recurs. If there is any evidence of respiratory embarrassment related to brain stem compression, continued tracheal intubation is appropriate and provides not only respiratory assistance but prevention of elevated intrathoracic pressure and subsequent compromise of cerebral venous drainage. Attention should also be paid to the risk of aspiration if the lower brain stem or lower cranial nerves are dysfunctional. Nasogastric drainage and feeding may be necessary during the recovery phase.

There are very few true neurosurgical emergencies. Epidural hematoma, impending spinal cord compression, and cerebellar hematoma are in this uncommon category. The least common, and therefore the most often misdiagnosed, is cerebellar hematoma. Early recognition and appropriate treatment bring their own rewards.

BRAIN STEM ISCHEMIA: RECONSTRUCTIVE OR BYPASS SURGERY

THORALF M. SUNDT Jr., M.D.

The technical advances in bypass surgery have recently enabled us to revascularize the posterior circulation. As a result, we are seeing an increasing number of patients with progressing symptomatology involving this system. In many instances patients have already undergone angiography prior to referral so that the population base from which this group of patients is drawn is essentially unknown. However, there is an increase in the numbers of patients being referred for this problem. This probably is related to increaed sophistication of generalists, internists, neurologists, and neuroradiologists in the identification of patients who would possibly benefit from a bypass procedure. All patients considered for bypass procedures have been actively suffering from ischemic symptomatology. In order to place this group of individuals in proper perspective it is necessary to review patterns of atherosclerosis in the anterior and posterior circulation along with the pathophysiology of occlusive cerebral vascular disease, the numbers of patients operated upon with this condition, a categorization of patients undergoing the procedure, the overall results of the operation, and an analysis of our results and experience to date.

PATTERNS OF ATHEROSCLEROSIS AND THE PATHOPHYSIOLOGY OF OCCLUSIVE DISEASE IN THE POSTERIOR CIRCULATION

The classic studies of C. Miller-Fisher over two decades ago clearly established that major cerebral infarctions in the posterior circulation attributable to atherosclerosis were, in general terms, related to intracranial atherosclerosis rather than extracranial atherosclerosis. This is a "flip-flop" of the anterior circulation, in which extracranial atherosclerosis is of seemingly greater importance. Atherosclerosis at the carotid bifurcations is a frequent source of intracranial embolic complications, and these plaques frequently lead to total occlusion of an internal carotid artery, producing infarction either from propagation of a clot from the site of the occlusion or from inadequate cross-flow from the opposite hemisphere. This is not so in the posterior circulation.

Although atherosclerosis at the origin of the vertebral arteries from the subclavian arteries is common (its frequency was documented by Stein and McCormick in the late 1960s), these plaques are not often the source of major intracranial ischemic events. This is not to say that these plaques are always asymptomatic, but merely to underscore the fact that they seldom lead to a major intracranial infarction. This is because plaques at the origin of the vertebral arteries are frequently fibrous and seldom the source for emboli. Although they can reduce flow, the vertebral artery is provided with adequate collateral circulation arising from the thyrocervical, transverse cervical, and occipital arteries so that collateral flow in the distal vertebral artery is frequently sufficient to maintain circulation through these vesels even after the vertebral artery occludes at its origin.

In contrast, large-vessel intracranial occlusive disease in the posterior circulation can be catastrophic in its consequences when there is inadequate collateral flow between the anterior and posterior cirulations. The exact frequency of adequate collaterals provided via the posterior communicating arteries between the anterior and posterior circulations is not established. Patients with adequate collateral flow do not come to angiography because they can undergo intracranial occlusive changes without symptomatology, and therefore the frequency of this pattern is unknown.

Strokes in the posterior circulation can be related to small-vessel occlusive disease, and lacunar infarcts in the pons are entirely analogous to lacunar infarcts which we see in the basal ganglia and internal capsule. Thus, it is important to distinguish between symptomatology possibly related to penetrating arteriolar disease and large-vessel occlusive disease when evaluating patients presenting with ischemic symptomatology in the posterior circulation.

SYMPTOMS OF LARGE-VESSEL INTRACRANIAL OCCLUSIVE VASCULAR DISEASE

Patients with large-vessel symptomatic intracranial occlusive vascular disease usually present with symptoms that are related to the upright sitting position or activity. They do not have a classic history of embolic events, and if one takes a careful history, one is usually able to establish a correlation between the onset of these symptoms and activity or position. In addition to brain stem signs and symptoms, a definite history of visual blurring and obscuration is frequently obtained. Vertical diplopia, vertigo, and light-headedness are classic symptoms. Not infrequently, patients have episodes of alternating hemiparesis involving the left and then the right side of the body. Dysarthria is classic for posterior circulation ischemia. Patients presenting with a constellation of these symptoms, variable in nature, are usually suffering from large-vessel occlusive disease rather than an isolated arteriolar sclerotic lesion. Occipital headaches, although a common complaint in the population at large, are particularly prominent in some of these patients. On physical examination, the most commonly producible finding is that of truncal ataxia. This seems to be particularly common in patients in whom the process involves the vertebral rather than the basilar artery.

BASILAR VERSUS INTRACRANIAL OCCLUSIVE DISEASE

Most patients currently seen with occlusive disease in the posterior circulation are suffering from basilar artery stenosis rather than from distal vertebral artery stenosis. Although an occasional patient has a stenosis proximal to the origin of the posterior inferior cerebellar artery, the lesion generally is distal to this location, so that an occipital to posterior inferior cerebellar artery bypass procedure is not as frequently indicated as a more distal graft.

OPERATIONS PERFORMED TO DATE

We have performed four general types of procedures for occlusive disease in the posterior circulation. These include (1) occipital to posterior inferior cerebellar artery bypasses, (2) transluminal angioplasties, (3) side-to-side anastomoses between the posterior cerebral artery and superior cerebellar artery in patients with fetal circulation, and (4) interposition saphenous vein grafts between the external carotid artery and the proximal posterior cerebral artery.

Patients have been categorized for surgery in two major groups: (1) those with multiple transient ischemic attacks, but with no fixed neurological deficit, who are stable on anticoagulant therapy in that they are able to ambulate without the development of ischemic symptomatology and (2) patients neurologically unstable who have either a progressing neurological deficit or deficit reproducible with activity and not controlled and prevented by anticoagulant therapy.

Occipital to Posterior Cerebellar Artery

We have thus far operated on 38 patients with intracranial vertebral artery stenotic lesions proximal to the origin of the posterior inferior cerebellar artery. Approximately half of these patients were considered to be category 1. The overall patency of grafts in these patients is about 80 percent.

Transluminal Angioplasty

Six patients have undergone transluminal angioplasty. All six patients were in category 2, with advancing and progressing neurological deficits while on anticoagulant therapy. Two patients had an excellent result with obliteration of the stenotic lesions. One patient had a vertebral occlusion that produced a lateral medullary syndrome from which he recovered. There were three deaths: one attributable to multiple emboli from the site of dilatation, one due to delayed rupture of the site of dilatation in an 84-year-old patient with a calcified basilar artery, and one due to an intraoperative rupture of the vertebral artery related to perforation of the basilar artery by the guide wire. Although these patients have represented an extraordinarily high risk group of individuals with adverse fixed risk factors related to both age and progressing neurological deficits, our current experience suggests that the procedure should be reversed for patients who are not considered suitable candidates for any form of bypass.

Side-to-side Anastomosis of Posterior Cerebral and Superior Cerebellar Arteries

Nine patients have undergone a side-to-side anastomosis between the posterior cerebral and superior cerebellar arteries. All nine patients were suffering from active ischemic symptomatology at the time of the side-to-side anastomosis. In these patients, a posterior communicating artery was constructed between the fetal circulation and the posterior circulation. There have been seven excellent results, one stroke from progression of the basilar stenosis to occlusion, and one death (related to myocardial infarction 3 days after operation).

Interposition Saphenous Vein Grafts—External Carotid Artery to Proximal Posterior Cerebral Artery

This is currently our procedure of choice in the management of patients with acute and severe ischemia involving the posterior circulation. To date we have performed 64 of these operations in the posterior circulation, with an overall patency rate of 92 percent. The vast majority of patients in this group were considered category 2 risks.

This operation is preferred because it provides immediate high flows to patients who are suffering from acute and severe ischemia. In our experience, the vein provides a better and more predictable bypass graft than does the temporal artery for this particular purpose. The distance between the temporal bone and the posterior cerebral artery makes it extraordinarily difficult to harvest a temporal artery pedicle with the required diameter throughout its length for a viable bypass. Nevertheless, this is an operation fraught with hazard and one in which meticulous attention to details is required.

There are many pitfals associated with the operative procedure, and thus we recommend that the following major points be observed:

1. The vein must be harvested in an atraumatic fashion and with sufficient length so that areas that tend to angulate or kink can be excised. The vein must not be overdistended when it is harvested, and to prevent this, a Shiley catheter is extraordinarily helpful. All small branches should be doubly ligated with 5–0 Prolene suture adjacent to the vessel wall. A slight amount of adventitia around the vein is preferable to having the vein harvested without adjacent soft tissue. For orientation, it is helpful to place a 5–0 Prolene suture in the adventitia while the vein is still in situ and prior to ligating the branches and rotating the vein. This provides unequivocal orientation for the vein and prevents angulation and twisting. We refer to this as a "Garrett line"

after the Memphis vascular surgeon from whom the trick was learned.
2. The intracranial anastomosis should be accomplished with either a running 8–0 Prolene suture or interrupted sutures placed close together. A 9–0 Prolene suture is too small for this type of bypass as the needles tend to bend in going through the thick-walled vein. The vein should be beveled and anchored at its base and apex for proper length.
3. The vein is brought through a previously prepared tunnel, which courses through the temporalis muscle to the subcutaneous tissue anterior to the tragus of the ear, where it follows a route that goes deep to the parotid gland to exit in the neck at the level of the carotid bifurcation. The vein should be brought through this path distended and then advanced and retracted several times to be certain that the orientation is correct and that there is no angulation or twisting.
4. The proximal anastomosis is best accomplished by performing an end-to-end anastomosis between the vein and the external carotid artery. This anastomosis can be dilated with an onlay saphenous patch graft, providing something of a bulb to the origin of the vein. The tendency is to underestimate the proximal anastomosis, but it is probable that the proximal anastomosis is the more critical of the two anastomoses.
5. The absence of a bounding pulse in the graft when flow is opened indicates a problem with the proximal anastomosis, and this should not be accepted. A weak pulse is synonymous with an occluded graft, and if a bounding pulse is not present, it is necessary to take the graft down and redo the anastomosis. On occasion we have used two vein segments anastomosed end-to-end to provide the proper length in patients in whom an adequate length of vein was not available from one leg or thigh. In order to have a viable bypass graft, one must first have an adequate vein, and the attempt to "get along" with less than an ideal bypass is ill-advised. The typical completed bypass vein graft measures 25 ± 5 cm. Thus, allowing for proper timing, a segment of vein approximating 35 cm should be harvested. This is a longer graft than is generally used in the heart for coronary bypass, and because the vein undergoes a number of bends and turns, it is absolutely imperative that it be prepared without error.

EVALUATION OF OVERALL RESULTS

The evaluation of results in these patients cannot be considered without viewing these results in the framework of the disease process. As stressed previously, patients accepted for surgery are individuals who have failed on anticoagulant therapy and who have angiographically isolated posterior circulations with no anastomoses through the circle of Willis to the anterior system. This is an extraordinarily high-risk category of patients, and the operative procedure in these patients carries with it the highest risk of any neurosurgical procedure at this institution. Nevertheless, when the procedure is successful, results are dramatic, and the follow-up has been excellent. The grafts, if they remain patent for one week, invariably remain patent. We have had two late graft failures, both early in our experience. These were related to dysproportion between the size of the vein and that of the recipient vessel. Thus it is important that the vein and the recipient posterior cerebral artery be carefully matched. One of these two failures followed a graft between the carotid artery and a branch of the posterior cerebral artery. Currently we always use the parent trunk of the posterior cerebral artery, which tolerates temporary occlusion quite well. The graft is placed in the P-2 segment of the posterior cerebral artery. Two of the graft occlusions occurred in patients in whom the proximal end of the graft was constructed to the subclavian artery.

ANEURYSMS AND ARTERIOVENOUS MALFORMATIONS

SUBARACHNOID HEMORRHAGE

NEAL F. KASSELL, M.D.
E. CLARKE HALEY Jr., M.D.

Aneurysmal subarachnoid hemorrhage is a vicious, devastating disease; only approximately 30 to 40 percent of patients who sustain rupture of an aneurysm are able to return to their premorbid condition. Most morbidity and mortality can be traced to vasospasm and rebleeding, events that are initiated or occur with the greatest frequency in the first several days following the initial bleeding. Although there is no constellation of signs and symptoms more pathognomonic for a specific disease in clinical medicine than those associated with a typical subarachnoid hemorrhage, the diagnosis of this disorder poses a persistent problem. This is due to at least two factors. First, there is a general lack of awareness of the clinical presentation of spontaneous subarachnoid hemorrhage. Second, in certain instances it is difficult to differentiate the signs and symptoms of subarachnoid hemorrhage from other common disorders such as migraine headache, particularly when the bleeding is minor. Owing to the gravity of subarachnoid hemorrhage, the surgical treatment, and emerging modalities for managing vasospasm and rebleeding, it is essential that the diagnosis be made promptly and that the patient be transferred as soon as it is feasible to facilities that are fully equipped and staffed to deal with these complicated and technically demanding disorders.

DIAGNOSIS

The patient with typical subarachnoid hemorrhage presents with a history of sudden or abrupt onset of headache, often described as the most severe headache in his life. In most instances, the patient can remember precisely the activity in which he was engaged when the ictus occurred. One-third of aneurysms rupture during sleep, one-third during sedentary activities, and one-third during vigorous activities. The headache is described by the patient as being unique in nature and severity, unlike any prior headache. Often, the headache is described as "bursting" or "exploding" and is associated with nausea and vomiting, loss of contact with the environment or frank loss of consciousness, a dimming of vision or hearing, and/or seizure activity. After the ictus, the patient is left with a severe headache and neck pain, and often develops fever, malaise, and photophobia.

When a patient presents with a clinical picture suggestive of subarachnoid hemorrhage, the diagnosis must be confirmed as expeditiously as possible. In the past, the method of diagnosis was examination of the cerebrospinal fluid (CSF) obtained by lumbar puncture. Although lumbar puncture remains the "gold standard" in the diagnosis of subarachnoid hemorrhage, it carries a small but definite risk of inducing rebleeding. Therefore, the initial approach for confirming subarachnoid hemorrhage is now CT scanning. The CT scan is positive for intracranial blood in 90 to 95 percent of patients if performed within 5 days of subarachnoid hemorrhage. Lumbar puncture should be performed directly only in those instances in which the story is suggestive of subarachnoid hemorrhage and the CT scan is negative or unavailable.

In undertaking diagnostic lumbar puncture for suspected subarachnoid hemorrhage, special care must be taken to avoid contamination of the CSF sample by blood introduced through a traumatic tap. Certainly the procedure should not be delegated to the least experienced member of the team. The patient should be placed in the decubitus position with nursing assistance to prevent excessive movement. If agitation is a problem, a short-acting sedative may be necessary. After the lumbar subarachnoid space is entered and a free flow of spinal fluid is established, sequential tubes of CSF should be obtained in the usual fashion for analysis. At least two tubes of fluid should be sent for cell count. If the CSF is examined shortly after the onset of bleeding (within 24 hours), red cell counts on sequential aliquots show little variability, and the supernatant fluid of a centrifuged specimen has a pink tinge related to the presence of oxyhemoglobin. If the specimen is obtained later than 24 hours after the ictus, centrifugation reveals a yellow-tinged, or xanthochromic, supernatant due to the presence of bilirubin.

Bloody fluid obtained from a traumatic tap, on the other hand, shows a rapidly decreasing red cell count in sequential tubes, and the supernatant is free of pink or yellowish coloration. The presence or absence of crenated red cells in the specimen is related to, among other things, the duration the cells have been suspended in the fluid, and thus is often an unreliable determinant, as when the specimen has been left standing before analysis or after recent subarachnoid bleeding.

After subarachnoid hemorrhage has been confirmed grossly by lumbar puncture, full spinal fluid analysis, including protein and glucose measurement, white cell count and differential, and culture and sensitivities, is recommended to help distinguish aneurysmal subarachnoid bleeding from other illnesses that may also present with red cells in the subarachnoid space (e.g., herpes encephalitis). Finally, if transfer to a regional center is planned, it is often useful to send a tube of CSF from the lumbar tap along with the patient so that confirmatory or supplementary studies can be performed if necessary.

MANAGEMENT

There has been a tendency to delay transfer of patients with subarachnoid hemorrhage until approximately the time of surgery (usually 7 to 14 days after aneurysm rupture) in most North American centers. This approach must be abandoned. Not only are certain patients candidates for early operation (to be discusssed), but modalities for managing vasospasm and rebleeding are emerging. These obviously must be instituted as soon as possible after bleeding. Furthermore, since patients with subarachnoid hemorrhage are extremely prone to neurological deterioration, they require intensive monitoring. There has also been a tendency to perform angiography to demonstrate the source of bleeding prior to referral of patients to neurosurgical attention. This approach should be discouraged for two reasons. First, scheduling and performing the angiogram often results in a delay of one or more days in transfer. Second, the angiogram is used by the neurosurgeon to plan the operative procedure, and not infrequently, the studies that arrive with the patient do not contain all the desired information since the neurosurgeon has not had the opportunity to interact directly with the neuroradiologist. Thus the angiogram, with its inherent risks of complication, must often be repeated.

On admission of the patient to the neurosurgical unit, angiography is performed to determine the source of the bleeding. Ultimately, both carotid and vertebral circulations should be studied, as multiple aneurysms are found in 20 percent of patients. Special views to delineate anatomic relationships and cross-circulatory capacity are often necessary, and require interaction between the neuroradiologist and the neurosurgeon while the study is in progress.

If the angiogram is negative, it should be repeated in approximately one week. By that time the vessel caliber usually has changed and occult aneurysms have become apparent. Attention should be concentrated on the arteries in the region of the most blood on the CT scan. For instance, if a thick layer of clot is present in the right sylvian fissure and only a diffuse deposition throughout other regions, the right middle cerebral artery should be examined most carefully. The yield from repeat angiography is low, approximately 2 percent, assuming that the initial study is of the highest quality. Nonetheless, the risks of leaving untreated a potentially lethal sac justify repeating the study in most instances. If angiography is negative, the patient is treated with bed rest, analgesics, sedatives, anticonvulsants, and gentle antihypertensives for a total of 21 days following the hemorrhage (to be discussed). If angiography demonstrates an aneurysm, a decision on when to operate on the patient must be made.

It must be recognized that the timing of aneurysm surgery is a major neurosurgical controversy. Precisely which patients in which circumstances will benefit from early surgery has not been fully defined. Factors that must be considered in selecting the time of operation for a specific patient include: the skill, experience, and availability of key members of the team; previous results with either late or early surgery; the neurological and medical condition of the patient; the configuration and bleeding history of the aneurysm; the number of days after subarachnoid hemorrhage; the amount of blood and brain swelling on CT scan; the degree of angiographic vasospasm; and, most importantly, the subjective feeling of the neurosurgeon for the status of the patient and the environment in which the patient is being managed.

It is our policy to proceed with surgery to obliterate the aneurysm at the earliest possible moment following diagnosis, provided (1) there is no severe vasospasm, (2) no infarction with mass effect by CT scan, (3) no prohibitive medical conditions, and the entire team, including neurosurgeons, neuroradiologistS, neuroanesthesiologists, and operating room nurses, is available and fit. In general, we tend to avoid operating in the middle of the night, assuming that the risk to the patient of rebleeding is overshadowed by the hazards of operating with a fatigued or less than optimally prepared team.

Preoperative management is oriented to preventing complications. Obviously, in patients who are desparately ill from subarachnoid hemorrhage with a severely impaired level of consciousness secondary to increased intracranial pressure, stabilization must be achieved. Mannitol, 1 g/kg, should be administered to decrease intracranial pressure. If there is any impairment of the airway, the patient should be intubated. Once the patient is stabilized, measures are instituted to minimize complications, primarily ischemic neurological deficits from vasospasm, seizures, and rebleeding.

REBLEEDING

There are two primary approaches for preventing rebleeding: minimizing the transmural or bursting pressure of the aneurysm and decreasing lysis of the clot sealing the rent in the sac.

The transmural or bursting pressure across an aneurysm is the difference between the systemic arterial pressure and the intracranial pressure. In this regard, the arterial pressure is of major concern. The objective is to obtain the lowest arterial pressure compatible with acceptable neurological function. The arterial pressure must be titrated to achieve a balance between minimizing rebleeding and development of ischemic neurological deficits. This is complicated by the changes of this set point during the first 14 days following subarachnoid hemorrhage due to the changes in cerebrovascular resistance resulting from vasospasm.

Arterial pressure can be elevated as a result of pain, anxiety, straining, or hypoxia to a level in excess of that required for cerebral perfusion. Likewise, essential hypertension may exist. Furthermore, arterial pressure may be elevated in response to cerebral ischemia. It may be desirable to decrease arterial pressure below normal levels in an attempt to minimize rebleeding.

To decrease arterial pressure related to pain, anxiety, straining, and hypoxia, the following measures should be employed. Headache and neck pain should be treated with acetaminophen, although frequently narcotic analgesics such as codeine are required. If the pain is particularly severe, intravenous or intramuscular morphine is appropriate. Anxiety and agitation are controlled with phenobarbital or diazepam. Phenobarbital also has good anticonvulsant properties. The patients are maintained at strict bed rest in a quiet, relatively dark room where the number and activity of visitors is limited. Soft, soothing music is permitted, but television is not. Only decaffeinated coffee should be allowed. Analgesia is provided by acetaminophen, codeine, or morphine. Straining is minimized by the use of stool softeners such as docusate sodium (Colace), 100 mg *bid* or the equivalent. It is probably judicious to avoid the use of flurazepam (Dalmane), which produces REM sleep with associated arterial hypertension, and vasoactive nasal decongestants.

Pharmacologic control of arterial pressure is achieved, in general, with short-acting agents that do not decrease cardiac output. We prefer to use hydralazine, either orally or intramuscularly, in doses up to 300 mg per day. Propranolol may also be efficacious, particularly in combination with hydralazine, in patients who develop tachycardia.

For patients who are seen in the first several days following the hemorrhage, i.e., in the period prior to the development of any significant arterial narrowing, intravenous sodium nitroprusside may be used to decrease arterial pressure to normal or hypotensive levels.

PREVENTION OF CLOT LYSIS

The role of antifibrinolytic agents in patients with ruptured aneurysms has not been fully defined despite the large number of clinical trials on the safety and efficacy of this therapeutic modality. The most recent evidence suggests that antifibrinolytic agents decrease rebleeding, but at the expense of increasing ischemic neurological deficits. Rebleeding is an abruptly devastating or fatal event in most instances. There is no opportunity for recovery. On the other hand, ischemic neurological deficits develop more gradually, and a variety of manipulations may be performed to prevent or reverse the ischemic consequences. Therefore, we continue to employ epsilon-aminocaproic acid in patients who are admitted within the first week following aneurysm rupture and in whom it is necessary to delay surgery for at least several days. The optimal dosage schedule for administration of epsilon-aminocaproic acid has not yet been established. We recommend a loading dose of 10 g intravenously followed by 48 g by continuous intravenous infusion for the first 48 hours, and then continuous infusion of 36 g per day for approximately the first 10 to 14 days following subarachnoid hemorrhage. These agents are discontinued 6 to 12 hours prior to surgery or angiography. In the not too distant future, the Cooperative Aneurysm Study is expected to develop information leading to a more rational basis for administration of antifibrinolytic therapy.

INTRACRANIAL PRESSURE

The intracranial pressure exerts a tamponade effect on the aneurysm. Accordingly, it is important to avoid abrupt or uncontrolled reductions in the intracranial pressure. Lumbar puncture should be performed only when absolutely essential for diagnosis. Likewise, ventriculostomy should be performed carefully, and the drainage level set at no less than 20 to 25 mmHg. CSF shunting in patients with ruptured aneurysms is hazardous owing to the difficulty in controlling the rapidity with which the intracranial pressure is decreased.

CEREBRAL VASOSPASM

There are five strategies for the management of patients with vasospasm: (1) prevention of the arterial narrowing, (2) reversal of the arterial narrowing, (3) prevention of ischemic consequences, (4) reversal of ischemic consequences, and (5) prevention of infarction. Many pharmacologic agents have been tried to prevent or reverse the arterial narrowing of vasospasm, but none have proved effective. An agent to block spasmogens awaits identification of the specific spasmogens. Mechanical removal of the hematoma at early surgery does appear to be effective in ameliorating the onset of vasospasm. A surprisingly large amount of clot can be removed through a unilateral pterional approach, for instance, but it is impossible to remove all of the hematoma, particularly that in the distal portions of the insular cisterns. Although removal of the blood does appear to decrease the incidence and severity of vasospasm, the effect of the inevitable bruising of the pial banks and damage to small vessels, particularly veins, produces some degree of complication which has yet to be quantitated.

Prevention of ischemic deficits is an area that is more promising. The calcium channel blocking agent, nimodipine, appears to be effective in preventing ischemic deficits, although the mechanism is unknown. Whether the action of this drug is exerted through hemodynamic effects, such as dilatation of leptomeningeal collateral circulation, or due to rheologic effects, such as changing red blood cell deformability or oxygen-carrying capability, remains unclear.

In patients who do develop ischemic deficits from vasospasm, assuming that therapy is instituted prior to frank infarction, approximately 70 to 80 percent of deficits can be reversed with a combination of hypervolemic and hypertensive therapy; the intravascular volume is increased with blood or colloid, and the cardiac output is increased either by blocking the vasodepressor response with atropine or by the use of cardiac stimulants such as isoproterenol. Controlled hypertension is achieved in certain instances with the use of drugs such as dopamine. According to our experience, therapy must be instituted promptly and continued for 12 hours to 2 weeks. The level of arterial hypertension and hypovolemia must be titrated to the patient's neurological status on a daily basis. Calcium channel blocking agents are probably effective in providing some degree of neuronal protection in circumstances of severe ischemia. Similarly, to protect the neurons, it is important in these situations to avoid hyperglycemia. If all other forms of therapy fail and neurological status continues to deteriorate, it may be worthwhile to use high-dose barbiturate therapy in an attempt to decrease cerebral metabolism to match the level of substrates provided by the compromised level of blood flow.

HYDROCEPHALUS

Following aneurysmal subarachnoid hemorrhage, hydrocephalus can be observed by CT scan in 15 to 20 percent of patients, is clinically evident in 10 to 15 percent of patients, and ultimately requires shunting in 5 to 10 percent of patients. In general, we attempt to avoid shunting preoperatively because, as previously mentioned, it is desirable to maintain the tamponade effect of the intracranial pressure to prevent rebleeding. In addition, the intraoperative drainage of CSF in the presence of hydrocephalus provides a more slack brain requiring less retraction.

SEIZURES

Seizures, in addition to those that accompany the ictus, occur in 3 to 5 percent of patients following subarachnoid hemorrhage. Preoperatively, we tend to use phenobarbital for both its sedative and anticonvulsant effects, except in those patients who have a compromised level of consciousness; in these circumstances, phenytoin is employed. Anticonvulsants are discontinued 3 months after the hemorrhage, assuming the patient has not developed a seizure disorder.

GIANT INTRACRANIAL ANEURYSM

ROBERTO C. HEROS, M.D.

Giant aneurysms have been arbitrarily defined as aneurysms larger than 2.5 cm in diameter. Although a somewhat arbitrary division, it has been useful in that the management of aneurysms larger than this size presents unique problems. With smaller aneurysms, the surgical results are generally determined by the general condition of the patient and the effects of a recent subarachnoid hemorrhage (SAH), which may result in brain swelling, cerebral vasospasm, or rerupture of the aneurysm as it is being approached. With certain exceptions, such as aneurysms of the basilar artery, the surgery of small aneurysms is now relatively safe with present surgical techniques. The surgical treatment of giant aneurysms, however, is frequently difficult and hazardous regardless of whether the patient has had a recent SAH. It is appropriate, therefore, to give separate consideration to the management of these lesions.

PREVALENCE AND INCIDENCE

The prevalence of intracranial aneurysms of all sizes appears to be about 5 percent in autopsy series. Of these, about 5 percent are giant. Intracranial aneurysms account for approximately 10 percent of all strokes, and there are approximately ten to fifteen thousand new cases diagnosed in the United States every year. The age at which giant aneurysms become symptomatic seems to be about the same as for intracranial aneurysms in general, with the peak during the fourth and fifth decades. Intracranial aneurysms are rare in children, but the percentage of giant aneurysms is slightly greater in children than in adults. Small intracranial aneurysms occur more frequently in females than in males; no such sex difference has been found for giant aneurysms.

SITES

In general, giant intracranial aneurysms occur with approximately the same frequency in the different arterial territories as do intracranial aneurysms of all sizes. There are specific sites, however, where giant aneurysms are unusually frequent. In descending order of frequency, these sites include (1) the internal carotid artery, (2) the middle cerebral artery, (3) the vertebrobasilar system, and (4) the anterior cerebral artery.

Internal Carotid Artery. The cavernous and the paraclinoid region of the internal carotid artery account for the largest proportion of intracranial giant aneurysms. The paraclinoid region includes aneurysms that originate from the internal carotid artery at the site of the origin of the ophthalmic artery, but also includes aneurysms of that general region that are not necessarily related to the origin of the ophthalmic artery. Giant aneurysms of the internal carotid artery may arise from the area of the posterior communicating artery and also from the carotid bifurcation, but these are less common.

Middle Cerebral Artery. After the internal carotid artery, the bifurcation of the middle cerebral artery is the second most frequent site of giant intracranial aneurysms.

Vertebrobasilar System. A high proportion of giant intracranial aneurysms are found at the top of the basilar artery. Most of these arise directly upward between the two posterior cerebral arteries, but a fair number of them arise in relation to the superior cerebellar arteries. There are also a number of giant intracranial aneurysms in the main trunk of the basilar artery and at the vertebrobasilar junction, as well as occasionally in the vertebral artery itself in the general region of the origin of the posterior inferior cerebellar artery.

Anterior Cerebral Artery. The least common site of giant intracranial aneurysms is the anterior cerebral territory. Most of these aneurysms arise in the anterior communicating artery complex; rarely do they arise more distally.

CLINICAL PRESENTATION

Giant intracranial aneurysms can present either with general symptomatology, which does not predict the site of the aneurysm, or with rather specific symptoms that occasionally allow for a clinical diagnosis of the specific site of the aneurysm.

General Symptomatology

About one-third of giant intracranial aneurysms present with SAH. In these cases the syndrome is indistinguishable from the syndrome of SAH due to rupture of smaller intracranial aneurysms. The history of a generalized headache of rather abrupt onset, sometimes followed or preceded by a short period of unconsciousness, is common to SAH from all sources. These patients are frequently found to have subhyaloid hemorrhages on funduscopic examination. When the patient is alert, the description of the headache is usually dramatic and leaves little doubt as to the diagnosis. Such descriptions as "the worst headache of my life", "like an explosion in my head", and "something burst in my head" are well known. If the patient has focal neurological deficits, the diagnosis of SAH may be a bit more difficult to make. In these patients, an intracerebral hemorrhage is frequently present and accounts for the focal neurological deficits. A history of catastrophic headache at the onset is the main clue; such a history is most suggestive of SAH. Frequently, the patients are obtunded or comatose at the time they are first seen. Under these circumstances, unless a history of a preceding severe headache is available, it is difficult to make the diagnosis. Again, the presence of subhyaloid hemorrhages can be helpful, and if they are present without a history of head trauma, SAH should be strongly suspected.

Other nonspecific presenting symptoms of patients with giant aneurysms may be the result of mass effect and include headaches in the absence of SAH, and signs of increased intracranial pressure, such as papilledema. Rarely, epilepsy can also be due to a giant aneurysm; if the seizures are of the "partial complex type" suggestive of temporal lobe epilepsy, a giant aneurysm of the middle cerebral artery complex may be suspected.

Specific Symptomatology

Petrous Portion of the Internal Carotid Artery. Aneurysms in this area sometimes cause a bruit that is audible only to the patient. Occasionally these aneurysms produce a variety of other otologic complaints. The alert otorhinolaryngologist may detect a reddish mass in the middle ear and then refer the patient for proper diagnostic studies. In the rare cases in which these aneurysms have produced a Gradenigo's syndrome, the patients have facial paresis, pain in the face, and objective evidence of decreased sensation in the distribution of the trigeminal nerve. This is due to involvement of the seventh and fifth nerves in the area of the tip of the petrous pyramid. The sixth nerve is occasionally involved in these cases.

Cavernous Segment of the Internal Carotid Artery. Aneurysms in this location can present with syndromes suggestive of disease in the area of the cavernous sinus. The third nerve is most frequently involved, but the sixth and fourth nerves can also be affected. The patient has mild proptosis and slight conjunctival injection, but usually does not have the pulsating exophthalmous, marked chemosis, and audible bruit that patients with carotid cavernous fistula have. Vision is involved when these aneurysms are large and erode the optic strut to involve the optic nerve in the optic canal or project intradurally to involve the intracranial portion of the optic nerve. The patient has retro-orbital pain which at times can be quite severe. Sympathetic fibers may become involved as they course through the cavernous sinus, resulting in oculosympathetic paralysis. The fifth nerve is variably affected. Jefferson's classic description contended that in aneurysms located in the initial segment of the cavernous portion of the carotid artery, all three divisions of the trigeminal nerve would be involved. Aneurysms of the midportion involved the second and the first divisions, and only the first division should be involved in aneurysms of the last portion of the intracavernous segment.

Paraclinoid Region of the Internal Carotid Artery. These aneurysms usually arise at the origin of the ophthalmic artery, but may also arise from the posterior aspect of the carotid artery or from its lateral wall. In some instances, it is not clear whether they arise in relation to any of the branches of the internal carotid artery. If they project posteriorly, they may present without specific neurological deficit. The laterally projecting aneurysms of this region usually involve the third nerve. When they project superiorly or medially under the chiasm, they usually involve the optic apparatus. Initially they present with signs of optic nerve involvement with decreased visual acuity in the ipsilateral eye and variable scotomata. As they grow, they involve the chiasm and may even project more posteriorly to present with hemianopic field defects. At times the syndromes exhibited by patients with giant aneurysms of this region are indistinguishable from symptoms of parasellar and suprasellar masses, such as those due to large pituitary tumors or meningiomas of that area.

Origin of the Posterior Communicating Artery. Aneurysms of the internal carotid artery at the origin of the posterior communicating artery or, less commonly, at the origin of the anterior choroidal artery usually project laterally or posterolaterally and involve the third cranial nerve. Most commonly they involve the pupil as well as oculomotor function. However, in some cases there has been pupillary sparing, so that the presence of a third nerve palsy with pupillary sparing by no means rules out the presence of an aneurysm in this region.

Bifurcation of the Internal Carotid Artery. Aneurysms in this region can present with signs of compression of the medial temporal lobe and temporal lobe epilepsy. They can simulate meningiomas of the medial sphenoid wing or basal ganglia tumors, since at times they project superiorly and back to involve the basal ganglia and internal capsule.

Middle Cerebral Artery. Most giant aneurysms of the middle cerebral artery occur in the region of the main bifurcation or trifurcation. They frequently grow to very large sizes. They often present with nonspecific signs of increased intracranial pressure including headaches and papilledema. Temporal lobe epilepsy occasionally results from these aneurysms. The frequently occurring ischemic symptoms are caused by (1) embolism from intra-aneurysmal thrombi, or (2) gradual occlusion of one of the divisions of the middle cerebral artery from either extension of thrombus into the lumen or gradual stretching of a major branch with eventual thrombosis.

Anterior Cerebral Artery. Most aneurysms of the anterior cerebral artery complex arise in the area of the anterior communicating artery. These aneurysms can compress the optic chiasm from above and present with unusual visual symptomatology. Frequently they grow superiorly and anteriorly and can reach very large sizes before becoming symptomatic. Occasionally they present with a progressive dementing syndrome like that caused by large subfrontal masses (i.e., olfactory groove meningiomas). I know of several older patients who were institutionalized because of "Alzheimer's dementia" who were eventually found to have a giant aneurysm of the anterior cerebral complex.

Basilar Artery. Aneurysms of the basilar artery can compress the third nerve. This is actually more common with aneurysms arising distal to the origin of the superior cerebellar artery as the third nerve courses forward from the brain stem between the superior cerebellar artery and the posterior cerebral artery. The "top of the basilar" aneurysms rarely compress the third nerve since they usually project superiorly. These aneurysms are more likely to project into the third ventricle and produce obstructive hydrocephalus. Occasionally, however, they compress the cerebral peduncle on one side or another and can produce a Weber's syndrome with a contralateral hemiparesis and an ipsilateral third nerve palsy. They can also project straight backward into the interpeduncular fossa and result in pseudobulbar palsy, ataxia, and quadriparesis. This also occurs with midbasilar aneurysms. Aneurysms at the vertebrobasilar junction and aneurysms at the origin of the posterior inferior cerebellar artery can compress the lower cranial nerves and the medulla, resulting again in medullary symptomatology, sometimes with hemiparesis or quadriparesis, difficulty in swallowing, dysphonia, and ataxia.

RADIOLOGIC DIAGNOSIS

Plain skull films occasionally are diagnostic of a giant intracranial aneurysm. The finding of "ring calcification" in a plain film is pathognomonic for these lesions. Less specific for giant aneurysms is bony erosion. Aneurysms of the internal carotid artery in its petrous segment can produce erosion of the tip of the petrous pyramid, which may be visible on plain roentgenograms. Aneurysms of the internal carotid artery in the distal portion of the cavernous segment can result in erosion of the optic strut, which is a rather specific sign of an aneurysm in this area. Paraclinoid aneurysms may deform the sella and erode the anterior clinoid as well as the posterior clinoid processes. They can also extend into the sella, produce sellar enlargement, and thus mimic a pituitary tumor.

The CT scan is almost invariably positive in cases of giant intracranial aneurysms. Recent SAH and secondary effects of giant intracranial aneurysms, such as intracerebral hemorrhage and hydrocephalus, can be readily diagnosed by CT scan. There are three general patterns of CT visualization of giant intracranial aneurysms:

1. Nonthrombosed aneurysms usually produce a slightly hyperdense shadow on the plain CT scan. They "light up" with a dense round uniform stain after contrast.
2. Partially thrombosed aneurysms produce an inhomogeneous pattern of variable density on the plain scans. There can also be ring calcification in these aneurysms in addition to variable degrees of intra-aneurysmal calcification. In general, it is said that there should not be significant perianeurysmal low density or edema around these lesions, but on several occasions we have noted massive amounts of cerebral swelling accompanying some of the larger partially thrombosed aneurysms. With contrast injection, these partially thrombosed aneurysms can present the pathognomonic "target sign" with a central or eccentric dense staining area surrounded by an area of no significant uptake and enclosed within a densely staining rim.
3. Completely thrombosed aneurysms present a variable picture depending on the "age" of the thrombus. A recent thrombus is seen as a hyderdense shadow on the plain scan. Later on they may be hypodense. No significant central uptake is seen after contrast enhancement, but rim enhancement continues to be visible for variable periods of time and occasionally indefinitely. Again, in

most instances, absence of surrounding brain edema differentiates these lesions from brain tumors, but occasionally, particularly in cases of recent thrombosis, significant edema may be present.

Angiography continues to be the definitive test in cases of giant intracranial aneurysms. However, the angiogram may be negative except for the mass effect in cases of completely thrombosed aneurysms. In cases of partially thrombosed aneurysms, only the portion of the lumen that remains patent is visible angiographically, but usually there is evidence of a larger mass effect such as displacement of surrounding vessels. Whenever treatment of these lesions is contemplated, angiography is essential in order to ascertain the vascular anatomy.

PROGNOSIS

The prognosis of symptomatic giant intracranial aneurysms is very grave. A review of several series indicates that approximately 80 percent of symptomatic patients who remain untreated are dead or totally incapacitated within 5 years of diagnosis. This includes both patients who present with SAH and patients who present as a result of the mass effect of the aneurysm. Patients who present with visual deterioration as a result of compression of the optic apparatus by a giant aneurysm usually continue to deteriorate steadily and, without treatment, almost invariably become blind within a few years. Patients presenting with brain stem compression progress even more rapidly to total disability and death, usually within months. Perhaps the most benign natural history is that of aneurysms in the cavernous portion of the internal carotid artery. These aneurysms are relatively protected against SAH, but the cavernous syndrome that they produce usually progresses to complete ophthalmoplegia and eventual blindness of the ipsilateral eye. Once a giant aneurysm results in SAH, the frequency of rebleeding is estimated to be similar to that of smaller aneurysms. Some series suggest that the incidence of rebleeding is higher with these aneurysms.

Less is known about the natural history of asymptomatic giant intracranial aneurysms. Many of these lesions are diagnosed when CT scans are obtained for unrelated symptoms. Not enough of these patients have been followed over the years to provide a clear understanding of their natural history. There is no reason to suspect that their natural history is any more benign than that of patients with asymptomatic smaller aneurysms which bleed at a rate of about 3 percent per year. Giant aneurysms bleed with at least as much frequency as smaller aneurysms in spite of earlier claims to the contrary, and they carry the risk of brain or optic compression as they continue to grow. Treatment is usually more hazardous once SAH or signs of brain compression occur.

Partial thrombosis of a giant aneurysm in no way protects against subsequent SAH. This has been documented repeatedly; as many as one-third to one-half of giant aneurysms that rupture do have evidence of partial intra-aneurysmal thrombosis. It is not clear how complete intra-aneurysmal thrombosis must be before a patient is considered "cured" from a giant aneurysm. Two of my patients who were considered "cured" because an angiogram showed that the aneurysm was completely thrombosed subsequently had a massive rupture.

At times patients with giant aneurysms present with abrupt clinical deterioration and evidence of recent intra-aneurysmal thrombosis. In a few of these cases, I have seen massive cerebral edema surrounding the partially thrombosed aneurysm. Such abrupt clinical deterioration has also been documented in cases in which the aneurysm is found to be completely thrombosed at the time of presentation. It appears that the aneurysm enlarges abruptly as it thromboses. It is also possible that this thrombosis represents intramural bleeding with aneurysmal enlargement. In any case, the development of intra-aneurysmal thrombosis is not always a benign clinical event.

TREATMENT

Because of the dismal prognosis of symptomatic giant intracranial aneurysms, an attempt should be made to treat these lesions. Whether asymptomatic giant intracranial aneurysms should also be treated is a different matter. As stated earlier, the natural history of these lesions when they are asymptomatic is not well known, and since the treatment is usually dangerous, careful clinical judgment must be exercised in each case. In general, it is my belief that when lesions can be treated with relative safety, they should be treated even if they are asymptomatic.

It is clear that direct clipping of the aneurysmal neck is the ideal form of treatment. When this is feasible, the results are generally excellent. If a study of the angiogram and the CT scan suggests that it may be feasible to place a clip directly on the neck of the aneurysm, an exploration should be carried out for such an attempt. Occasionally, even very large aneurysms can be clipped satisfactorily if they have a relatively narrow neck. This may be true for as many as 20 to 30 percent of all giant intracranial aneurysms. Intracavernous aneurysms obviously cannot be clipped directly, and an indirect method of treatment must be used.

When direct clipping is not feasible, the surgeon must decide between an indirect approach and aneurysmorraphy. Aneurysmorraphy usually involves excision of the bulk of the aneurysm, which is likely to be partially thrombosed, and then reconstruction of the neck of the aneurysm, usually with a continuous suture, so as to re-establish near-normal anatomy of the parent vessel. This procedure needs to be carried out while the vessel is temporarily occluded both distal and proximal to the origin of the aneurysm. Several adjuncts have been suggested to protect the brain during the time of temporary vessel occlusion. The parent vessel usually needs to be occluded for a minimum of 20 minutes, and occasionally for an hour or longer. The type of brain protection used depends on the vessel involved and the potential for collateral circulation. The internal carotid artery frequently can be trapped for a significant period of time without the need for any adjunctive measure because of the excellent potential for collateral circulation across the circle of Willis. This is not the case when the middle cerebral artery or the basilar artery is involved. Protection by barbiturates, mannitol, or hypothermia is useful, and if the contemplated timing of occlusion is longer than 1 hour, the operation needs to be done under cardiopulmonary arrest. This represents a major endeavor with significant added morbidity and mortality. Occasionally one can perform an extracranial-to-intracranial bypass graft to protect the distal territory of the involved artery, but only after careful study of the properative angiogram with a view to the potential for collateral circulation. Sometimes this can be ascertained angiographically by temporarily occluding the vessel involved while other vessels are injected.

Proximal ligation or trapping can be accomplished, particularly in cases of aneurysms of the internal carotid artery, when the potential for collateral circulation is good. This also may be feasible after a bypass graft, in cases of middle cerebral or basilar artery aneurysms, but in these cases the potential for collateral circulation is more limited and one must depend primarily on the bypass graft as a source of distal circulation. In cases of carotid aneurysms, the most conservative form of treatment is common carotid occlusion. Internal carotid ligation would seem intuitively to be more effective than common carotid ligation in reducing intra-aneurysmal pressure. A careful review of the literature, however, indicates that no difference in effectiveness has been documented between internal and common carotid ligation. Both seem to be as effective in preventing aneurysmal rehemorrhage or enlargement and both seem to be as effective in inducing intra-aneurysmal thrombosis. It also appears that the rate of complication for internal carotid ligation is higher than for common carotid ligation. Even though the natural assumption is that gradual occlusion is safer than acute occlusion, the literature does

not bear this out. There does not seem to be much difference between abrupt and gradual occlusion. The fact remains, however, that about 20 percent of the patients do not tolerate acute occlusion, and in these cases gradual occlusion with a clamp may be necessary.

It has been claimed that internal carotid ligation now has become relatively safe when preceded by a bypass graft. However, there is a striking incidence of thromboembolic complications related to the thrombus that forms invariably in the internal carotid artery after ligation of this artery at its origin. These thromboembolic complications are not prevented by a bypass graft. For this reason I have increasingly used internal carotid occlusion right at the site of origin of the aneurysm by a detachable balloon. Even with this method, however, I have seen thromboembolic complications. The incidence of complications from indirect methods of treatment of giant intracranial aneurysms is higher than when direct clipping is feasible.

Other less available and more specialized forms of treatment for giant intracranial aneurysms involve the induction of intra-aneurysmal thrombosis by injections of hair or copper wire or needles into the aneurysm. This can be done under direct vision or by stereotaxis. Occasionally this is accompanied by the induction of an electric current, which promotes thrombosis. In general, these methods have not found general application since the rate of complication has been relatively high and the techniques are very difficult. They are best considered innovative in nature, and their continuing development should be left to the few investigators who have special expertise in this area.

There are no general rules or guidelines for treating giant intracranial aneurysms. These lesions are all different from one another and an individual judgment is necessary in each case. The complications and morbidity of treatment vary with each lesion, but it is clear that treatment is much more dangerous for giant aneurysms than it is for smaller aneurysms. Nevertheless, their grim natural history warrants a surgical attempt.

GIANT ANEURYM OF THE BASILAR ARTERY

CHARLES G. DRAKE, M.D., F.R.C.S. (C), F.A.C.S.

Giant intracranial aneurysms have been defined as those reaching 2.5 cm (1 inch) in size and make up about 5 percent of all aneurysms. Since only about 14 percent of aneurysms arise on the vertebral-basilar tree, the occurrence of giant aneurysms on this circulation is unusual. However, because of a special interest, our

surgical experience has consisted of over 450 giant aneurysms, of which 246 were on the posterior circulation. Most presented as mass lesions, but about 40 percent of our cases were recognized only after recent subarachnoid hemorrhage, and another 6 percent have a history of remote bleeding, presumably when the aneurysm was small. The diagnosis in a few cases with slowly deteriorating neurological function, thought to be of other cause, has come to light suddenly after a spontaneous rupture of the sac.

Headache is frequent, but poorly localizing for these masses. Various degrees and levels of brain stem compression make up the clinical picture, depending on the site and projection of the aneurysm. Those at the basilar bifurcation commonly present with gait disturbance, a faint hemiparesis, diplopia, and then confusional or amnestic syndromes. Only rarely are the visual fields involved with compression of the optic apparatus by a forward projecting sac. Transient visual field involvement may be due to ischemic episodes related to small emboli emerging from mural thrombosis within the sac. The giant aneurysm arising from the basilar artery at the origin of the superior cerebellar artery classically produces Weber's syndrome, a third nerve palsy with contralateral hemiparesis from hemi-midbrain compression. Truncal and vertebral aneurysms produce varying pontine and medullary compression syndromes including those of the cerebellar pontine angle. Strangely, severe degrees of obstructive hydrocephalus are unusual.

The bleeding from rupture of a giant aneurysm differs little from subarachnoid hemorrhage from smaller aneurysms except that more neighborhood signs may be evident. Plain skull films are rarely diagnostic for giant posterior aneurysms unless classic curvilinear calcification in the wall is seen. CT scanning, which is now the primary diagnostic study, is done before and after contrast. Before enhancement, the outline is circular, sometimes with curvilinear calcification previously unseen. After dense enhancement, the lumen either conforms to the circular wall or may be smaller and irregular because of mural thrombosis. Overlying such thrombosis, the wall of the sac is enhanced in curvilinear fashion. Final definitive diagnosis of course remains with angiography.

Follow-up of a few untreated giant aneurysms suggests that the future for these patients is bleak, most suffering severe disability or death from bleeding or mass effect within a few months or years.

When our surgical adventures with giant aneurysms began, there was little recorded experience except for carotid ligation for giant aneurysms of that artery. However, since experience has increased, it has been learned that most are now surgically treatable. On our unit, the therapeutic options have been reduced to neck clipping or hunterian ligature of the parent artery, sometimes with trapping, if opening and evacuation of the sac is essential to relieve brain stem compression. Other methods to obliterate the sac by promoting intraluminal thrombosis, such as by the infection of thrombogenic wire, have been found wanting in our three attempts because the neck of the sac has remained open and subject to the pounding axial stream and gradually dilated to produce another dangerous aneurysm beneath.

Most giant aneurysms result from the growth of small saccular aneurysms arising at the typical arterial branchings in both the anterior and posterior circulations and have been so named. As the region of the neck expands, it begins to incorporate the parent branching, often creating broad globular necks with the branches well separated from each other out on the neck or even on the waist of the sac. In experimental aneurysms, mural thrombosis tends to begin when the length of the sac begins to exceed twice the diameter of the ostium. In large aneurysms, much of the sac may be obliterated by mural thrombosis, leaving only a small cavity. Extent of the mural thrombosis can be accurately assessed by comparing the angiographic cavity with the mass in the CT scan. Even massive mural thrombosis does not appear to be a deterrent to further enlargement. Mural thrombosis involving the neck region makes this structure stiff and difficult to clip. Furthermore, atheroma is prone to develop in the walls of giant aneurysms including the neck region and is not infrequently calcified.

NECK OCCLUSION

It is surprising how often the necks of giant aneurysms are small enough, or can be made so, for a strong spring clip to be applied. Neck clipping in this series was accomplished in 91 of 246 cases. Great care must be taken that severe stenosis or occlusion of the parent artery, a major branch, or vital perforating vessel does not occur from a sliding clip or crimping of the neck tissue. Temporary occlusion of the parent artery or even trapping during the dissection around the neck and clip application is helpful. We have found that the use of modern gentle temporary clips has not produced arterial injury sufficient to promote occlusive thrombosis in any of over 100 patients, all of whom have had postoperative angiography. Temporary clipping is only undertaken with mannitol, 2 g/kg, in the circulation as some protection against cerebral ischemia. Ordinarily the occlusion time is only for 2 or 3 minutes, during which much dissection can be accomplished. For any but smaller neck occlusion, the Drake clip is commonly used so that either an adherent vessel may be accommodated in the aperture at its base or in tandem for larger necks. This clip may be used to occlude the far half or so of the neck while another straight clip is added to occlude that portion of a large neck remaining in the aperture. This avoids the problem of using long clip blades, which are often held open at the tips by the bulk of the neck at the fulcrum near the handle. Once the orifice is closed, the aneurysm may be aspirated or opened to evacuate the contents to relieve mass effect. Of the 91 giant aneurysms that could be clipped, 61 percent had good results, but 11 percent died and 27 percent had poor results (Table 1). However, when only patients in good condition are considered, 80 percent had good results.

TABLE 1 Results of Clipping of Giant Vertebral and Basilar Aneurysms

	No.	Excellent	Good	Poor	Dead
Basilar bifurcation	48	17	13	13	5
SCA	24	4	8	7	5
Trunk	3	2		1	
V-B junction	3	1		2	
Vertebral	2	2			
Posterior cerebral P1	5	3		2	
Posterior cerebral P2	6	4	2		
Total	91	33	23	25	10

Unfortunately, the necks of the majority of giant aneurysms are impossible or dangerously possible for clipping without great risk because either too much of the parent artery is incorporated into the neck or the bulbous steep slope of a firm neck will not prevent the closed blades of the clip from sliding in to occlude the parent artery or major branch, particularly when it is stiffened with atheroma or mural thrombosis. Occasionally with temporary occlusion of the parent artery, an aneurysm may be opened and thrombus evacuated to make the neck clippable. In a few pliable broad-necked aneurysms, the tandem clip principle using multiple Drake clips, as modified by Sugita in various angles, in tandem or in parallel, an be used to reconstruct the arterial lumen; this procedure has been very successful for giant carotid aneurysms.

PROXIMAL PARENT ARTERY OCCLUSION

For unclippable necks, the current best option is occlusion of the parent vessel as near to the aneurysm as is feasible to stop the high pounding axial flow into the sac. The stagnant flow in the sac thus isolated usually promotes intraluminal thrombosis, which obliterates all or most of the aneurysm. This maneuver obviously requires adequate circulation into the territory of the obliterated artery by communicating arteries or leptomeningeal collateral. Unfortunately, in contrast to the carotid circulation, there is no safely reliable extracranial-intracranial bypass to the basilar artery via the posterior cerebral or superior cerebellar arteries. However, it has been found that when posterior communicating arteries exist, even of modest dimensions, occlusion of the upper basilar artery is usually possible for aneurysms in the region of the basilar bifurcation. Even the lower basilar or both vertebral arteries have been occluded successfully.

The presence and caliber of the posterior communicating arteries may not be known from routine carotid and vertebral studies. However, these vessels can be opacified routinely by using Allcock's method, first right then left carotid compression during vertebral angiography. Clip occlusion of the basilar or both vertebral arteries may be used when one or both communicating vessels are obviously sufficient to carry the basilar circulation above the point of occlusion. Clip occlusion of the basilar artery in 33 patients resulted in 69 percent good results with a 9 percent mortality and 21 percent poor results. Again, if only patients in good condition are considered, the results were very much better. Complete thrombosis of the aneurysm, or virtually so, has occurred in two-thirds of these patients.

If the circulation is marginal, a tourniquet has been developed to test the adequacy of the collateral circulation when the patient is conscious. During operation, when it is discovered that the aneurysm cannot be clipped, a snare consisting of a plastic suture around the basilar or vertebral artery is placed and brought out of the head in small polyethylene tubing through a stab wound. Later, when the patient is awakened, the tour-niquet can be closed by hand during angiography, and the closure maintained by a small artery forcep while the patient is carefully monitored for any ischemic deficit. If none appears after 30 minutes or so, the stem of the tourniquet may be clipped to hold the occlusion while the patient is kept under close observation. The snare can be quickly opened by means of clip-removing forceps if ischemia develops. After 24 hours, the stab wound is enlarged under local anesthesia, the tourniquet can be reclipped as deeply in the wound as possible to maintain the occlusion, and the end is cut off so as to be buried subcutaneously. Tourniquet occlusion of the upper basilar artery in 32 patients with presumed marginal collateral effected good results in only 50 percent of these cases. However, patients in good condition fared much better. Remarkably, in a study of the number and size of the posterior communicating arteries, it was found that there was little correlation with subsequent ischemia; sometimes tiny vessels were able to maintain the upper basilar circulation.

Occlusion of the lower basilar artery, or of one or both vertebral arteries, has been used for giant sacs arising from the trunk of the basilar artery at or above the V-B junction. In 17 lower basilar and two solitary vertebral artery occlusions, the results were good in 14 patients. In eight other basilar artery occlusions for smaller unclippable aneurysms, the results were good in seven patients.

Giant aneurysms on the trunk of the basilar artery have been trapped on six occasions for evacuation of the aneurysm, which was considered essential to relieve critical brain stem compression. There were four excellent results, one poor, and one death. In four, the anterior inferior cerebellar arteries and some perforators undoubtedly were included in the trapped segment, and in two of these, there was sufficient collateral circulation to the region of these vessels bilaterally. In three of the trappings, the tourniquet was used to test the collateral flow in the awake patient.

For giant unclippable aneurysms arising at the vertebral basilar junction or the vertebral artery, occlusion of one or both vertebral arteries is necessary. This can be done extracranially, but intracranial vertebral occlusion is preferable to avoid reconstitution from rich cervical collateral. One vertebral artery may be occluded beyond posterior inferior cerebellar artery (PICA) almost routinely as long as the other exists and fills the basilar artery. Occlusion proximal to the PICA risks medullary infarction, although it is remarkable how often PICA fills retrogradely through a channel underneath the thrombosed aneurysm or by collateral from anterior inferior cerebellar artery (AICA). Complete thrombosis of an aneurysm restricted to one vertebral artery is usual.

Similarly, where one vertebral artery is atretic or ends in PICA, giant lower basilar trunk aneurysms can be treated by occlusion proximally of the only vertebral artery filling them, but this requires sufficient posterior communicating collateral, which may have to be tested with the tourniquet. Detached balloon occlusion of an intracranial vertebral segment is undoubtedly dangerous because the ostia of perforating branches may be occluded as well. All eight unilateral vertebral occlusion procedures for giant vertebral aneurysms produced good results and complete obliterative thrombosis. Unilateral occlusion for 14 giant basilar trunk and vertebral-basilar aneurysms was very satisfactory in 10 patients, but two worsened and two died from brain stem ischemia.

Ordinarily, bilateral vertebral occlusion is necessary for most giant vertebral-basilar junction aneurysms, but requires sufficient posterior communicating collateral. Clip occlusion of one with placement of the tourniquet on the other during the initial exploratory craniotomy has merit in marginal situations. Occasionally, one vertebral artery has been clip-occluded intracranially and the other in the neck by a detached balloon where collateral circulation is deemed or shown to be marginal.

Huge vertebral-basilar junction aneurysms, which involve a considerable segment of the basilar artery with its branches, especially AICAs, are particularly dangerous since bilateral vertebral occlusion is very efficient in promoting complete thrombosis within the sac, which may result in severe brain stem infarction from occlusion of important branches arising from the sac. Recently, severe stenosis of the second vertebral artery by means of a Drake clip has been used to promote collateral development over a period of months. Bilateral vertebral artery occlusion has been done in 16 patients, and good results were obtained in 11. The three poor results and two deaths were clearly related to brain stem infarction after branch occlusion from massive thrombosis within the aneurysm.

Only a few giant posterior cerebral aneurysms are clippable whether they arise on the first (1 of 4 on P1) or second (1 of 3 on P2) segments. Many tend to be fusiform. However, the results with P1 and P2 occlusion have been excellent in promoting complete obliterative thrombosis, but without occipital infarction. Occipital infarction did not occur after any of 15 P1 occlusions, but occurred in only three of nine P2 occlusions; the aneurysm was trapped for evacuation in five of these nine P2 occlusions. Although the posterior communicating artery may confer some protection for P1 occlusion, this is seldom the case for these aneurysms since the communicating artery may be occluded by aneurysmal thrombosis. In cases in which no field defect occurred, leptomeningeal collateral from A2 and M2 branches has been spectactular, even filling P2 retrogradely nearly as far as the aneurysm. The results in all 15 P2 aneurysms were good whether neck occlusion (6), proximal clipping (4), or trapping (5) was used. P1 occlusion (10) or trapping (7) was used in 17 of 22 giant P1 aneurysms, with only two poor results from midbrain ischemia because of perforator isolation. Another patient died, however, when the proximal P1 trapping was improperly placed or slipped, and the previously intact aneurysm burst.

In contrast to giant aneurysms on the anterior carotid circulation, where 85 percent have successful outcomes, only about two of three patients with giant aneurysms arising on the basilar artery fare well. Posterior cerebral and vertebral giant aneurysms have an 85 percent and 90 percent surgical success rate respectively. Sixty percent of the patients with poor results were in poor condition before operation and, even though the aneurysm was obliterated, remained unchanged.

It is hoped that earlier recognition of giant aneurysms with CT scanning for fleeting or vague neurological syndromes will reveal a larger number of patients in whom the neck may be occluded more safely.

SUBARACHNOID HEMORRHAGE FROM AN ARTERIOVENOUS MALFORMATION OF THE BRAIN OR SPINAL CORD

BENNETT M. STEIN, M.D.

Vascular malformations of the brain and spinal cord comprise a heterogeneous group of lesions including those that are entirely venous or arterial and those that are a combination of both elements. Although in the eyes of the pathologist, the most common lesions are the small telangiectasia or cavernous type of malformation, the surgeon is most commonly called on to treat arteriovenous malformations (AVMs) of the brain and spinal cord. It would appear that telangiectasias or cavernous malformations are pathologic curiosities and do not appear clinically with the frequency and devastation that is common to AVMs. Arteriovenous malformations are thought to be congenital and therein lies the enigma of these lesions. If this presumption is correct, they are present in infancy and adolescence, but rarely become symptomatic until the second, third, or fourth decade. Their most common presentation in the brain is with hemorrhage (75%) and seizure disorder (25%). The presumed congenital origin of these lesions is reconciled to the onset of clinical features in midlife by assuming that the malformation causes progressive damage to adjacent neural tissue and in itself undergoes gradual attenuation of its vascular channels, leading to hemorrhage during this period of life.

Arteriovenous malformations of the spinal cord have somewhat different features. They tend to become symptomatic later in life and are not identified with the frequency of hemorrhage that is seen in AVMs of the brain. In fact, only 10 percent of spinal AVMs present with subarachnoid hemorrhage (SAH).

In planning any treatment program for neurological disorders, it is preferable to have statistical information available on the natural history of a disease process so that the results of medical or surgical treatments can be compared with the course of events that might be expected to occur should no treatment be instituted. Unfortunately, these data are not readily available in terms of AVMs of the brain and spinal cord. These lesions are uncommon. The AVMs of the brain are one-tenth as common as intracranial aneurysms, and AVMs of the spinal cord are about one-tenth as common as their cerebral counterparts. Furthermore, the clinical syndrome of these disorders spans many years, if not decades. Therefore, it has been impossible to assemble a large number of patients who have been followed for 2 or 3 decades without medical or surgical intervention. Most of the statements relative to the natural history of these two disease processes fall into the realm of anecdotal comments or comments about selected cases. However, in dealing with patients, certain presumptions must be made:

1. The younger the patient when symptoms occur, the greater the risk to the patient. It is easy to see how a patient in the midtwenties who presents with a hemorrhaging AVM will be at greater future risk than an individual who presents in this fashion at age 65. It is also known that patients are most frequently seen with symptomatic AVMs in the middle decades. It is also presumed that individuals with AVMs do not generally attain old age since symptoms from these lesions after age 60 are uncommon, and the incidental finding of AVMs post mortem is rare.
2. Approximately 80 percent of cranial AVMs present with major parenchymal or subarachnoid hemorrhage. These hemorrhages result in death in an unknown percentage of patients and significant handicap from the initial hemorrhage in approximately 25 to 30 percent.
3. Hemorrhages are often recurrent, sometimes separated by decades, and although on many occasions associated with spectacular neurological recovery, they appear to result in cumulative neurological deficit over the passage of time with recidivous hemorrhage.
4. Patients who present with a seizure disorder as the initial manifestation of an AVM are not immune from future hemorrhage. Approximately 10 to 15 percent of hemorrhages are clinically silent and are discovered at operation without an antecedent history typical of hemorrhage. Perhaps some seizures are a manifestation of these hemorrhages.

Conjoined with these conjectures must be a broad surgical experience with all types of malformations located in different portions of the brain. Considering the meager data available, I tell a young patient with a cranial AVM, whether it has created hemorrhage or seizures or is relatively asymptomatic, that they have a 40

to 50 percent risk factor of incapacitating neurological deficit or possibly death during what might be expected to be their normal life span.

In terms of AVMs of the spinal cord, although these are rarer than cranial AVMs, it would appear that deterioration after the onset of primary symptoms is more rapid (averaging 6 years) than the course of cranial AVMs. Paradoxically, they are not as commonly associated with hemorrhage, but rather with a progressive neurological deterioration and a background of pain. Again, it is necessary to compare the experience without treatment with a broad surgical experience in decision making so that the patient may understand what the risks are of a do-nothing course versus interventional treatment.

THERAPY

It should be kept in mind that a high percentage (75 to 80%) of AVMs of the brain present with hemorrhage, whereas only 10 percent of those located in the spinal cord present in this fashion. In both instances, i.e., the cerebral and the spinal AVMs, the hemorrhage can be parenchymal, subarachnoid, or even subdural. The ratio between intra- and extra-axial hemorrhage depends on the size and location of the malformation. In most instances, the hemorrhage is a significant mass in the parenchyma. This often creates neurological deficits, some severe enough to cause death immediately. In most instances, when the patient has weathered the effects of the initial hemorrhage, even though the parenchymal hematoma may be large, there is a gradual recovery, perhaps to a normal neurological status. Rarely is it necessary for the surgeon to intervene in the acute phase of hemorrhage. Such intervention in the acute state would be indicated if there is progressive neurological deterioration or evidence that the hematoma located in a critical location is causing impending brain herniation. In such instances, the surgical intervention may be lifesaving. However, no serious attempt should be made to remove the vascular malformation at that point, and only decompression of the hematoma should be performed to permit the patient to recover gradually on his own.

The incidence of vasospasm following subarachnoid hemorrhage from vascular malformations is considered to be low. It has remained unexplained why subarachnoid blood from an AVM should not produce spasm, whereas with a ruptured cerebral aneurysm, spasm occurs in a high percentage of patients. There may be other factors unique to the hemorrhage from an AVM which create what may be an illusion. Consider that the hemorrhages from AVMs have greater volume in the parenchyma than in the subarachnoid space, that the hemorrhage uncommonly breaks into the large CSF cisterns and therefore does not spread in great quantity throughout the CSF spaces. Finally, the hemorrhage is slower in nature and less cataclysmic than that from a ruptured cerebral aneurysm. These factors result in less blood entering the subarachnoid space over a given period of time and in total quantity and also result in a delayed recognition of the clinical events. I have seen patients with subarachnoid hemorrhage from AVMs, usually in relation to a large CSF cistern, in which spasm of all of the intracranial arteries, even those far removed from the AVM, has been intense and, in some patients, has lead to tragic neurological deficits. Without statistical information to support these assumptions, I believe that given similar circumstances in relation to the hemorrhage, i.e., location and amount of blood, spasm will occur with the same incidence following hemorrhage from an AVM as from a ruptured cerebral aneurysm. If spasm does occur secondary to the subarachnoid hemorrhage, it should be managed with a generally accepted protocol, such as careful monitoring of circulation parameters, blood volume, and blood pressure. I have not found the various "cocktails" useful in reversing spasm. Similarly, operation on an AVM when spasm is present would be expected to produce unsatisfactory results.

The main aim, therefore, in treating AVMs of the brain and spinal cord, is to deal with them in an effective way that obliterates their contents and therefore negates the possibility of future hemorrhage, either parenchymal or subarachnoid, from these life-threatening lesions. Other than doing nothing, there are three basic methods of treatment. Only one (surgery) will lead to complete obliteration of the malformation. Embolization, by various techniques, has been most useful as an adjuvant to surgery. When used as a primary therapy, it cannot reliably be expected to obliterate the lesion. Radiotherapy in the form of proton beam therapy is high-dose radiation and, although focused, has resulted in significant radiation damage to normal brain. Furthermore, it rarely obliterates the lesion, and its ability to protect the patient against future devastation from the AVM is in question. It should be reserved for patients who have small inaccessible AVMs fed by numerous small arteries. The inoperability of these lesions suitable for proton beam therapy should be determined by a neurosurgeon with extensive operative experience.

In deciding whether an AVM is operable with acceptable mortality or morbidity, one should consider the following:

1. *Age of the patient.* Patients over 55 years of age do not tolerate major AVM surgery as well as younger individuals.
2. *Location of the AVM.* Those that are located deep within the diencephalic region, brain stem, or basal ganglion region are generally inoperable regardless of their size. The problem here is that adequate exposure cannot be obtained without violating essential cerebral tissue.
3. *Size of the AVM.* A large extensive AVM that encompasses a number of lobes, perhaps close to a whole hemisphere, is generally considered inoperable. It appears in these cases that the theory of displacement of function based on the fact that these lesions are congenital is no longer tenable under such circumstances. Ordinarily,

AVMs appear to displace functioning cerebral tissue to their margins and contain little viable neural tissue. Because of this it is theoretically possible to remove an AVM from any region and not produce a permanent neurological deficit. This is contingent on excellent exposure of the AVM and experience that permits the surgeon to work close to the margin of the lesion without violating it.

Between cases meeting the foregoing criteria and the very small discrete malformations located in polar regions of the brain, which are easy to remove, lies a group of cases in which a decision can only be based on a broad surgical experience. It is now possible, in many of the cases, to equate the features of an AVM with those of patients previously treated surgically, and therefore to give the patient a more realistic appraisal of the risks of the surgery.

The overall treatment plan often involves more than surgery, and here we must consider modification of the AVM by embolization in order to make it easier to resect. At The Neurological Institute, we prefer to use Silastic pellet embolization. The primary purpose of this embolization is to attain the following:

1. Reduce the size and blood flow of the malformation while eliminating a number of major feeding arteries.
2. Occlude deep relatively inaccessible arteries that feed the apical parts of the AVM. Such arteries include the lenticulostriate arteries and branches or main divisions of the posterior cerebral arteries.
3. Gradually reduce the major artery-to-vein shunts within the malformation so that the final removal does not create an intolerable load for the vasculature of the adjacent normal brain. This refers to the theory of perfusion-pressure breakthrough, which is akin to congestive heart failure when a large systemic AV shunt is suddenly obliterated.
4. To occlude, in a step-wise fashion, major arteries that not only nourish the AVM, but pass through it to supply the normal surrounding brain. We have not used this in the management of acute hemorrhage from an AVM.

In determining the usefulness of embolization as a preoperative adjuvant to accomplish the aforementioned objectives, one must evaluate the anatomy of the vascular system to determine the following points: (1) the ratio between the feeding arteries and the arteries that nourish normal brain, which, for the AVM to attract emboli, should be 3 to 1 or greater, and (2) the anatomic contour of the vessels supplying the AVM. Generally a smooth course from the parent vessels, whether it be the internal carotid or the vertebral artery, is necessary to ensure that the pellets will go directly to the malformation and not lodge in normal cerebral arteries. This presumes that the angulation of the arterial tree supplying the malformation is marked by smooth contours. It is now possible, by means of specialized balloon catheters placed at critical junction points of normal vessels, to redirect emboli into arteries that arise at acute angles from the parent artery.

At our Institution, Hilal has used this technique in embolizing the more difficult malformations, especially to occlude deep branches that supply the apical portion of the malformation. With these considerations in mind and comparing them with a broad experience, it is now possible to recommend, in certain selected cases, the use of embolization, and certainly the smaller malformations, which are located at polar regions of the brain or at the end of a tortuous arterial supply, are not ideal for embolization.

If the AVMs have been embolized prior to surgery, some of the emboli back up proximally into the feeding arteries. It is not necessary to remove these at the time of resection of the malformation. Generally, most of the pellets are removed along with the AVM, but the patient should be cautioned that some residual pellets may be seen on postoperative skull films.

In cases in which embolization is not expected to be effective in making a lesion operable or in which the lesion appears to be inoperable from the start, I have used embolization as the only treatment. In these cases it is extremely difficult to obliterate the entire malformation, but marked reductions of 70 to 80 percent in the size of the malformation and the feeding vessels can be accomplished by this technique alone. Embolization is relatively safe, with approximately a 1 to 2 percent incidence of serious complications, and when surgical obliteration is impossible, it may be the only reasonable form of treatment. I have recommended it to patients with the qualification that we have no statistical evidence at the present time to indicate that it will protect the patient against future hemorrhage, reduce the incidence of seizures, or improve progressive neurological deficits. However, in a relatively short 10- to 15-year follow-up, it would appear that the incidence of recidivous hemorrhage has been lessened and that headaches and seizures as a manifestation of the AVM have been reduced. I still consider the greatest usefulness of embolization to lie in its ability to prepare malformations for surgery and to make the task of the neurosurgeon easier.

When considering surgery, personal statistics should be considered. Cumulative experience with a large number of these difficult and uncommon lesions has convinced me that the results of surgery are proportionate to the surgeon's experience. In treating almost 200 patients with AVMs of the brain, 135 were operated on, and of these, 129 patients had total removal of their AVMs. Five patients underwent two operations for a total of 140 operations. In the six cases of partial obliteration of the malformation, partial obliteration was unintentional in only one. In the other cases, because of the magnitude of the malformation, in conjunction with embolization only ligation of major arterial feeders was carried out. I am still following these patients to determine whether this form of treatment can be recommended for others. The cases in which total surgical resection of the malformation was carried out represent a broad spectrum of malformations located in all areas of the brain, including the cerebellum, brain stem, caudate nucleus, and the various lobes, both superficial and deep. There were two deaths, representing a 1.4 percent mor-

tality. In terms of morbidity, I consider it significant if it includes hemiparesis, hemisensory loss, aphasia, or mutism. These complications were noted in 12 patients or 9 percent. In all but one of these patients, the deficits were noted. Hemianopsia in varying degree was seen in 12 percent of the cases and was related to those lesions resected from the visual cortex or radiations. It was difficult to avoid some degree of hemianopsia when the lesions were located in the aforementioned areas. Fortunately, the visual defect, whether to the left or the right, partial or complete, was not felt to be a disabling complication by any of these patients after a period of approximately 3 months of adjustment. The malformations of the cerebral hemispheres were located in or encroached upon motor, sensory, and speech areas. The cases were selected for operation by aforementioned criteria, and whether or not the malformation was located in an eloquent area of the brain was not necessarily a determinant of its operability. The results appear to support the contention that an AVM, being congenital, displaces cerebral function to its margins, and if the malformation can be exposed and dealt with at the time of surgery, it can be removed from almost any region of the brain.

The surgery of AVMs of the brain entails long tedious operations which require the use of the operating microscope in most instances and specialized surgical instrumentation and anesthesia. Hypotension is frequently used during the removal of the deeper portions of the malformation, and care must be taken that hemorrhage, especially uncontrollable hemorrhage, does not occur from the malformation during the operation. The patients are prepared for surgery with loading doses of anticonvulsants and corticosteroids. The management prior to surgical incision includes spinal drainage in order to maximize brain relaxation; wild swings of blood pressure during the induction of anesthesia are avoided by the use of appropriate antihypertensive agents and an open airway, and excellent oxygenation must be ensured by the anesthesiologist. The patient's head is positioned so that the malformation will be above cardiac level and, whenever possible, will be easy to expose because of the parallel position of its surface to the floor. In this manner, the surgeon is able to approach the malformation at a perpendicular, ensuring that the margins of the malformation may be separated from the normal brain as the cortical relationships are developed, and the arteries that feed the malformation over the surface of the cortex or deep in the sulci may be identified and divided. It is important to have stereoscopic angiograms available during the operation. Some of the more treacherous areas of the malformation are in the deep white matter, especially in the region of the ependyma, where large draining veins course through the ependyma and may be difficult to control, leading to serious intraventricular hemorrhage. Many of the deeper malformations or those that extend deep from the surface are related to the choroid plexus of the lateral ventricle. This must be anticipated from the preoperative angiogram and every possible measure taken to prevent hemorrhage from this area.

Special note should be made regarding surgery of

three groups of AVMs. The first are those malformations which are located intrinsic to deep structures such as the basal ganglion thalamus or brain stem; second those located in the posterior fossa and third, those located on the medial aspect of the cerebral hemispheres - often intimate to the limbic system.

Small discrete malformations that are located in the deep diencephalic or basal ganglion regions, if they reach the surface, such as the sylvian fissure in relation to the lenticulostriate arteries or the ependyma in relation to the choroidal arteries, may be resectable, depending on their size and blood supply. Some malformations located in relation to the brain stem may be accessible on the surface of the stem or via the fourth ventricle. If exposure can be gained to these malformations, it is possible to remove them. Much information can be obtained in terms of resectability by stereoscopic angiograms of these special cases.

Malformations that are located in the posterior fossa, in my experience, occur in an older age group. They are associated with hemorrhage to a slightly greater extent than those malformations located in the hemispheres. They are often related to a specific distribution of the three major cerebellar arteries, or in some cases they may receive blood supply from all three. These are some of the most difficult malformations with which to deal because of the problem in gaining adequate exposure, especially of the larger ones, and the threat of brain stem injury as the malformation encroaches on the fourth ventricle or brain stem. Indirect brain stem injury can result from interruption and retrograde thrombosis of some of the major arteries supplying these malformations.

Malformations located on the medial aspect of the hemisphere are unique in that they are more difficult to expose than those located on the convexity. The surgeon often attains the surface of the malformation with a tangential view, making definition of the anatomy more difficult. With experience, one can operate on these and obtain excellent results. However, one must consider potential injury, either by hemorrhagic onset or by surgery, to portions of the limbic system. We have found in three cases of left-sided malformations, located in proximity to the posterior caudate nucleus, fornix, and portions of the corpus callosum that a recent memory deficit was a prominent part of the clinical syndrome both after hemorrhage and after surgery. The same phenomenon has not been observed in similar cases in which the malformation was on the right side. Different surgical approaches are used for malformations located in different portions of the medial aspect of the hemispheres. In general, the malformations which are most difficult to deal with on the medial aspect are those located medial to the trigone of the lateral ventricle. These may be approached interhemispherically, adjacent to the parietal lobe, under the temporal lobe along the tentorium, or transcortically through the temporoparietal junction.

The results of surgery on these three unique groups of malformations have been gratifying and comparable to those of the series as a whole.

The postoperative management of these patients is unique and requires special expertise. The two catastrophic phenomena that are most likely to occur in the postoperative period are recurring seizures and hemorrhage into the area of resection. Everything is done to prevent postoperative seizures including: (1) loading of the patient with a standard anticonvulsant; if the patient has been on Dilantin previously we give a booster dose; and (2) addition of phenobarbital during the operation and immediately postoperatively. In spite of these measures, because of the sensitivity of the cortex and potential for a spreading cortical vein thrombosis in the postoperative period, some patients undergo focal status or have recurring seizures. It is necessary to control these immediately by intravenous injection of anticonvulsants. I prefer to use phenobarbital, titrating it to stop the seizures. To avoid hemorrhage into the area of resection, the blood pressure is always returned to normal or above normal level while the area of resection is inspected at the termination of the operation. Hemostatic agents must also be utilized about the cavity. Close monitoring of the blood pressure while the patient is being extubated and transported to the recovery room, as well as 24-hours afterward, is mandatory. If there is a hint of hypertension, antihypertensive agents given intravenously are instituted immediately. The worst thing that can happen is brief but severe hypertension associated with extubation of the patient or the transfer of the patient from the operating room to the ICU. Therefore, intra-arterial pressure monitoring must be continued until the patient is secure. Even though immediate postoperative seizures and postoperative hemorrhages are significant complications and have had serious import, early control of these situations often prevents serious permanent complications. Seizures, when controlled early, do not lead to permanent deficits. If they are the manifestation of a postoperative hemorrhage, one must deal directly with the hemorrhage. The larger hemorrhages must be evacuated immediately and a search made for any residual malformation that may be the cause of a postoperative hemorrhage. It may be necessary, in serious cases, to keep the patient relatively hypotensive for 48 to 72 hours after one of these events.

In all cases except one, I have performed postoperative arteriography to ensure complete obliteration of the malformation, if that was the goal of the operation, and also to observe dynamic changes that appear in the arteries that previously supplied the AVM.

The management of AVMs of the spinal cord is based on different factors than the management of intracranial AVMs. These lesions become apparent at a somewhat later age and therefore we have not been so stringent about age guidelines. Although embolization using liquid embolic material has been successful in some cases of spinal AVMs, it is not so important in the preparation of the lesion for surgical resection. These lesions are "slow-flow" as compared to cranial malformations. They are frequently located on the dorsal pial surface of the cord, where their whole extent may be visualized. Those that are obscure and intramedullary, with which I have experience, are also slow-flow, and it is virtually impossible to embolize these without interrupting the arteries that feed normal portions of the spinal cord. Therefore, I do not rely extensively on preoperative embolization when I am contemplating surgery of a malformation of the spinal cord. More important in the preoperative evaluation is some indication as to the location of the malformation. Generally, AVMs of the spinal cord can be divided in four major anatomic groups: (1) the long extensive dorsal malformation composed of coils of arterialized veins which receive their blood supply from numerous small radicular arteries; (2) the dorsal nidus malformation, which is located over a limited portion of the spinal cord fed by one or two major arterial feeders and associated with a number of arterialized draining veins; (3) the malformations that permeate all aspects of the spinal cord and have sometimes been labeled the "juvenile type", for which there are no surgical possibilities, and (4) a group of AVMs, primarily of the nidus type, which are located partially or wholly intramedullary and are often associated with the mass effect of a concomitant venous aneurysm.

Information as to the configuration of these malformations is therefore critical. Unfortunately, spinal angiography has not attained the degree of clarity and sophistication that one sees with cerebral arteriography in dealing with AVMs. Paradoxically, a myelogram may be more helpful in locating the position of the malformation, its extent, and the presence of associated globular defects indicating venous aneurysms. At present, I use both myelography and selective spinal angiography in the preoperative evaluation of these lesions. However, I do subscribe to the philosophy that the exact location, extent, and nature of the malformation cannot be determined without surgical exploration. Therefore, in all cases of AVMs of the spinal cord, I have advised surgical exploration to include laminectomy over the entire area of the malformation, as identified on the myelogram.

It has been presumed, and this is supported by surgical experience, that these malformations are separable from the normal or critical circulation of the spinal cord. Therefore, at the time of surgery, when exposure is adequate, the malformation may be removed from the dorsal portion of the spinal cord using the operation microscope and microdissection. Microsurgical techniques are utilized, interrupting and dividing the feeding arteries while the involved arterialized veins are peeled away from the dorsal surface of the spinal cord, leaving intact the circulation to the normal spinal cord. Using these techniques, malformations involving extensive areas of the spinal cord can be removed in single or multistage operations.

The lesions that are intramedullary and fed by perforating branches of the anterior spinal artery may also be removed by the techniques of intramedullary spinal cord surgery. The results have been most gratifying in these lesions, with greater improvement in neurological deficits than noticed in the dorsally situated AVMs.

Unlike surgery on their cerebral counterparts, this surgery is aimed at improving neurological deficits rather than preventing future hemorrhage. Since less than 10 percent of the spinal malformations have hemorrhage as the initial presentation, by operating and obliterating the lesion, we are not protecting the majority of patients from hemorrhage. Unfortunately, we have not obtained postoperative angiography in the majority of the cases because of the lack of detail and difficulty in performing this procedure. However, follow-up indicates that most of the patients have been stabilized. In the presence of intramedullary AVMs, especially those with large venous aneurysms (which is common), there has been remarkable improvement following removal of the lesion. However, one problem with these vascular malformations, especially with intramedullary ones, is a postoperative pain syndrome that is probably related to injury in the dorsal root entry zone. These pains may be focal, radicular in nature, or diffuse involving the entire body below the level of the lesion. The pain syndromes have been difficult to treat, but fortunately, with the passage of time, they appear to lessen in severity.

TRAUMA

MONITORING THE CRITICALLY ILL PATIENT

DANIEL F. HANLEY, M.D.
CECIL BOREL, M.D.

Neurosurgical intensive care has evolved from a need to localize special care skills that are appropriate for patients with severe neurological impairment. Special nursing care, frequent neurological assessment, advanced cardiopulmonary life support treatments, and specialized monitoring techniques for the neurosurgical patient all must be combined to attain the best possible recovery of neurological function. The frequent assessment of intracranial pressure (ICP), auditory evoked potentials, somatosensory evoked potentials, and the serial assessment of the neurological examination are the important variables that we follow in our neurological intensive care unit.

INTRACRANIAL PRESSURE MONITORING

Lateral ventricular catherization is the ICP monitoring modality of choice. This technique was developed by Lunberg. It allows access to the ventricular CSF for therapeutic withdrawal and produces a high-quality pressure recording. Intraventricular administration of antibiotics is also feasible. Disadvantages of this technique include the risk of infection particularly in the lateral ventricular space, occasional cerebral hemispheric hematomas related to the catheter placement, and the inability to use this technique when ventricular collapse or displacement is a significant problem. The lateral ventricular catheter is placed through a posterior frontal bur hole. We use a site anterior to the coronal suture approximately 3 cm from the midline. The catheter is passed and directed centrally toward a point midway between the outer canthus of the eye and the external auditory meatus and medially toward the inner canthus of the ipsilateral eye. The lateral ventricle is usually cannulated with 6 cm or less of catheter. Entry into the ventricular space is confirmed when CSF returns through the catheter. We usually tunnel the catheter about 5 cm beneath the galea to emerge from a separate scalp inci-

sion. This seems to reduce the risk of infection. Nondistensible tubing is connected from the catheter to a pressure transducer. With a three-way stopcock, we connect a sterile bile bag to the system by means of nondistensible tubing. This serves as a reservoir to collect CSF when ventricular drainage is used as a therapeutic modality. The height of this reservoir can be varied depending on the clinical condition of the patient. It is usually set at 15 to 20 cm above the auditory meatus. A sampling port is often added to the system to facilitate collection of CSF for chemical and microbiologic testing. We administer prophylactic nafcillin intravenously for the duration of the intraventricular monitoring. Careful attention to sterile technique is important. The wound site is treated with topical antibiotic ointment and frequent dressing changes. The connecting tubing is changed every 48 hours under gown-and-glove conditions. The risk of contamination probably increases with duration of catheterization; for this reason we attempt to remove the catheters as soon as possible, preferably within 5 days. However, when required by the patient's condition, they can be maintained for a longer period of time with the appropriate care and surveillance.

Subarachnoid Screw

The subarachnoid screw is well suited for situations in which the ventricular anatomy is significantly altered. This method is quickly used in emergency situations and has the advantage of not directly communicating with the brain parenchyma and the ventricular spaces. Serious infectious complications occur less frequently than with the intraventricular catheter. The screw is particularly well suited for monitoring patients with closed head injury. Disadvantages include the inability to aspirate significant amounts of CSF through the screw. The CSF pressure wave derived from the screw is occasionally damped, particularly at high intracranial pressures. Under these conditions, quantitation of intracranial pressure is not so accurate as with the intraventricular drain.

The screw is inserted through a skin incision made in the frontal area, usually 3 cm anterior to the coronal suture in the midpupillary line. A quarter-inch bur hole is made in the frontal bone with a hand-held twist drill. Bone fragments and debris are removed from this hole, and the screw is advanced through the bone until it penetrates the intracranial space approximately 3 mm. The dura is widely incised or repeatedly punctured with a small-gauge needle through the bolt opening. In this way, the bolt provides a continuous fluid connection between the subarachnoid space and the attached fluid-filled pressure tubing. The tubing and transducer are similar to those previously described.

Clinical Indications for ICP Monitoring

Elevated ICP is often associated with central nervous system damage. The degree of ICP elevation is similarly associated with the severity of damage. The effective treatment of intracranial hypertension correlates with good clinical outcomes for three different illnesses: closed head injury, acute noncommunicating hydrocephalus, and Reye's syndrome. For each of these illnesses the earliest indication of physiologic abnormality should be accompanied by ICP monitoring and aggressive intervention aimed at maintaining a normal ICP (less than 15 mmHg). Another group of illnesses are those that are sometimes associated with ICP abnormalities: cerebral hemorrhage, cardiac arrest, near drowning, meningitis, encephalitis, and cerebral mass lesions such as abscess or tumor. The degree of the ICP abnormality in these illnesses does not seem to relate as directly to the severity of illness and the likelihood of successful clinical outcome. For patients with these diagnoses, we choose to monitor and/or treat ICP when the clinical course suggests a possible benefit, specifically if the patient has a progressive neurological disability and signs of intracranial hypertension. For such patients the type, intensity, and duration of therapies can often be simplified by intracranial pressure monitoring. This is particularly true of illnesses in which the risk of dehydration, diuresis, and corticosteroid effects might outweigh the benefits. Monitoring provides the needed measurements of ICP that allow the clinician to decide how vigorously to treat intracranial hypertension and to balance these treatments with their systemic effects on the cardiovascular, renal, and gastrointestinal systems. Monitoring ICP is helpful in predicting impaired cerebral perfusion and in defining shifts of intracranial contents. We look carefully at the wave form of ICP induced by pulsatile and tone blood flow, the trend of pressure values, and the (absolute) mean intracranial pressure. Normal CSF pulse pressures range from 1 to 2 mmHg for subarachnoid screws. This pulse pressure is usually 1 to 5 mmHg with the intraventricular drain. As ICP rises the CSF pulse pressure also rises, reflecting compromised intracranial capacitance. An increase in the size of the pulse pressure is often an early indication of rapidly rising ICP or so-called "plateau waves". The trend of ICP measurements is perhaps the best indication of the underlying state of the patient. With subarachnoid screws, when the absolute value of ICP may be underestimated, a rising or falling trend is particularly important. Similarly, in patients with temporal lobe mass lesions, a progressive trend of small increases in ICP may signal incipient uncal

herniation. These mass lesions are eccentrically placed and often produce pressure gradients capable of shifting intracranial contents, but do not always elevate the absolute intracranial pressure above 15 mmHg. The absolute value of the ICP is the most commonly followed measurement (normal 5 to 10 mmHg). Sustained elevations over 15 mmHg can be considered abnormal. For acute closed head injury patients, the degree of elevation of intracranial pressure correlates with likelihood of meaningful recovery. In this group of patients undergoing aggressive therapy for elevated ICP, persistent elevation of this pressure above 60 mmHg is associated with exceptionally high mortality. When the ICP can be maintained between 40 and 20 mmHg, there is approximately 50 percent mortality. With effective ICP control (less than 20 mmHg), mortality is approximately 20 percent. For head trauma in particular, but also for other causes of elevated ICP, we use a calculated cerebral perfusion pressure (CPP) to follow the effects of treatment. CPP can be calculated by subtracting the mean ICP from the mean arterial pressure. Physiologic studies of cerebral circulation suggest that the regulation of the cerebral blood occurs effectively until a calculated CPP of 40 to 60 mmHg is reached. However, this picture is greatly influenced by the effects of disease on brain vessels: as both head trauma and ischemia are known to be accompanied by decreased cerebral vascular response. For this reason, we ask that our treatments maintain a CPP greater than 60 mmHg. We frequently add either pressor agents or supplemental fluids when the treatment for intracranial pressure lowers mean arterial pressure and adversely affects the CPP. Intracranial pressure monitoring is always incomplete without an independent assessment of neurological function. It is only by integrating the data derived from ICP monitoring with the physical examination and the natural history of the patient's illness that diagnostic and therapeutic decisions are made (Table 1).

PHYSICAL EXAMINATION

For the critically ill neurosurgical patient, a physical examination of neurological function is an important monitoring technique. The usual clinical examination has to be adapted for the intensive care unit setting, the patient's condition, and the confounding influences of anesthetics and sedatives. We believe that a short examination assessing the level of consciousness and the motor system gives the examiner the most accurate picture of neurologic function, particularly if it is repeated frequently. We placed the greatest emphasis on the trend of several examinations rather than on the location of any lesion that might be postulated from a single examination. This examination is best performed at least once a day at a time when all physicians and nurses caring for the patient can be present. By doing this, we eliminate much confusion about the actual findings and find that communication is improved by focusing on specific areas of concern.

TABLE 1 Clinical Use of ICP Monitoring by Diagnostic Category

	Monitor		Treatment		
	When	What	Mode	Until	Goals
Head Trauma	Glasgow Coma Scale < 7	ICP (screw); MAP; ABG; neuro exam	P_{CO_2}; barbiturates; dehydration	$P_{CO_2} \le 25$; burst suppression; serum osm ≤ 320	ICP < 15; CPP > 60
Reyes syndrome	Lethargy (Stage II to III)	ICP (screw); MAP; ABG; glucose	P_{CO_2}; mannitol; barbiturates	$P_{CO_2} < 25$; serum osm ≤ 320; serum glucose 300 mg/dl	JCP < 15; consciousness
Acute hydrocephalus	Ventricular dilation; obtundation; intraventricular blood clot	ICP (drain); MAP; CT	P_{CO_2}; remove CSF	$P_{CO_2} < 25$; CPP > 60	ICP < 15; normal ventricles; consciousness
Focal mass lesions Abcess Tumors Herpes encephalitis Hemorrhage	Incipient uncal herniation	ICP (drain); MAP; LOC; Pupils; CT	P_{CO_2}; steroids; dehydration; remove CSF; barbiturates	$P_{CO_2} < 25$; clinical response; serum osm ≤ 325; ICP stable and < 10; burst suppression	ICP; free parasellar cisterns; resolved mass
Sagittal sinus occlusion	Lethargy; focal deficits	ICP (drain); MAP; ABGs; Coagulation; Angio	P_{CO_2}; barbiturates; hydration; anticoagulants	$P_{CO_2} < 25$; burst suppression; Hct 25 to 30; normal platelet count	ICP < 30; patent sinus

ICP = intracranial pressure; MAP = mean arterial pressure; ABG = arterial blood gases; CT = computerized tomography; CPP = cerebral perfusion pressure; LOC = Level of consciousness

We start our examination by assessing the level of consciousness. Patients who do not respond to voice or deep pain are said to be unresponsive; they then undergo an assessment of brain stem reflexes and are rated with the Glasgow Coma Scale (Table 2). Pupillary size and reaction to light are recorded, and the vestibulo-ocular reflex and the corneal response are examined closely. The absence of these reflexes suggests either primary brain stem dysfunction or a secondary process leading to brain stem dysfunction such as any of the herniation syndromes. The Glasgow Coma Scale is particularly useful for these patients and for those who are stuporous but arousable. This scale allows a uniform rating of eye opening, verbal response, and motor responses to either command or pain. For patients who are stuporous but arousable, examination of cognitive, visual, and somatosensory functions is not possible. Instead we concentrate on evaluating the motor system. This group of patients are those who localize pain well to an extremity and are capable of obeying simple motor commands. For this group the highest level of performance can often be defined by the evaluation of more complicated movements. Resting position of extremities should be evaluated and observed closely for external rotation of the leg, finger flexion with thumb adduction in the hand, and/or flattening of the nasolabial fold. Examination for the presence or absence of pronator drift (arms abducted anteriorly with palms supine), dorsiflexion drift (ankle dorsiflexed at 0° of hip internal rotation), and fine motor movement of the fingers and oral musculature provides for a thorough assessment of motor performance. When examining for fine motor coordination, we concentrate on sequential finger opposition with the thumb as well as

rapid tapping of the index finger against the interphalangeal joint of the thumb. Grimace, lip pursing, and rapid side-to-side motion of the tongue should be noted in the evaluation of oral musculature. Because of the large cortical representation of these oral and hand-related tasks, they are particularly sensitive to mild degrees of focal brain impairment. These tests can be performed rapidly with only a minimal amount of the patient's cooperation. They rarely provoke pain in the postoperative setting, and do not require the patient to be moved when this might be contraindicated. No matter what the level of consciousness, the neurological examination should always be focused toward the area of greatest known pathologic involvement. This is most easily done on the alert patient, in whom language function, memory, visual fields, and somatosensory function can also be assessed. Even though we try to perform a small number of bedside tests in as unfiorm a manner as possible, significant small variations occur in the results of these examinations. For this reason, we put greatest emphasis on changes of status that occur at the extremes of performance. Improvements above the best previously noted performance should be carefully noted. Such changes in status often require the use of other diagnostic assessments such as CT scanning or angiography and occasionally require operative intervention. The best and worst levels of neurological performance are reviewed daily by all physicians and nursing staff caring for any given patient. For patients in deep coma, for those who have had drug overdoses, and for those whose therapy requires large doses of sedatives or anesthetics, the neurological examination frequently is not helpful. In these situations, we rely on electrophysical monitoring.

TABLE 2   Glasgow Coma Scale

	Notation
Eyes open	
Spontaneously	4
To sound	3
To pain	2
Not at all	1
Verbal response	
Oriented	5
Confused conversation	4
Inappropriate words	3
Incomprehensible sounds	2
None	1
Best motor response	
Obey commands	6
Localize pain	5
Normal withdrawal	4
Abnormal flexion	3
Extend	2
None	1
	15

ELECTROPHYSICAL MONITORING

The auditory and somatosensory evoked responses provide a specific assessment of central nervous system integrity for patients who cannot reliably be monitored with physical examination because of the presence of barbiturates, anesthetic agents, or neuromuscular blockade. Useful information is derived from comparing the latencies and amplitude of a patient's potential with those of normal individuals and by following the trend of changes in latency and amplitude while the patient is in the intensive care unit. Either failure to transmit electrical potential past a specific electrode or an increased latency at a specific electrode indicates functional injury to neural tissues. Normal values for amplitude and latency must be established for each laboratory or intensive care unit and preferably for each patient during a period of relative normal function. However, even without such information, trended evoked potential data correlate well with local pathologic conditions.

Auditory Evoked Response

The brain stem auditory evoked response (BAER) is derived from the sequential activation of the peripheral and central auditory pathways. Repeated clicks are delivered to an ear piece in one ear while the contralateral ear does not receive these clicks, but rather is masked with "white noise". The clicks are delivered at an intensity of about 60 to 70 decibels and a frequency of 10 Hz. Five positive peaks (depolarization) are commonly identified: these are produced by sequential stimulation of the auditory apparatus, cochlear nucleus, superior alive, lateral lemniscus, and inferior colliculus. The time measured from peak to peak is called the interpeak latency and is essentially unaffected by changes in either stimulus intensity or the peripheral apparatus that transduces auditory impulses into neuro-excitation. The auditory evoked response is relatively unaffected by large doses of barbiturate and thus serves well to monitor brain stem integrity during drug overdose or therapeutic barbiturate coma. Disappearance of wave 5 (inferior colliculus) has been observed with increased intracranial pressure and probably represents progressive central herniation. Changes in the interpeak latency from wave 1 to 5 have also been associated with brain stem ischemia or physical compression during operative positioning. Changes in wave 1 are seen under conditions of severe brain stem damage. In this situation the potentials derived from the peripheral auditory apparatus and the auditory nerve are frequently lost because of local ischemia. When wave 1 is not present, any inference about the integrity of the central nervous system pathways of audition cannot be made. However, in the opposite situation, in which there is progressive loss of waves 5, 4, 3, and 2 with preservation of wave 1, the BAER strongly suggests midbrain and pontine dysfunction. In our experience, this pattern correlates well with the clinical diagnosis of brain death.

Somatosensory Evoked Potential

Electrical depolarization of sensory nerves generates potentials which can be recorded not only along the peripheral course of these nerves, but at the cervical-medullary junction and over the scalp. Depolarization in this pathway occurs sequentially in either the median nerve or tibial nerve, the dorsal column nuclei and the cervical-medullary junction, and at the ventroposterior thalamus and its frontoparietal cortex. The stimulus intensity is adjusted to excite the largest myelinated fibers in the peripheral nerve. A stimulus rate of 5 Hz is used with electrodes placed over the scalp, the second cervical vertebra posteriorly, and either the contralateral brachial plexus or cauda equina, depending on the peripheral nerve stimulated. Since the absolute latency (time from stimulus to peak) is affected by limb temperature and peripheral neuropathy, interwave latencies are best described. This is done by subtracting the scalp and cervical latency from either the brachial plexus or cauda equina latency. If dorsal column nucleus stimulation can be identified, but depolarization of the contralateral sensory cortex cannot be identified, then a lesion causing conduction blockade between the lower medulla and the cortex must exist. The potentials measured by stimulating these sensory pathways cross a larger portion of the cerebral hemisphere than those measured in the BAER. For this reason, the somatosensory evoked potential is particularly sensitive to local hemispheric mass lesions and vascular events. We follow the trend of both latency and amplitude of these potentials. The absence of a scalp potential correlates closely with severe hemispheric damage and can be noted in brain-dead individuals. The cervical potentials are often preserved when the clinical diagnosis of brain death is made. In our experience, a trend showing prolongation and absence of the scalp potential when there is serious hemispheric dysfunction and other evidence of probable herniation is almost always associated with a poor outcome.

Currently available technology offers a dynamic insight into the management of the critically ill neurosurgical patient. Each of the modalities described here fulfills criteria for accurate assessment of a portion of brain function. When these techniques are used together, a more complete picture of brain function and response to therapy can be obtained. We believe that the application of appropriate monitoring techniques improves therapy and outcome in the critically ill neurosurgical patient.

CLOSED HEAD INJURY: MANAGEMENT DILEMMAS

CHARLES J. WROBEL, M.D.
LAWRENCE F. MARSHALL, M.D.

The basic pathophysiologic mechanisms at work in head injury, and the therapeutic options available, are now well known to most physicians engaged in trauma care. Prompt identification of mass lesions and control of increased intracranial pressure represent the standard of care in most centers, although techniques employed may differ. Obtaining the optimum "yield" of patients with good functional recovery further requires aggressive attention to subtle phenomena and seemingly trivial details. This chapter reviews the diagnosis and management of head injury as practiced at the University of California San Diego Medical Center, with particular emphasis on recent observations and changes in our thinking.

DIAGNOSIS AND EARLY MANAGEMENT DECISIONS

Decision making is fairly straightforward in trauma victims with Glasgow Coma Scores (GCS) below 9, with or without injuries to other organ systems. It must be assumed that all such patients have suffered a severe head injury, physical appearances notwithstanding. Following initial resuscitative efforts, a noncontrast CT scan of the head is obtained. If the scan demonstrates a surgical lesion, the patient is taken immediately to the operating room. In patients without a surgical lesion, a frontal ventriculostomy is usually placed within one hour of admission. A Richmond bolt is used when (1) the ventricles are so small that they cannot be cannulated (less than 10% of cases); (2) the patient has an initial normal CT scan, without compression of the basal cisterns or lateral ventricles; and (3) the patient has not suffered hypoxia, hypercapnia, or multiple trauma along with the head injury.

A few patients arrive in extremis and require immediate operative intervention for extracranial injuries. These patients are vulnerable to neurological catastrophe from a mass lesion or uncontrolled intracranial hypertension. Where there is no time for a CT scan, an air ventriculogram can be easily obtained through the ventriculostomy and offers diagnostic information as to the extent of midline shift. In patients where the shift exceeds 5 mm, a craniotomy is performed because the overwhelming majority of these patients will have a surgical mass.

Patients suffering moderate head injury, which is defined as a Glasgow Coma Scale score of 9 to 12, usually require a CT scan. It should be performed with more urgency if the patient has focal neurological deficit or has deteriorated. Intracranial pressure monitoring usually is not necessary in patients with moderate injuries, unless the CT scan demonstrates evidence of compression or absence of the basal cisterns, or there is some shift of the midline. The following CT findings presage elevated ICP: compressed basal cisterns, slit-like or asymmetric lateral ventricles, multiple small white matter hemorrhages suggesting a major shearing injury, and hemorrhagic contusions, particularly in the context of established diffuse intravascular coagulation or hypothermia and its attendant disturbance of coagulation. Clinically, hypoxia, hypercarbia, or shock occurring early in the trauma victim's course can be associated with serious ICP elevations days later, even in patients whose ICP is normal during the first 24 hours after injury.

Patients with minor head injury (GCS 13 to 15) constitute the majority of neurotrauma cases in most centers. Essentially, the problem is to detect a low probability event, epidural hematoma, in a heterogenous population. The presence of a skull fracture increases the chances of a mass lesion significantly, and for this reason plain skull films are obtained. A CT scan follows for patient with significant nonvertex skull fractures. Patients manifesting focal deficits (aphasia, motor weakness) clearly need a CT scan, but such cases are unusual. A normal scan performed shortly after injury can be falsely reassuring. Certain clinical signs such as tachypnea, episodic bradycardia, and restlessness are ominous irrespective of earlier neurodiagnostic findings (or lack thereof) and should be pursued.

OPERATIVE INDICATIONS

Extra-axial hematomas (subdural or epidural) associated with a midline shift of 5 mm or more must be rapidly evacuated. The size of some hematomas can be underestimated owing to the partial volume effect inherent in CT scanning; these "small" collections with disproportionate shift constitute no less an emergency.

The hematoma found at craniotomy is usually larger than expected. Bilateral balancing lesions or hematomas with minor degrees of shift should be evacuated if the basal cisterns are compressed or if there are other factors conducive to later increases in ICP. Cerebral contusions smaller than 30 ml are not primarily debrided, with the notable exception of contusions bracketing the sphenoid wing, i.e., posterior, frontal, and temporal tip. These lesions are tracherous by virtue of location rather than sheer bulk. As these contusions swell, the vector of forces is largely directed mesially, and we have seen several patients herniate despite genuinely low ICP measured by ventriculostomy.

MEDICAL MANAGEMENT OF INTRACRANIAL HYPERTENSION

Therapy directed at controlling ICP begins ideally at the accident scene. In San Diego County in recent years we have witnessed a decline in the incidence of uncontrolled ICP (above 40 mm Hg) which, is probably explained by the development of a rapid-response Emergency Medical System. Field neuroresuscitation of the patient with severe head injury includes endotracheal intubation and controlled hyperventilation, prophylactic anticonvulsants, and mannitol, 1 g/kg, provided the patient is not in shock. Further in-hospital therapy is outlined as follows:

1. Head up 30 degrees and in neutral position.
2. Hyperventilation to $PaCO_2$ of 25 to 30 torr.
3. Maintain PaO_2 above 80 torr.
4. Maintain adequate sedation (morphine) and muscle relaxation (Pavulon).
5. Maintain systolic arterial pressure between 100 and 160 mm Hg.
6. Normothermia.
7. Maintain hematocrit above 35.
8. Prophylactic anticonvulsants.
9. Maintain fluid balance with 0.5 normal saline.

Long-term, hour-to-hour ICP management is largely a matter of attention to details. Monitoring system integrity is assessed routinely. Gentle jugular venous compression should elevate ICP modestly in healthier patients and dramatically when autoregulation is deranged.

The neurosurgeon's greatest concern is that a sudden upward change in ICP is secondary to a delayed intracranial hematoma, which reflects brain swelling directly related to the intracranial injury or secondary to changes in pulmonary function. The mechanism underlying these sudden changes is not entirely clear, but in some patients this relationship is so tight that the ICP monitor can almost be used as a mechanism to detect inapparent pulmonary problems. Since arterial blood gas analysis is seldom obtained more often than every 2 to 4 hours, substantial intervals of hypoxia or hypercarbia would otherwise go undetected.

The osmotic diuretic mannitol is a mainstay of ICP management. In the intensive care unit setting usually we reserve mannitol for patients where ventricular drainage no longer reduces the ICP to less than 20 mmHg. Mannitol must be given in adequate doses, and in general, doses of less than 0.25 g/kg are not effective. In some patients up to 600 g mannitol per day may be required to control elevated intracranial pressure. As long as the serum osmolarity can be maintained below 330 m Osm, we have not found a deleterious effect from this management scheme.

PREDICTING INTRACRANIAL PRESSURE TRENDS

Abnormal ventricles and/or hypotension on admission are associated with future ICP elevations. The highest ICP during the first 24 hospital hours is predictive of future elevations in ICP. The presence of a large area of hemorrhagic contusion at the time of first CT scan and the development of pulmonary failure will increase the likelihood that prolonged therapy for elevated ICP will be required. Low intracranial compliance is also a bad sign. Some centers test intracranial compliance by intraventricular saline challenge, but we have found simple bedside observation of the ICP waveform just as useful. The development of a steep and wide pulse pressure waveform which resembles the arterial trace indicates low compliance in patients who are at significant risk for precipitous rises in ICP. Such patients tolerate adverse events, such as inappropriate head position, very poorly.

BARBITURATE COMA

In the early 1970s, high-dose barbiturate therapy was demonstrated to be effective in treating intracranial hypertension that occurred during elective neurosurgical procedures. This treatment modality soon found wider application, and our group has published two clinical series describing its use in severe head injury. Although barbiturate therapy is clearly effective in many patients whose intracranial hypertension is refractory to conventional therapy, its overall impact on outcome is not yet well defined. To this end, we and others are now participating in a randomized controlled clinical trial on a nationwide scale. Patients with ICP elevations who meet certain pressure criteria, who have received maximal conventional therapy as previously described, and who have no untreated surgical mass lesions are randomized either to barbiturate therapy or to further conservative therapy. ICP is considered uncontrolled by conventional means if ICP is 25 mmHg for 30 minutes, 30 for 15 minutes, or 40 for 1 minute; or for patients who have undergone decompressive surgery if ICP is 15 mmHg for 15 minutes, 20 for 10 minutes, or 30 for 5 minutes. Patients are randomized to barbiturates or to a continuation of conventional therapy if they meet these criteria. As of this time, outcome data are not available, but it is apparent that early concerns about the complications of the use of high doses of barbiturates appeared to be unfounded. The incidence of pulmonary failure, for example, was just as severe in patients suffering severe head injury who were treated conservatively as in those who had received high doses of barbiturates. Systemic hypotension, which appears to be related primarily to poor cardiac filling pressures from progressive mannitol dehydration rather than from barbiturates, also occurred as commonly in patients randomized to nonbarbiturate therapy.

The rapid removal of surgical mass lesions, coupled with meticulous detail in the medical management of the airway and of ICP should mitigate the deleterious response of the brain to secondary insults and poor cerebral perfusion.

HEAD INJURY IN THE CHILD

BENJAMIN S. CARSON, M.D.

The unbounded curiosity and energy of children unfortunately places them in a number of precarious positions daily. Small children seem to have a particular affinity for moving objects, whether large or small, so that head injury is a common problem in children. Many children seen in emergency rooms as accident victims have multiple system trauma. In nearly one-third of such children, craniocerebral cerebral injuries constitute their most significant problem.

MANAGEMENT OF SPECIFIC LESIONS

Concussion

The diagnosis of "concussion" should be made in a situation in which trauma has resulted in a brief loss of consciousness from which the patient makes a total recovery and has a normal neurological examination. In addition, in the older child or the adult, a history of retrograde amnesia can usually be obtained. In the immediate postconcussive period, the patient frequently complains of headache, dizziness, nausea or vomiting, and sometimes lethargy. Usually these symptoms resolve quickly and permanently. It is not unusual for some patients to subsequently develop the same symptoms days and sometimes even weeks later. They can also develop visual blurring, photophobia, weakness, and/or personality disturbances. Extensive work-ups, including skull films, CT scans, metabolic screening, and lumbar puncture, usually are not fruitful, but probably should be undertaken once if symptoms persist for more than a few weeks after the trauma. If there is any evidence of focal disturbance, the patient should be admitted to the hospital and intensively investigated at once.

The emergency room or office management of children who have sustained a concussion depends on the physician's index of suspicion concerning the degree of cerebral trauma. If a loss of consciousness has extended beyond 5 minutes or if, for some other reason, the examiner suspects a skull fracture, skull films should be obtained. If a fracture is demonstrated overlying a venous sinus or the middle meningeal artery, consideration must be given to inpatient observation for a period of 24 hours. If no fracture is revealed in a child who is otherwise neurologically normal, one can feel free to discharge such a patient to the care of responsible guardians, with a pre-printed form explaining concussion in layman's terms and indicating danger signs that should be brought to the immediate attention of a physician. It is neither wise nor correct to prognosticate about the significance of the concussion on the child's neurological or intellectual future because, although the overwhelming majority of patients have no further sequelae, reports of long-term complications have been made. In cases of serious recurrent vomiting, clearly the patient should be admitted to the hospital for intravenous fluid administration.

Cerebral Contusion

Cerebral contusion, like concussion, also causes loss of consciousness which may be transient or prolonged. Unlike concussion, however, contusion causes actual disruption of cerebral tissue to varying degrees. Frequent accompaniments are parenchymal hemorrhage and focal edema, which can generalize to involve an entire hemisphere and, eventually, the entire brain, producing "malignant cerebral edema", for which children seem to have a particular proclivity.

Focal neurological deficits localizing themselves to one or both cerebral hemispheres and/or to portions of the brain stem are usually present. A variety of patterns can be found on CT scanning in these patients. The most common pattern manifests multiple small hemorrhages surrounded by varying degrees of edema. These lesions can be found virtually anywhere within the cranium, but tend to be most frequent along the basal anterior frontal lobes, the temporal lobes, and the occipital lobes in a "coup-contracoup" distribution. The important thing to remember about patients with cerebral contusions is that, owing to the disruption of cerebral tissue, local alterations of blood-brain barrier and autoregulatory functions are likely to occur. This can eventually result in significant increases in intracranial pressure caused by ischemia and edema. Compression of the adjacent normal cerebral tissue causes extension of the abnormality. One must be particularly cautious of this extension of the lesion when the contusion has occurred in the temporal lobes since significant progression could result in uncal herniation.

The management of patients with cerebral contusions depends on whether they are conscious or unconscious. Patients in both categories should be admitted to the hospital. However, the conscious patient requires only mild fluid restriction and careful observation until the neurosurgeon is satisfied that his condition is stable. It must be kept in mind that the maximal manifestation of edema caused by cerebral contusion can sometimes occur as late as 7 days after the trauma and that the phenomenon of delayed intracerebral hemorrhage can occur in these patients. This usually happens 36 to 72 hours after the trauma, but can occur even 1 to 2 weeks later. The unconscious patient or the patient who is deteriorating must be treated aggressively to maximize chances of recovery. These patients should be in the intensive care unit and, if unable to respond to commands, should be mechanically ventilated. In addition, it is imperative that their intracranial pressure be monitored on a continuous basis. Once again, the method of intracranial pressure monitoring should depend on the equipment available to the neurosurgeon and his expertise in the management of this device. Therapeutic maneuvers aimed at controlling intracranial pressure should progress logically from head elevation to radical resection of brain, depending on the effect of the last modality used to control ICP. Before embarking on many therapeutic maneuvers to control the intracranial pressure, one must ascertain that cardiovascular monitoring is accurate. The intracranial pressure monitoring device should be placed on the same side as the lesion, and one should be able to affect the pressure reading by changing the head position or by compressing the internal jugular veins transiently. An arterial line should be in place for continuous blood pressure monitoring and frequent arterial blood gas determinations. A method of central venous pressure monitoring should be established. In addition, any metabolic abnormalities should be addressed quickly. Respiratory acidosis or alkalosis can result from inappropriate respirator settings. When hyperventilation is being used as a method of controlling intracranial pressure, care should be taken not to depress the carbon dioxide tension below 25 mmHg. While the CO_2 tension is dropping, attention must be paid to the pH as well, which should not be allowed to rise beyond 7.55 since the resultant electrolyte disturbances might precipitate seizure activity. Seizure activity can also be precipitated by severe hyponatremia resulting from the syndrome of inappropriate antidiuretic hormone secretion (SIADH). Both SIADH and diabetes insipidus can result from traumatic neuroendocrinologic disturbances and can manifest themselves in the acute or late phases of craniocerebral trauma. Their management in the traumatic setting is virtually the same as their management in

the postoperative setting. It should be kept in mind that diabetes insipidus seen in the traumatic setting is associated with hypothalamic dysfunction secondary to progressive rostrocaudal herniation. In addition to treating the underlying cause of the dysfunction, it is important to begin immediate control of massive diuresis. This can be achieved with a continuous intravenous Pitressin drip. If blood gases, serum electrolytes, glucose metabolism, and serum and urinary osmolality can be maintained within normal range, the physician gains a significant advantage in his attempts to control intracranial pressure.

The use of steroids in the treatment of massive head injury remains a controversial issue. Certainly in the case of pediatric head injury with the demonstrable CT scan evidence of hemorrhagic contusions, there is much agreement that steroids are appropriate since the surrounding progressive edema is vasogenic in origin. If steroids are used, an intravenous loading dose should be given early in the course of treatment, followed by regular 6-hourly maintenance doses, according to the patient's size. There is no hard evidence that administration of antacids when steroids are used is beneficial in preventing gastric ulceration. However, whenever the possibility of emesis and aspiration exists, it is wise to try to maintain gastric pH in a neutral range. Both loop diuretic and osmotic diuretics have a role in the control of intracranial pressure, when all the aforementioned steps have been tried successfully. However, their use must be accompanied by diligent monitoring of serum electrolytes and osmolality.

If, in addition to the aforementioned modalities, the patient is normothermic and is not convulsing, and continues to manifest a rising intracranial pressure, one must seriously consider operative intervention. If a focal area of hemorrhagic contusion can be identified in a nonvital area of the brain, resection of this area can frequently be undertaken with no extension in neurological deficits. The goal of resection is to provide room for viable brain tissue by sacrificing tissue of doubtful viability. After resection, if surrounding brain tissue immediately fills the cavity and no cerebral pulsations can be observed, it is likely that either an inadequate amount has been resected or there has been a complete loss of cerebral autoregulation. In either case, if further resection can be carried out safely, it should be done immediately. In addition, at this point it is often wise to divide the falx anteriorly in order to more evenly distribute the intracranial pressure. No attempt should be made to close the original dura, but rather a generous dural graft should be placed. It is probably wise to leave out the bone flap to provide additional room and to provide an easily accessible means of monitoring cerebral pulsations and tension. Finally, if all else fails, pentobarbital coma can be induced. Before proceeding with full pentobarbital coma, one should probably observe the effect of a few periodic treatments with thiopental. If no improvement is observed with thiopental or if there is a paradoxical reaction producing increased intracranial pressure, it is unlikely that pentobarbital coma will be useful. Pentobarbital is by no means a benign treatment and should be employed only in patients with uncontrolled intracranial pressure who have some neurological function. Such patients should clearly have a means of cardiac output monitoring since many require pressors in order to sustain adequate cardiac output and systemic blood pressure.

Cerebral contusion is a serious lesion and can produce progressive neurological dysfunction. This lesion is as serious as an acute epidural hematoma or acute subdural hematoma, and indeed frequently accompanies these lesions.

Skull Fractures

Simple Linear Fractures

The vast majority of skull fractures are linear in nature and may assume a variety of patterns: single fractures, stellate fractures, circular fractures, diastatic fractures, or multiple nontransecting fractures. The significance of these lesions depends largely on their location on the skull. If they overlie a major branch of the middle meningeal artery or a venous sinus, the potential for underlying bleeding is magnified, and such patients should probably be admitted to the hospital for a period of observation. When these fractures do not overlie such structures, but the physician is uncomfortable with the child's home situation, level of consciousness, or other neurological manifestations, he is perfectly justified in admitting such a patient for observation. Sometimes it is difficult to determine whether a line on the skull film represents a fracture or a vascular marking. This problem tends to dissipate as the examiner becomes more experienced in reading skull roentgenograms. However, when doubt exists two clues can be helpful: the presence of an overlying scalp hematoma and tenderness to palpation over the area of concern are confirmatory signs of a fracture. In the case of a simple linear fracture in which there was no significant loss of consciousness, if the patient is intact neurologically with no symptoms and has a reliable family, the patient should be sent home with a printed list of signs and symptoms to which the guardian should be alert.

The potential for the development of a "growing fracture of childhood" or "leptomeningeal cyst" must be recognized with any fracture, particularly if it extends into a suture line. Whether such a lesion should be explored depends on the feasibility of careful follow-up by a physician who recognizes the development of this entity.

Nondepressed Compound Skull Fractures

The same principles of treatment that apply to simple linear skull fractures also apply to these fractures, except for the additional problem of a potential communication into the central nervous system from the outside environment. The laceration must be meticulously cleaned after adequate local anesthesia is adminis-

tered, and the underlying skull should be palpated. If there is no depression, the scalp should be closed after copious irrigation, in such a way that both the galeal layer and the skin are well approximated, but not strangulated. Although the scalp has a rich vascular supply, making infection less likely, the potential for CNS infection is considerable in such cases. Therefore, the patient should be admitted to the hospital for at least 48 to 72 hours of observation and given appropriate antibiotics for a length of time commensurate with the examining physician's index of suspicion for infection. Such patients should be seen weekly on an outpatient basis for 3 or 4 weeks to rule out any late complications, and the patient should be seen once again after a couple of months to rule out the possibility of osteomyelitis.

Depressed Skull Fractures

All skull fractures in which a depression of bone fragment which is equal to or greater than the full thickness of the skull has occurred must be operatively explored and debrided. If these fractures are compound, the risk of meningitis or local infection is high, and the urgency to the exploration and debridement increases significantly and probably should be done within 12 hours. In addition, appropriate antibiotics should be given intravenously immediately, and the wound should be assessed as soon as possible by someone experienced in asessing craniocerebral trauma. It is important that no attempt be made to remove bone fragments outside the operating room, since they frequently act as tamponade against potentially serious underlying bleeding. During operative management of the lesion, the surgeon should have available a complete set of skull films or a CT scan, which will guide him to the most effective scalp opening and craniectomy for dealing with the underlying lesion. After the wound is carefully irrigated and the patient has been properly shaved and prepped for surgery, the scalp should be opened in such a way as to provide maximum exposure of the depressed fracture. It is usually necessary to place a bur hole adjacent to the depressed area and perform a controlled craniectomy around the involved bone. When the depression occurs over a venous sinus or over the distribution of the middle meningeal artery, it is imperative that a controlled craniectomy, starting away from the depressed segment, be carried out to ensure adequate exposure of the underlying dura and/or brain, before trying to unwedge the depressed fragments. If this is not done and the depressed bone fragment is forcefully extracted before adequate exposure has been achieved, massive bleeding may make subsequent backtracking to achieve such exposure much more difficult. When the wound is compound and there is gross evidence of contamination, it is probably unwise to replace bone fragments. However, if the wound is simple or not grossly contaminated, these can frequently be replaced with good results and little chance of infection. If the periosteum is intact over the depressed fragments in a compound wound, it is usually possible to reuse the bone fragments in reconstruction of the skull, even in a grossly contaminated wound, provided adequate debridement of the external wound has been achieved. Such patients should receive continuous antibiotic coverage for at least a week postoperatively. In the case of a simple depressed skull fracture in which bone fragments cannot be reutilized, the surgeon can proceed immediately with a cranioplasty.

In addition to the more traditional types of depressed skull fractures, the pliable nature of an infant's skull makes it susceptible to the so-called ping-pong fracture. This is a rounded depression that occurs in the skull and looks very much like the depression that occurs in a ping-pong ball when one forcibly pushes his thumb into it. When the infant is otherwise neurologically normal, and this lesion does not overlie a particularly epileptogenic region of the brain, it is not important that the fracture be elevated immediately. However, if such lesions do not revert to a normal state after a couple of weeks, it is wise to elevate them since the depression can increase with skull maturation. The elevation is a simple procedure that requires a small craniectomy next to the depression and passage of an instrument, such as a Penfield elevator, into the epidural space beneath the depression, followed by a prying motion until the normal contour of the skull has been restored. It should be remembered that the principal reason for repair of significantly depressed skull fractures of all types is not to achieve a cosmetic result, although is is important, but rather to prevent future development of seizures or infection.

Basilar Skull Fracture

Basilar skull fractures are common, but not necessarily serious. They should be suspected in patients who have sustained head trauma and present with periorbital and/or lid ecchymoses without a history of direct orbital trauma, CSF rhinorrhea or otorrhea, acute loss of smell, acute loss of hearing in one or both ears, Battle's sign, hematympanum, or laceration of the external auditory canal without a history of direct trauma to the ear. Since a significant amount of force is necessary to crack the skull base, all such patients should be admitted for observation. Occasionally a patient with a basilar skull fracture, particularly when CSF rhinorrhea or otorrhea is present, develops meningitis. For this reason, some people place patients with basilar skull fractures on antibiotic coverage routinely. This is a reasonable practice, at least until the leakage is controlled. In addition, antibiotics should be given if pneumocephalus is noted on skull film or CT scan, since there is clearly a basal skull aperture permitting the entrance of air into the cranium. When there is evidence of compromise of the functions of the seventh and/or eighth cranial nerve in patients with basilar skull fracture, the otolaryngologist should be notified early in the course of treatment. If there is clinical evidence of a basilar fracture, radiographic evidence is not crucial. It is difficult to detect most such fractures with plain skull films, CT scanning being much more sensitive.

Epidural Hematoma

Because the dura is tightly adherent to the inner table of the skull, particularly at the suture lines in infants and young children, epidural hematomas are relatively rare in this group. In children under the age of one year, one must be suspicious of this lesion or any other expanding intracranial lesion when the initial post-trauma assessment reveals widened sutures and/or a tense fontanelle. This lesion need not always be associated with a skull fracture, although when such a fracture is present it usually overlies a major segment of the middle meningeal artery or a venous sinus.

The degree of trauma necessary to create such a lesion varies markedly, and sometimes there is not even a loss of consciousness initially. The classic "lucid interval" only occurs in approximately 50% of cases, and the interval usually is not completely lucid since there are residual complaints of headache or dizziness or lethargy. Unfortunately, the vast majority of these lesions occur in the temporal region, producing medial displacement of the temporal lobe with eventual transtentorial uncal herniation if the process is not arrested in time. The patient who manifests a progressive downhill course with gradual loss of consciousness, focal motor weakness, and possible pupillary changes along with other signs of increased intracranial pressure should be intubated and hyperventilated at once. In this situation, it is appropriate to do anything possible to decrease the rising intracranial pressure. This includes the administration of mannitol, usually in a bolus of 0.5 to 1 gram per kilogram. The effect of the mannitol should be documented in terms of the patient's neurological status. If there is a transient improvement, the chances of achieving a good surgical result with removal of an epidural hematoma are enhanced. It is not appropriate to wait for long periods if a CT scan cannot be obtained immediately on these patients. Instead, they should be taken directly to the operating room and a bur hole should be placed over the area of the suspected hematoma. If skull films have been obtained, this area usually corresponds to the area where the fracture crosses the middle meningeal artery. If no fracture is present, the bur hole should be placed on the side ipsilateral to the affected pupil or contralateral to the side of hemiparesis. If pupillary changes and hemiparesis are on the same side, the pupillary changes are the more reliable sign 90 percent of the time.

Placement of a bur hole over the clot is really more a diagnostic than a therapeutic maneuver since a great deal of the clot will have reached a currant jelly consistency by the time exploration takes place. This means that a craniectomy or craniotomy has to be performed in order to remove the clot and in order to gain visualization of the bleeding vessel and control it. There is usually no indication to open the dura if the underlying brain remains relatively relaxed after the clot has been removed. If, on the other hand, there is much tension beneath the dura after removal of the clot, an intradural exploration should be undertaken at once with removal of any blood clot or any severely damaged brain tissue. In addition, if a CT scan has not been obtained, one has to consider the possibility of a contralateral clot and seriously consider exploration of the contralateral side. Once the hematoma is adequately evacuated, it is imperative that the dura be stitched to bone or to temporalis muscle to prevent reaccumulation of the blood clot. Drainage of the epidural space through a catheter usually is not a reliable method of preventing accumulation of the blood clot.

Quick and effective action in the diagnosis and treatment of epidural hematomas in children usually results in a relatively good outcome, with less than a 30 percent mortality rate. This lesion should therefore always be ruled out in any case of craniocerebral trauma.

Acute Subdural Hematoma

Acute subdural hematomas in childhood are associated with a high morbidity and mortality rate. This is secondary to the fact that the lesion is usually caused by disruption of a cortical artery or large bridging vein, which requires a tremendous amount of force. In addition, there is frequently associated severe contusion of underlying brain. The combination of these two potentially lethal processes acts synergistically to usually produce an undesirable outcome. As in the case of epidural hemorrhage, a skull fracture need not be present and in fact is less frequently present, as might be expected, since skull fractures serve as a means of dispersion of energy. It is the lack of dispersion of disruptive energy that results in both the disruption of surface blood vessels and the cerebral contusion.

The downhill course is rapid and progressive and usually requires immediate action. If time permits, an emergency CT scan should be obtained since severe underlying parenchymal brain damage may make localization of disease based on neurological signs difficult. The administration of mannitol is a useful adjunct that may provide enough time to obtain a CT scan prior to operative intervention. Ventricular drainage is seldom helpful for supratentorial rapidly expanding mass lesions since the CSF is usually displaced from them already. In the case of expanding mass lesions of the posterior fossa, however, ventricular drainage can provide dramatic transient relief if the fourth ventricular flow has been obstructed. However, it must be kept in mind that when pressure in the posterior fossa vastly exceeds supratentorial pressure, as might be the case after ventricular drainage in such a situation, the possibility of upward herniation of the brain stem does exist.

The most effective treatment is rapid craniectomy with dural opening and extraction of the clot followed by control of any bleeding sources. Severely contused brain in nonvital areas must also be considered for resection since this tissue invariably eventually results in massive edema. The dura should be closed or patched in such a way as to prevent sharp dural edges from lacerating the swelling brain. If the bone flap is not left out, a method should be established for constant monitoring of intracranial pressure and the patient should subsequently be treated in the same way as a patient with a severe cerebral contusion.

The clinical picture at the time of arrival in the emergency room has considerable bearing on the eventual prognosis even if the lesion is rapidly diagnosed and treated. However, regardless of the patient's clinical condition at the time of emergency room evaluation, it is important to realize that the eventual outcome is potentially devastating, and an optimistic picture should never be painted during the course of early therapy.

In the case of infants with subdural hematoma, it is sometimes possible to perform a subdural tap through the coronal suture and remove enough blood to alleviate symptoms. A subdural tap set should be kept in the emergency room for this purpose. More commonly, however, in the acute situation, such taps only buy time, and a more definitive procedure becomes necessary.

Intracerebral Hematoma

The occurrence in young children of traumatic intracerebral hematomas is rare, except in the case of penetrating injuries to the brain. Today, most such hematomas are discovered by CT scanning. When the hematoma is causing significant mass effect and is surgically accessible, it should be removed. Traumatic intracerebral hematomas are usually associated with surrounding contusion of the brain. Their treatment frequently is identical to that for hemorrhagic intracerebral contusion.

In the case of a penetrating injury to the brain, if the foreign object is still present at the time of initial assessment, it should not be removed until a CT scan has been obtained and the patient is in the operating room with the neurosurgeon since the penetrating object often acts as a tamponade against bleeding. All such wounds must be explored and dural integrity ensured. It usually is not appropriate to simply extract the foreign object and treat with antibiotics.

The advent of CT-guided stereotactic aspiration technology in recent years provides the neurosurgeon with yet another weapon to combat deep-seated intracerebral clots that are producing mass effect. When this technique is employed, the neurosurgeon must be prepared to spend a number of hours irrigating the aspiration cavity in case fresh bleeding is encouraged by the procedure.

Birth Trauma

Although birth trauma is a frequent cause of pediatric craniocerebral damage, it is a large and complex topic that deserves a separate discussion, and therefore will not be addressed in this chapter.

CLOSED HEAD INJURY

JOHN D. WARD, M.D.

Head injury is a common emergency. In 1976, there were 1,255,000 severe head injuries including concussion, skull fracture, intracranial hematoma, cerebral laceration, and cerebral contusion. Damage to the brain is present in 75 percent of fatal accidents; in 80 percent of multiple-injury patients, the head is injured. Proper and detailed care of the head-injured patient is demanding but can improve the prognosis significantly, even in patients with very severe injuries. If these patients are to receive optimal treatment, the persons charged with their initial care should be skilled in the evaluation and management of head injury. Although there are many grades of head injury, the focus here is on the more severe types. Several concepts are fundamental to the care of head-injury patients: (1) every effort should be made to protect the brain from ischemia and hypoxia that may result in further damage; (2) accurate diagnosis and rapid removal of mass lesion are mandatory once the patient has arrived at the hospital; and (3) good intensive monitoring and care are vital.

The rationale for treatment follows from the pathophysiology of head injury. Brain injury can be classified as primary, that which occurs on impact, and secondary, that which occurs as a result of some insult subsequent to the original trauma. The main primary injuries to the brain are contusions, lacerations, shearing injuries, hemorrhage, and swelling. Contusions occur typically over the frontal and temporal poles of the brain, regardless of the cranial site of impact. Brain lacerations occur with or without associated fractures and are usually located in the central areas adjacent to the floor of the anterior and middle fossae, corpus callosum, and pontomedullary junction. Shearing injuries occur at the time of impact after sudden, angular rotation of the skull. Hemorrhage can range from small intracerebral collections to large intra- or extracerebral clots that cause deterioration by mass effect on the brain. Swelling occurs around areas of contusion or throughout large areas of white matter.

Secondary damage results from physiologic insults to an already damaged brain, and includes hypoxia, ischemia, and mechanical distortion. Hypoxia is seen in at least 30 percent of severely injured patients on arrival at the hospital; hypotension, which also can further injure the brain, is seen in approximately 15 percent. Adequate perfusion can take place in a properly autoregulated brain even with a significant drop in arterial blood pressure, but in a patient with impaired autoregulation from brain injury, perfusion may be totally dependent on systemic blood pressure. If the blood pressure drops, there is no mechanism to maintain perfusion, and a secondary ischemic insult can develop.

Brain shifts and distortions occur when there is an enlarging mass lesion or swelling. These lead to a rise in intracranial pressure (ICP), resulting in ischemia and a shift in brain structures that causes tearing and compression of vascular and neural structures. Although the brain is of obvious importance, primary injury is difficult to treat once it has occurred. It is in the prevention and treatment of hypoxia, ischemia, and mechanical distortion that the physician can play a role in the care of head injury.

EVALUATION

The initial evaluation of the patient is straightforward. All patients seen in the emergency room have their vital signs stabilized. If the patient is unable to follow commands, a central venous line and a Foley catheter are inserted. The patient is promptly intubated if comatose, usually after being paralyzed with pancuronium. It is preferable that this be done by an anesthesia team if one is available; if not, someone accomplished in smooth endotracheal intubation is required. It is imperative that the patient be paralyzed during this maneuver to prevent coughing, bucking, and unnecessary delay that might aggravate brain damage if a mass lesion is present. Furthermore, it is important that this be done smoothly and quickly to avoid hypoxia. If the patient has extensive facial injuries that preclude intubation, tracheostomy is warranted. Having established an adequate airway and good IV access, a blood sample is obtained for type and crossmatch, CBC, electrolytes, coagulation studies, and blood gas analysis. A urinalysis is also performed. Fluid, blood, and blood products are given as indicated to maintain normal blood pressure. There is no indication for fluid restriction in these patients; hypotension further aggravates brain damage. During resuscitation, a cross-table lateral cervical spine x-ray is done to rule out a cervical spinal injury. If this is normal, a chest film is obtained, as well as other requisite films. The indications for skull films are discussed below.

A brief but adequate neurological examination is done. The neurologic examination should answer the following questions: What is the extent of neural damage? Does the patient have a mass lesion? Is the patient getting worse, better, or staying the same? The examination consists of determining the patient's response to pain; checking for eye opening, verbalization, and pupillary, oculocephalic, and oculocaloric response and assessing the motor power of each side. This examination is usually carried out prior to the administration of paralyzing drugs and intubation. Stabilization of the airway, however, should not be postponed.

Once the patient's respiratory and cardiovascular status has been stabilized and the neurological examination completed, the next step is a prompt evaluation for the presence of a mass lesion. A CT scan is the procedure of choice. I routinely call in the CT personnel as soon as it is evident that the patient is neurologically damaged. This way, the patient can be taken to the CT-scan center as soon as his vital signs are stabilized.

The use of skull films is controversial. I obtain skull films if there is an open wound to the scalp, the possibility of any type of fracture or of an intracranial foreign body or penetrating wound, or significant soft-tissue injury. I do not postpone the CT scan, however, to get skull films; the CT scan can be utilized to look at the cranial vault. If CT scanning facilities are not available, ventriculography or angiography can be employed, although these procedures are inferior to the CT scan.

Whether and which medications and fluids to administer depend upon the patient's condition and the extent of damage. In mild head injury, no medications are given. For the patient with a severe head injury, the role of Decadron is controversial. If given, it should be administered in equivalent doses of 10 to 20 mg IV initially, then 4 to 6 mg IV every 4 to 6 hours. Anticonvulsants, usually phenytoin or phenobarbital, are also administered to those patients with significant neurological deficit. If there is any question as to the presence of a mass lesion prior to CT scanning or if the patient's neurologic status worsens, 20 percent mannitol is administered rapidly in doses of 1–2 g/kg. Fluid management of the patient consists of the use of crystalloid, usually normal saline or Ringer's lactate, in quantities sufficient to maintain normal blood pressure. Blood and blood products are also administered as needed.

After the CT scan is obtained and if a decision is made that surgery is needed, mannitol is given, the hyperventilation initially started in the emergency room is continued, and the patient is promptly taken to surgery. If no surgical mass is present, the patient is moved to the intensive care unit for proper care, management, and monitoring.

Multiple Injuries

In treating patients with multiple injuries, cooperation should exist among surgical services. If the patient has a life-threatening abdominal or thoracic injury and cannot be stabilized, immediate surgical intervention is indicated and the patient is taken directly to the operating room prior to any neurological studies. Exploratory burr holes or ventriculography is performed if one thinks that an intracranial mass lesion may be present. If in the presence of systemic injuries the patient can be stabilized, a CT scan should be obtained prior to other surgical procedures. Again, it should be emphasized that there should be good cooperation among those caring for the patient's various injuries.

MONITORING

Adequate monitoring is essential in the patient with a severe head injury. I routinely monitor arterial blood pressure via an arterial catheter for the first 24 to 48 hours. Ischemia must be prevented. Therefore any significant hypotension (blood pressure <90 mmHg) should be treated vigorously. Arterial monitoring provides a prompt warning if such hypotension should occur. Arterial blood gas samples, as well as materials for frequent analysis of electrolytes, osmolality, BUN, and glucose, can also be drawn via the arterial catheter.

Perhaps the most important aspect of monitoring of the head-injured patient is ICP monitoring. I routinely insert an ICP monitor in all patients who have severe head injuries, that is, all patients who are unable to obey commands. I do this because there is a significant risk (30–70%) of intracranial hypertension depending on the type and extent of head injuries. I employ a ventricular catheter under most circumstances. However, if the ventricles are small and cannot be cannulated, I use a subarachnoid bolt (screw).

I try to maintain the ICP between 20 and 25 mmHg. Any elevations above this are treated; at the same time, investigations as to possible causes are carried out. Elevated intracranial pressure is treated sequentially as follows. The patient is hyperventilated to a PCO_2 of 25 mmHg with a volume ventilator at volumes of 12 to 15 cc/kg. Sedation with morphine (1–2 mg/hr) or paralysis with pancuronium is also used as needed. After an initial loading dose of pancuronium of 0.1 mg/kg, often only 1 to 2 mg per hour are required to keep the patient adequately phased into the ventilator. End-tidal CO_2 monitoring is done via a capnometer, which permits immediate assessment of the adequacy of hyperventilation. If elevated ICP is still a problem, ventricular drainage is carried out as often as necessary. If ICP still cannot be controlled at desired levels, mannitol is administered in doses of 0.25 to 2 g/kg. The basic principle is to use as much as is needed and no more. Mannitol is given until serum osmolality exceeds 320 mm. If mannitol cannot control the ICP, barbiturates (either phenobarbital or pentobarbital) are used. I routinely use pentobarbital in doses of 5 to 10 mg/kg in a bolus of 50 to 100 mg up to blood levels of 35 to 45 mg percent. Care must be taken not to cause hypotension, which can be detrimental in the presence of an elevated ICP. Either a CVP line or a pulmonary artery catheter should be used so that an accurate assessment of vascular volume is available. Central venous or pulmonary capillary wedge pressure should be kept between 10 and 15 mmHg. I do not perform large, decompressive craniotomies routinely for control of intracranial hypertension.

Head injury increases nitrogen loss and seems to increase caloric expenditure. Head-injured patients have a correspondingly higher risk of becoming malnourished, which may result in an increased rate of infection and poor wound healing.

In general, if the patient with only a head injury has not had a laparotomy, bowel sounds should be audible within 48 to 72 hours. When these are present, a small feeding tube can be placed and the patient started on enteral nutrition. Enteral feedings must be administered slowly and in small amounts to avoid diarrhea and volume overload. In addition, stomach contents should be aspirated periodically to ensure proper emptying. If the patient cannot take enteral feeding within 48 hours, hyperalimentation is begun.

Respiratory problems in the head-injured patient with elevated ICP may require the use of paralysis with hyperventilation. Small (1–2 mg) doses of morphine administered each hour just prior to suctioning may help to decrease afferent stimulation and may prevent secondary increases in ICP. Lidocaine also has been proposed for this.

High levels of positive end-expiratory pressure (PEEP) sometimes are required if significant atelectasis and shunting that cause severe hypoxemia occur. Although some authorities feel that PEEP levels of up to 20 cm H_2O have virtually no effect on ICP, this is not universally accepted. If high levels of PEEP are needed in patients with severe head injury, ICP should be closely monitored. Positive end-expiratory pressure should be applied gradually and should be discontinued as soon as a rise in ICP is noted. In addition, care must be exercised to ensure that PEEP not precipitate hypotension, which can further aggravate a head injury. Should hypotension occur, normovolemia must be restored. The patient who is being hyperventilated with PEEP should be allowed to resume normal respiration before ICP monitoring is discontinued. Hyperventilation should be discontinued slowly until CO_2 levels are at least normal; then PEEP should be discontinued slowly. If there is no subsequent rise in ICP, ICP monitoring can be discontinued.

LONG-TERM MANAGEMENT

Hydrocephalus

Ventricular dilatation is one problem that can occur after the acute phase of head injury. The dilatation is due either to atrophy secondary to loss of brain tissue or to communicating hydrocephalus. The distinction is important; the latter is treatable, and when it is treated the outcome may be more promising. Hydrocephalus usually occurs between two weeks and two months after the injury. It is usually accompanied either by a leveling off of neurologic recovery or by loss of previously restored function. The condition can be detected on CT scan; however, at times the distinction between hydrocephalus and atrophy is very difficult. Occasionally it is impossible to tell the difference, and

shunting may have to be carried out in the hope that improvement will occur. This is preferable to allowing a chance for further recovery to slip away.

Seizures

There is controversy concerning the use of prophylactic anticonvulsants in patients with severe head injury. I use them under the following circumstances; (1) when there is major neurologic deficit, (2) when there have been penetrating injuries to the brain, and (3) when there has been a seizure in the early post-traumatic period. The anticonvulsants are continued for two years. At the end of this period of time, an EEG is performed. If there is no indication of an active focus and the patient has not had a seizure, the medication is discontinued slowly.

Rehabilitation

I believe rehabilitation begins immediately after a head injury. Consequently physical and occupational therapy should be started as soon as possible. Care must be taken not to aggravate acute situations such as elevated ICP; however, active and passive range-of-motion exercises and proper pulmonary physiotherapy are important and are employed whenever possible. As the acute phase of the patient's illness recedes, the patient undergoes a more active and aggressive rehabilitative program that is gradually phased into a return to as normal a living situation as possible. I have noted, as have others, that these patients usually have profound neuropsychological abnormalities. Therefore it is important that objective neuropsychological testing be performed to define the extent of damage, to document progressive improvement, and to provide clues as to how patients can cope with a permanent deficit. It should be remembered that the patient's illness is not over once he leaves the hospital. Oftentimes, lengthy vocational and rehabilitative programs are necessary before the patient is able to resume anything resembling his normal activities. During the patient's illness his family should not be forgotten; they often require intensive counseling and encouragement.

SUBDURAL HEMATOMA IN THE ADULT

KEITH ARONYK, M.D., F.R.C.S. (C)
BRYCE WEIR, M.D.

Subdural hematomas are commonly encountered in adults and are generally best treated surgically. Collections of blood or blood-derived fluid easily open up the potential space between the arachnoid and the inner surface of the dura and cause compression of the underlying cerebral cortex with varying degrees of midline shift (subdural hematoma).

These subdural hematomas may accumulate rapidly in the absence of severe cerebral injury or may be associated with cerebral contusions and/or lacerations. Alone or in combination, they can lead to an acute rise in intracranial pressure. Subdural hematomas usually result from head trauma, and those that present within the first 48 hours are referred to as *acute subdural hematomas*, whereas those presenting between 2 and 14 days following injury are referred to as *subacute subdural hematomas*.

For various reasons, the collection of blood may not be clinically significant at the time of injury, but may slowly enlarge over time and present later as the cortex is compressed and brain shifted. If this delay measures at least 14 days from the inciting event, or if, as in many cases, no specific event can be remembered, this hematoma is referred to as a *chronic subdural hematoma*. These clearly represent two different situations, with the acute and subacute hematomas associated with relatively severe trauma and significant cerebral injury and the chronic subdural hematomas associated with minor or even no trauma and an insignificant cerebral injury. The great majority of subdural hematomas occur over the convexities of the cerebrum, although a very few in adults occur below the tentorium. The same general principles of accurate localization, adequate exposure, early drainage, and decompression using the simplest procedure apply to the management of all subdural hematomas.

ACUTE AND SUBACUTE SUBDURAL HEMATOMAS

These are more common than chronic subdural hematomas and usually represent an urgent management problem. Whether these occur secondary to head trauma or spontaneously (coagulopathy, meningeal tumor/inflammation, arachnoid cyst), the patient usually presents with a depressed level of consciousness and hemispheric localizing signs. Signs of rostral-caudal deterioration may rapidly supervene and require the urgent institution of medical means to control intracranial pressure. This almost always provides enough time to obtain a CT scan to define the nature of the intracranial lesion. Emergency "blind" bur holes should rarely, if ever, be required in an institution where a CT scanner is available.

Rapid control of intracranial pressure (ICP) is attempted by:

1. Early airway control established with a cuffed endotracheal tube and positive pressure ventilation with large minute volumes. This usually requires the use of a muscle relaxant (nondepolarizing) and intravenous sedation (ultra short-acting barbiturate).
2. Maintenance of a normal or slightly elevated blood pressure.
3. Diuretic therapy using a combination of an osmotic diuretic (mannitol) and a loop diuretic (furosemide).
4. Measures to ensure optimal cerebral venous drainage.

Before the patient leaves the emergency department, routine blood tests including arterial blood gases and a blood crossmatch are requested, and measures to correct specific problems such as coagulopathy are initiated.

The CT scan is the diagnostic procedure of choice and, in most cases, gives a rapid and unequivocal diagnosis of a subdural hematoma. In a few cases, the hematoma may have become isodense during its resolution, but associated changes in ventricular configuration and cortical sulcal pattern usually justify the use of intravenous contrast to increase the diagnostic yield.

Acute subdural hematomas require urgent surgical intervention since the time of compression is definitely inversely related to the overall prognosis. These patients are transported immediately to the operating room, where the light neuroleptanalgesia is continued and the patient is positioned supine with the head immobilized in a pin-fixation head rest. Using the CT scan as a guide, a large free bone flap is removed and the dura rapidly opened to provide decompression. In the setting of trauma, brain contusion hematomas are often noted in association with the subdural hematoma, and the craniotomy is fashioned in such a way that large intracerebral hematomas or areas of "pulped brain" can be removed. The hematoma is removed as completely as possible, and obvious sources of bleeding are controlled. Vigorous attempts are not made to locate bleeding sites in the parasagittal area and basal skull area since these can usually be better controlled by gentle pressure with hemostatic materials and/or bone wax. A small fluid-filled catheter is left beneath the dura to act as an ICP monitor, and the dura is closed using dural substitutes if necessary. The dura is not usually sutured to the bone edge in this setting. The bone flap then is replaced and wired securely before the scalp is closed in two layers.

In the neurosurgical intensive care unit, management is directed by serial neurological examinations, ICP measurements, and CT scans. ICP control is often a problem requiring continuation of medical means and, on occasion, institution of CSF drainage with an external ventricular drain. Ultra-short-acting barbiturates are used to avoid or treat acute rises in intracranial pressure, but barbiturate therapy for sustained increases in intracranial press has not been found to be of value in this setting.

These are major management problems, and the overall prognosis remains poor with a mortality rate ranging from 50 to 90 percent.

Subacute subdural hematomas are intermediate in severity as well as in time of presentation. They also usually occur in a setting of trauma and present as mass lesions with raised intracranial pressure requiring urgent surgical intervention. The surgical management is similar since formed clot is still usually present and a craniotomy is required for complete removal of the hematoma. However, this is the situation in which only one limb of the proposed incision is opened to initially place a single bur hole in the event that the hematoma has liquefied sufficiently to be drained completely. The postoperative course is much better in this group, and the overall mortality is lower at 20 to 25 percent.

CHRONIC SUBDURAL HEMATOMA

A collection of blood in the subdural space may not be large enough to cause symptoms or signs of brain compression or shift. This collection of blood incites a reaction in the overlying inner dural surface, which is normally a vascular membrane, but results in very little reaction in the much less vascular underlying arachnoid membrane. Cells and blood vessels from the inner dural surface begin to permeate the blood clot as it begins to resolve. If the clot is small, it is largely organized by the infiltrating granulation tissue, and the small amount of liquefied blood is absorbed by the neovascular membrane on the dural side. This results in conversion of the clot to a thin fibrotic layer, which is not clinically significant. The liquefying hematoma, however, is rich in fibrinolytic activity and can incite an inflammatory response from the already "leaky" neovascular membrane. The neovascular membrane may leak small amounts of blood and fluid into the hematoma cavity, but this is likely to be greatly intensified by the presence of the fluid itself. Recurrent hemorrhages within, and fluid loss across, the neovascular membrane may contribute to a gradual expansion of the hematoma over time. This then results in delayed compression of the underlying brain with late signs of raised intracranial pressure and hemispheric signs. The clinical presentation is not dramatic, and the underlying cause may not be immediately obvious. Head trauma can still be related to about half of chronic subdural hematomas, although factors that decrease brain volume (CSF shunting, atrophy) or the effectiveness of the coagulation cascade may be even more important in some. Other important etiologic considerations are alcoholism (poor nutritional state and hepatic coagulopathy), structural and vascular abnormalities of meningeal neoplasms or infections, arachnoid cysts, and elevated central venous pressure (chronic obstructive pulmonary disease with paroxysmal coughing). As the hematoma slowly enlarges, most adults complain of increasing headache and drowsiness associated with confusion and often nausea and vomiting. Examination usually reveals a depressed level of consciousness with defective higher mental functioning as well as at least a minor upper motor neuron motor deficit. There is no typical clinical picture, and often the diagnosis is made incidentally during a neurological work-up.

The most important diagnostic procedure again is the CT scan, and again the picture is virtually diagnostic. Radionuclide brain scanning is helpful if a CT scanner is not readily available.

Once an extra-axial mass lesion suggesting a chronic subdural hematoma is discovered, surgical evacuation should be considered. This is imperative in the presence of signs or symptoms suggesting raised intracranial pressure or cortical dysfunction. If the lesion is completely silent clinically and especially if it is bilateral, it may be related simply to a decrease in brain volume with fluid filling a widened subarachnoid space or passively filling a dilated subdural space. This situation usually does not require surgical drainage, but does require careful follow-up. In the presence of clinical signs or symptoms, the fluid should be evacuated and the brain decompressed. Since the fluid itself is thought to be a major factor in the persistence and growth of the hematoma, any surgical therapy must remove the fluid to allow the subdural membranes to gradually resolve by fibrosis. This may be achieved safely and effectively under local anesthesia at the bedside with a twist drill craniostomy and insertion of a subdural catheter (to gravity drainage). However, in this situation, a bur hole under general anesthesia is preferable since the dura is visualized and can be opened to allow limited inspection of the subdural membrane and subdural space. Under direct vision, a pliable, wide subdural drain (Jackson-Pratt) can be placed into the subdural space while fluid is still spontaneously draining. The suction drain is then brought out through a separate stab wound and sutured in place at this location. The subdural space is not flushed, and the brain is not artificially "inflated". The incision is then closed primarily with buried absorbable sutures and skin tapes, and the subdural drain is connected to gentle suction, which is maintained for 24 to 48 hours. Large collections of subdural air are avoided by placing the subdural drain in the subdural space quickly, while fluid is still spontaneously draining, and maintaining gentle suction for the prolonged period. No more than "thumb print" pressure should be used on the drainage bulb. The drain is removed within 48 hours, but unless recurrent symptoms or signs appear, a follow-up CT scan is usually not obtained for at least 10 days. If the hematomas are bilateral, they are drained simultaneously by means of the same technique. Intraoperative antibiotics are used on all cases and are continued until the subdural drain has been removed.

Many neurosurgeons achieve satisfactory results without the use of drains, but we believe that they produce a more rapid and dependable clinical improvement.

The outlook with this limited surgical approach is excellent since recurrence rates are very low (about 2%), and brain injury is not usually a factor. Mortality rates for chronic subdural hematomas are falling and are now probably below 5 percent.

Adult subdural hematomas behave as mass lesions which in most cases require surgical evacuation. A chronic subdural hematoma requires only a minor intervention to drain the fluid that is preventing the natural resolution of the hematoma, whereas an acute subdural hematoma requires major medical and surgical intervention to evacuate an expanding mass lesion and support an injured brain.

EPIDURAL HEMATOMA

HOWARD M. EISENBERG, M.D.

The epidural hematoma, an intracranial collection of blood superficial to the dura, almost always occurs as the result of a head injury, usually with skull fracture. The force precipitating the injury is generally of low velocity, as opposed to the high-velocity forces that produce diffuse white matter injury or the acute subdural hematoma. The most common cause, as with most head injuries in this country, is a motor vehicle accident. The significance of the distinction between high- and low-velocity forces is that the epidural hematoma is the one kind of severe head injury that is likely to occur without primary focal or diffuse brain injury, the reverse being true of the acute subdural hematoma. In most cases then, complete recovery is possible without persistent behavioral sequelae.

The clot is generally due to arterial bleeding, typically from a bony laceration of the middle meningeal artery. The primary injury is frequently a fracture of the squamous portion of the temporal bone, the bulk of the clot lying adjacent to the anterior temporal lobe. However, other locations are not uncommon. Epidural hematomas can occur frontally, occipitally, and in the posterior fossa. The vertex hematoma is frequently difficult to diagnose and can be missed on CT scan unless the higher views are carefully inspected. Venous bleeding is a less common cause of epidural hematoma than arterial bleeding, but may account for relatively more cases when the presentation is delayed 2 or more days after impact. In rare instances, epidural hematomas are found in patients in whom there is no history of trauma and in whom even careful inspection of the scalp and skull (at operation and by x-ray examination) reveals no evidence of a blow. The cause of bleeding in these rare cases is difficult to explain. Rupture of an occult dural arteriovenous malformation is a possible cause.

While epidural hematoma is relatively uncommon, accounting for less than 10 percent of the primary diagnoses in patients with severe head injury and perhaps less than 5 percent of patients with head injury admitted to a hospital, it is considered a topic of educational importance. Virtually all medical students have heard the familiar scenario: The victim who, after sustaining a blow to the head, immediately but briefly loses consciousness, recovers (the lucid interval), later lapses again into coma with a dilated pupil, and is then saved when the correct diagnosis is made with the aid of skull films, which show a temporal fracture traversing the groove of the middle meningeal artery, and an urgent operation is performed. This "classic" story, while not representative in detail of most cases, stresses the most important features which are the absence of an important primary brain injury, the risk of temporal lobe herniation, and the need for urgent treatment. In approximately 75 percent of the reported cases, there is little or no primary brain injury, and loss of consciousness at impact is frequently a transient event (concussion). Pupillary dilatation and secondary coma are generally the results of temporal lobe herniation with injury to the underlying third cranial nerve and secondary brain stem compression. However, the lucid interval occurs only in approximately 25 percent of cases, either because the primary injury is not severe enough to cause concussion or because secondary brain stem injury supervenes before resolution of concussion. Nonetheless, delayed alteration of consciousness after injury is an important indication of mass lesion. Dilatation of the pupil is also an important sign indicating deterioration and is reliable in aiding in lateralization of the mass. In some cases, the pupil may take on an ovoid appearance, like a football held horizontally, before actually dilating. Although the skull film is considered useful, in centers with CT scanners, the time required for this examination is generally not considered worthwhile, and patients are taken directly for CT scanning, whereby both the hematoma and the fracture, if present, can be seen. The CT scan is also important for detection of other concomitant lesions such as subdural hematomas, contusions, and intracerebral hematomas. The most important point regarding treatment, which cannot be emphasized enough, is the need for urgency. Virtually all patients who are awake immediately prior to operation survive, whereas patients in coma prior to operation are at considerably greater risk; their mortality in some large and carefully studied series is greater than 40 percent. Patients who are not in coma should have CT scans and operations carried out without delay and under continuous and careful observation. Patients who are already in coma require resuscitative measures prior to CT scan or operation. These include endotracheal intubation with hyperventilation, maintaining a high PaO_2, and a $PaCO_2$ below 30 torr, and IV mannitol, 1 to 2 g/kg. A Foley catheter is inserted in all patients who are given mannitol. Both hyperventilation and osmotic diuretics are potent measures for reducing increased intracranial pressure and retarding herniation. While there is the unknown risk that relaxation of the brain may reduce whatever tamponade effect is present, the risk is clearly worth taking since progressive brain stem compression can rapidly lead to irreverisble injury and death. When shock is present it should be attributed to some cause other than the head injury unless the patient is flaccid owing to advanced brain stem compression. Other injuries should be identified and the shock should be treated. If the systolic blood pressure is less than 90 mmHg, mannitol should be withheld. X-ray studies of the cervical spine are important to rule out unsuspected cervical dislocation before the patient is moved, but obtaining these studies should not cause a delay in diagnosis or therapy. Although CT scans are of obvious importance, there is a small percentage of patients in whom the diagnosis is reasonably certain and in whom operation is particularly urgent, for example, patients with a history of an obvious blow to the temporal region, a clear history of a lucid interval and later progressive coma and pupillary abnormalities. In these patients, operation without CT scan should be considered, averting even the small delay required for scanning.

OPERATIVE TECHNIQUE

When the hematoma is in the temporal region, the typical location, the operation consists of splitting the temporalis muscle just anterior to the ear and just above the zygoma. Bur holes are made in the underlying temporal squama and clot removed through these bur holes by suction. Even removal of small amounts of clot may be helpful in urgently reducing intracranial pressure. A craniotomy incorporating these bur holes is then extended to the floor of the temporal fossa. The remaining clot is then removed. The point of bleeding is sought, and this may require exposure of the foramen spinosum. This bleeding can be brisk and difficult to control, and the foramen may need to be packed with bone wax or other materials. In the older literature, packing the foramen with a sterile wooden matchstick was recommended when persistent bleeding was difficult to control. In all cases, there should be an effort to have blood available for transfusion, but the operation should not be delayed while typing and cross-matching are awaited.

It is important to decide whether the clot extends under the temporal lobe. This determination may be difficult to make with CT scans when cuts are made in the standard orientation. Extradural temporal lobe retraction is usually the most efficient way to answer this question. Clots in locations other than the temporal area may be removed by craniotomy rather than craniectomy because the former is a faster and less cosmetically disfiguring procedure. However, as in the temporal approach, removal of a small amount of clot through the bur holes may be helpful in urgently dealing with raised intracranial pressure while the flap is being turned. In patients with large or relatively longstanding clots (several hours), particularly patients who are comatose, the brain may swell after removal of the clot, even when the brain appears slack at operation. An intracranial device (Richmond bolt) inserted on the same side as the lesion to measure intracranial pressure may be helpful in later management.

Since CT scanning has become routine in the diagnosis of head injuries, an increasing number of patients have been found with epidural hematoma in whom the clot seems to produce little in the way of symptoms or signs. Obviously, without CT scanning these clots would have gone undetected. In most of these cases the hematoma is small, and there is little reason to consider removal. However, in a few of these cases a surprisingly large clot may be found. The appropriate stance with regard to operation in these patients has not been determined. However, when the risk of herniation is great, particularly when the clot is in the temporal location or when observation would require prolonged hospitalization and frequent CT scans, operative risk is generally low and operation may be warranted even in these asymptomatic patients.

SUBDURAL HEMATOMA IN THE PEDIATRIC AGE GROUP

DAVID C. McCULLOUGH, M.D.

Subdural hematomas continue to represent a serious neurosurgical problem in children and provide a diagnostic challenge to pediatricians, especially in early infancy when the history of a traumatic incident is often obscure. Although the majority of hematomas are subacute or chronic and may be managed with serial subdural needle taps, nearly half of the operations performed for pediatric central nervous system injuries still are done for subdural collections.

DIAGNOSIS

Clinical Presentation. Subacute or chronic liquid hematomas comprise the majority of subdurals in the childhood years, most occurring in the first 2 years of life. Peak incidence is at about 6 months of age. The most common symptoms are macrocephaly and convulsions, each occurring in approximately 50 percent of cases. Recurrent vomiting, irritability, fever, developmental delay, and chronic nutritional deficit or failure to thrive are frequently observed.

Although less than half the patients have a convincing history of head injury, about one-third have been delivered traumatically or following a prolonged labor. The incidence of child abuse, which is often suspected, is very difficult to ascertain. Among all patients admitted to pediatric services for head injuries, about 5 percent are victims of abuse. Shaking probably causes a high proportion of subdurals in the cases of "battering".

About 5 percent of children treated for hydrocephalus with cerebrospinal fluid diversionary shunts may harbor symptomatic or occult subdurals. The risk increases with age and with the severity of the initial hydrocephalus.

Examination of the infant often discloses an abnormally large head circumference. A full anterior fontanelle and widened cranial sutures, although common, do not invariably appear. Familiar nonspecific signs of childhood illness such as fever or anemia are at least as common as neurological signs such as paresis or developmental delay.

It is incumbent upon the physician to inspect the optic fundi of infants because subhyaloid (preretinal), dense, round-to-oval hemorrhages frequently accompany subdural blood collections. The discovery of subhyaloid hemorrhages may preclude the potentially dangerous lumbar puncture when bacterial meningitis is originally suspected. Papilledema is observed in a minority of infants with subdural hematomas. External evidence of abuse such as echymosis, limb deformities, and burns dictates careful inquiry and future protective measures.

Subdural hematoma of significant volume is occasionally seen in the newborn, usually after a frankly traumatic delivery. The acute lesion in the middle or posterior fossa or around the tentorium cerebelli may be associated with hypovolemic shock, signs of transtentorial herniation, or acute hydrocephalus requiring expeditious intervention.

Acute interhemispheric subdural hematoma of infancy is frequently a consequence of child abuse, and acute convexity subdurals of later childhood are usually associated with recognized severe traumatic episodes such as motor vehicle accidents, falls, or "battering". Impaired consciousness and hemiparesis or signs of impending transtentorial herniation (anisocoria, decerebrate posturing) are quite as common as the less alarming symptoms, headache and vomiting.

Differential Diagnosis. During infancy the differential diagnosis of subdural hematoma requires particular consideration of conditions that produce macrocephaly and seizures. The most common patient referred for evaluation of a large head has constitutional macrocephaly, a benign familial condition. A developmentally and neurologically normal infant with slack fontanelle and a parent with a head circumference greater than the 98th percentile seldom requires diagnostic studies. However, one must consider hydrocephalus, various intracranial cysts, and anomalies in the symptomatic child and bacterial meningitis in the acutely ill infant with fever and nuchal rigidity. A careful examination of the eyegrounds may prevent injudicious diagnostic intervention.

Diagnostic Tests. Computed tomography (CT) has dramatically improved our ability to detect and treat subdural hematomas, but has also produced some dilemmas of interpretation because of its extreme sensitivity in disclosing subdurals. With CT available, skull radiography is seldom useful or necessary. Cranial sonography with the current generation of real-time scanners is less sensitive than CT for imaging lesions near the cerebral surfaces, but some high-quality transducers may readily detect subdural collections. As the fontanelle closes, the procedure is nullified.

Diagnostic subdural taps in the infant and radionuclide brain scanning or arteriography for older children are no longer required because of the efficiency of CT.

Present generation CT scanners seldom fail to disclose the lesion, although the problem of collections isodense with brain requires careful evaluation of images. Infants usually show bilateral collections which are either more or less dense than the underlying brain. The subarachnoid spaces may be dilated. If normal subarachnoid sulci extend to the inner table of the skull on plain CT scan, isodense collections can be excluded. When diagnostic problems arise, contrast medium enhancement may contribute by disclosure of subdural membranes.

Interhemispheric subdurals are seen in association with lesions of the cerebral parenchyma, reflecting contusion or ischemic infarction. Acute and subacute hematomas in older children are usually unilateral, dense (white on the gray scale), and crescentic in outline on CT.

A special clinical problem of the CT era is the so-called "benign" subdural collection of infancy. The scan discloses small deposits of low-density bilateral extracerebral fluid. Often the subarachnoid sulci and cerebral ventricles are enlarged, suggesting the image of low-grade communicating hydrocephalus. In fact, the differentiation of these conditions may be quite difficult. Contrast scanning for evidence of membranes and radionuclide cisternography may contribute to a correct diagnosis. Alternatively, serial CT provides evolutionary data depicting enlargement of the collections (confirming a subdural location), resolution, or the development of a progressive hydrocephalus.

NATURAL HISTORY AND PATHOPHYSIOLOGY

For an individual infant presenting with subdural hematomas, unless unconsious with signs of herniation, the outlook is conjectural. In many cases the collections have been reported to resolve with negligible morbidity. However, in the symptomatic patient, including the neurologically normal infant with macrocephaly, spontaneous resolution cannot be predicted or assumed.

Hemorrhage into the potential space between dura and arachnoid results from rupture of cortical "bridging" veins between the hemispheric surfaces and dural venous sinuses. The inner dural surface becomes irritated and cells proliferate, producing a discernible outer membrane within a week. The membrane is granulation tissue consisting of fibroblasts and capillaries. Collagen gradually appears as the membrane thickens. Later an inner membrane develops. The capillaries proliferate rapidly. They are incompetent and fragile, breaking down or leaking, thus contributing volumetric increase of fluid as the cranium expands. The dynamic character of the enlarging subdural collection has been described. Albumin, water, and red blood cells move in and out of the space. In many patients in whom subdural collections spontaneously subside, there is a rapid turnover of albumin between subdural spaces and plasma. In others, with expanding heads, the turnover appears to be slower. Red blood cells eventually disintegrate and their components are absorbed, resulting in relatively clear fluid, forming the hygroma.

Aside from the evidence of small collections which may spontaneously resolve or the absence of serious symptoms, the fate of subdurals is unpredictable, except that the expanded head with disproportion between brain and calvarium seems to promote a net gain of fluid in the subdural space, making cure difficult. When cerebral atrophy occurs in the presence of a large calvarium, spontaneous resolution is rare. Conventional surgical therapy may be ineffectual. The existence of vascular membranes within a large calvarium may predispose to recurrent frank bleeding with minor trauma, leading to the rare but unfortunate cases of multilayered "geologic" subdural hematomas. In neglected patients, diffuse dense calcifications may ultimately develop.

THERAPY

Symptomatic infants with subdural hematomas or hygromas 1 cm thick or greater and seizures, developmental delay, neurological signs, or progressive abnormal increase in head size should be treated. Pharmacologic therapy with diuretics, osmotic agents, or corticosteroids has been advocated, but has not been well accepted, perhaps because the collections may expand as brain volume diminishes.

The therapist has multiple surgical options including daily needle taps, burr holes with external drainage, subdural to pleural or peritoneal shunting, and craniotomy for lysis and stripping of membranes.

Subdural Taps

Daily subdural taps represent the cornerstone of therapy because they are safe and effective when performed by experienced physicians. The majority of patients are cured by daily taps over a 2-week period.

Technique. The infant is held horizontally, firmly wrapped, crosswise on a treatment table. The head is shaved bilaterally to a plane well back of the anterior fontanelle. After sterile scrubbing and antiseptic painting, the 20-gauge, 3.8 cm, short-bevel spinal needle is introduced through the skin at the lateral angle of the fontanelle, walked forward 2 to 3 mm, and "popped" perpendicularly through the periosteum and dura. The

physician holds the needle firmly, stops immediately after the needle pops through, and makes no attempt to twist or probe the needle horizontally, medially, or laterally. The subdural fluid varies considerably, ranging from clear to frankly bloody. Fluid is allowed to drip from the needle hub. Suction aspiration should be avoided. No more than 20 ml is drained from either side the first day. Puncture sites are sealed with small cotton balls dipped in colloidion solution. Fluid from each side is analyzed for cells, protein, and bacterial culture the first day and periodically thereafter. Part of the samples may be saved for daily visual comparisons. As serial tapping proceeds, larger volumes of fluid may be gradually removed from each side. Fluid ceases to drip from the needle as intracranial pressure equilibrates with the atmosphere. For this reason, the initial tap should be performed on opposite sides on alternate days. Tapping should be discontinued on any side from which a dry puncture is obtained on 2 consecutive days. Weekly CT scans suffice to monitor the therapy. Complications in well-selected patients are miniscule, but include infections and exacerbation of subdural bleeding.

Subdural-to-Peritoneal Shunting

Because of the prolonged time in hospital, the anguish and expense involved, the patient who fails to respond to a series of 14 taps should be treated with a subdural-to-peritoneal shunt. This method has supplanted pleural diversion in most clinics. It is an extremely effective method of evacuating a chronic hematoma if tapping fails (or if the fontanelle is closed). After 2 weeks of tapping, the red cell and protein concentrations have usually declined sufficiently to promote adequate shunt diversion with minimal irritation of the peritoneal contents.

Technique. Correct positioning of the patient on the operating table for access to both sides of the head may be absolutely critical to the successful placement of subdural catheters and smooth subcutaneous tunneling of the peritoneal arm of the system. For bilateral collections, the patient is placed supine, horizontally on the table with the axis of the head, neck, and trunk hyperextended. Both sides of the top of the head should be well exposed by turning the head sharply to one side and using a head holder with skull pins or a firm small pad to elevate the top of the head from the surface of the table. If a unilateral shunt is required, patient positioning is obviously less complicated. After sterile scalp, neck, chest, and abdominal skin preparation and draping, bilateral linear incisions are performed at appropriate marked sites on the scalp. Self-retaining retractors are placed and the bur holes are drilled. The dura at the lowermost hole is first incised. Multiperforated, soft, 10 or 12 size silicone catheters are introduced immediately after incising dura and subdural membranes. Gentle irrigation at body temperature helps to clear the cavities and confirm patency of the tubing. The catheter from the "down" side is threaded under the scalp, cut to appropriate length, and attached through a Y connector to the trimmed catheter from the uppermost side. An open-ended silicone peritoneal catheter is placed into the abdominal cavity via trochar or open peritoneostomy. The proximal end is tunneled under the skin to the level of the Y connector at the upper burr hole incision, filled with irrigation saline and attached to the connector. After the tubes are secured to the connector with firm 2–0 silk ties, the connector complex is advanced subcutaneously just beyond the incision and sutured to the periosteum. After final inspection for kinks and other irregularities, wounds are closed firmly in two layers. Adhesive pressure dressings are applied to scalp wounds. Progress of therapy can be monitored by fontanelle examination and CT. Within 6 to 8 weeks the entire catheter system can usually be removed through a single incision placed over the site of the Y connector. Gentle, steady tugging should be exerted to remove each limb of the device without disrupting tissues or catheters.

Other Surgical Measures

Formerly, craniotomies with stripping of subdural membranes were effective measures for treating chronic subdural hematomas in infants. However, the excellent results of subdural-to-peritoneal shunting, especially with the monitoring capabilities of CT, have rendered craniotomies unjustifiable except in isolated cases of neglected and thickened membranes in which cerebral growth may actually be restricted. These cases may comprise a tiny minority of the infants treated unsuccessfully with shunts.

Older children with extreme macrocephaly, recurrent bleeding episodes from retained multiple membranes, reasonable mental capacity, and neurological function may be considered for the extensive surgery required to effect control or cure. Generous craniotomies, craniectomies, and calvarial reduction procedures necessitate careful planning and judicious staging as well as excellent anesthesia and transfusion capabilities. Thick, calcified subdurals ordinarily should not be resected.

The subdural effusions in shunted hydrocephalic patients often abate spontaneously. If symptoms such as head pain, seizures, dullness, and cognitive abnormalities develop, burr hole drainage to external reservoirs usually suffices. If brain re-expansion fails to occur after 7 days, subdural shunts should be inserted.

The acute or subacute unilateral or interhemispheric hematoma in infants and older children requires expeditious wide craniotomy to evacuate the solid clot. Acute cerebral swelling, which often accompanies the more severe injuries, may be extremely difficult to manage even by standard methods of controlled hyperventilation and osmotherapy with intracranial pressure monitoring.

COMPLICATIONS AND PROGNOSIS

Even though some chronic subdural hematomas spontaneously subside and most are relieved successfully by serial tapping or peritoneal diversion, a persistant intellectual and neurological morbidity of about 25 percent pertains after successful resolution of the condition. A portion of the deficit may be attributed to cerebral injury in association with the initial trauma, but some of the survivors are victims of herniation or deficits of cerebral perfusion in relation to progressive brain swelling. A minority have complications of seizures such as anoxic brain damage or infections related to therapy. Hydrocephalus also occasionally follows successful evacuation of subdurals.

After treatment of acute solid subdural hematomas of childhood, approximately 20 percent of patients expire of multiple trauma, associated cerebral injury, or uncontrolled intracranial hypertension. Thirty percent of survivors suffer irreversible and severe neurological impairment including hemiparesis, hemiplegia, intellectual deficit, or a vegetative state.

BRAIN AND SPINAL WOUNDS CAUSED BY MISSILES

MICHAEL E. CAREY, M.D., M.S.

BRAIN WOUNDS

Surgical debridement of a missile wound in the brain is usually undertaken to remove necrotic brain, indriven bone, and foreign bodies and to close the dura in order to prevent late infection.

Mechanism of Injury

When a missile (usually a bullet in the civilian milieu, but either a shell fragment or a bullet in the military) enters the brain, it transfers kinetic energy from itself to adjacent brain molecules. These adjacent molecules are set in motion away from and perpendicular to the path of the missile. They then collide with brain molecules slightly further away. Energy is thereby transfered to these more distant molecules, setting them in motion also, again at right angles to the missile track. These further molecules then collide with even more distant ones, repeating the process and transfering energy and motion to more and more distant brain molecules about the missile track. Energy transfer to the molecules of brain sets them in motion and causes them to move very rapidly away from the missile track. This movement of brain particles away from the missile path creates a subatmospheric void along the path of the missile which is called the "temporary cavity", which is several times larger than the diameter of the missile itself. Tissue molecules moving rapidly away from the missile track cause shearing and disruption of tissue adjacent to the track and also create an overpressure in the surrounding brain. When the kinetic energy of the brain molecules moving away from the track is dissipated, they cease moving outward and then fall back toward the track. This movement toward the track obliterates the temporary, subatmospheric cavity and reduces the overpressure in the surrounding brain. When tissue movements have ceased, there remains a permanent missile track in the brain owing to some frank tissue destruction by the missile. The track is surrounded by a variable zone of more severely and then less severely damaged brain. The severely damaged brain is pulped and necrotic and would provide an excellent culture medium for any indriven bacteria.

Overpressures in the brain elevate the intracranial pressure and may cause fracturing of the skull. Severe skull fractures associated with a missile wound to the brain indicate extremely high increases in intracranial pressure consequent to the deposit of missile energy. Such cases are usually fatal owing to severe brain disrup-

tion and brain stem effects. The usual, nonfatal missile wound deposits much less energy in the brain, causes far less brain damage, does not severely affect the brain stem, and does not usually create large skull fractures. If energy deposit within the brain is low, brain stem effects may be minimal, and the individual sustaining a hemispheral brain wound may not even lose consciousness. If sufficient energy is transmitted to the brain stem, a nonfatal hemispheral brain wound may be associated with varying degrees of unconsciousness.

Preoperative Assessment

In the military setting, those with brain wounds often have other wounds as well. There may be associated hypoxia consequent to hemopneumothorax or hemorrhagic shock from a major vascular injury. Either hypoxia or hemorrhagic shock in themselves may cause severe neurologic dysfunction. I have seen several instances in which patients with brain wounds were *in extremis*, it was initially believed that the brain wound was responsible. Upon proper evaluation, however, it was ascertained that their dire straits resulted from hypoxia, hemorrhage, or both. With correction of these conditions, it was appreciated that their brain wounds were relatively minor and that their neurological function was actually quite good. Although this situation is more likely to arise in combat, the civilian physician should be acutely aware that hypotension and hypoxia may severely depress neural function. An extreme amount of blood loss is unusual with most civilian bullet wounds to the brain, but aspiration is not uncommon.

Once hypotension and hypoxia have been excluded or have been diagnosed and corrected, a proper neurological evaluation can be performed to ascertain whether the brain stem is neurologically viable and what specific neurologic deficits exists. In this regard, the history is very important, especially if the patient is drowsy or frankly comatose. If the patient is seen to be alert after sustaining the brain wound, this indicates that the missile did not damage the brain stem. If he subsequently becomes comatose, one must suspect an intracranial clot and rapid surgical decompression is indicated. If, on the other hand, the patient is noted to be deeply comatose from the time of wounding, one should suspect that the bullet or concomitant energy deposit has damaged the brain stem. In this case, surgery may or may not be worthwhile.

In the awake, brain-wounded individual, one can undertake a rapid but comprehensive neurological examination, documenting hemiparesis, aphasia, visual defects, and even somatosensory loss. In the increasingly obtunded patient, the neurological examination is more and more pointed toward evaluating brain-stem function because in the individual with brain trauma, this indicates the limits of brain stem viability. In comatose patients, my decision to operate is based on brain-stem viability tested by the usual reflexes: pupillary, corneal, vestibular, eye responses and spinociliary.

It is well known that the respiratory pattern varies

with the level of brain-stem function. In my opinion, in the face of adequate mean arterial pressure and oxygenation, apnea is an absolute contraindication to surgical debridement of a brain wound. Surgery is also contraindicated if neurologic tests indicate that the brain stem is nonviable, but other, disorganized breathing patterns persist. My Vietnam neurosurgical experience provided a unique opportunity to follow up seven individuals who presented with severe brain-stem dysfunction following a cerebral hemisphere missile wound. All subsequently died 7–30 days after debridement. In the civilian setting, operating on those with nonviable brain stems for "humane reasons", though futile, may not be of critical import. In a military or mass casualty situation, expending time and resources on doomed individuals is not prudent. The best time to make the decision either for or against brain debridement is at the time of initial neurological evaluation done when the patient has adequate oxygenation and cerebral perfusion.

Preoperative Care

Following or even simultaneously with initial neurologic evaluation, immediate care includes an intravenous infusion and possibly an endotracheal tube, urinary catheter, and nasogastric tube. If blood loss has been a problem, a central venous pressure line may aid in determining blood volume replacement. I have no personal experience with the Swan-Ganz catheter, but the usual patient with a brain wound can be managed without this device. Plain skull roentgenograms allow one to estimate missile trajectory and predict with fair accuracy what brain area has been damaged. This aids in planning the surgical approach. The number and position of indriven bone fragments can be seen as well. In the civilian setting, a CT scan is often done, but this test is not really necessary. A main rationale for performing CT is that an associated intracranial blood clot can be quickly identified. With brain wounds, clots greater than 50 ml occur in only 5 to 10 percent of cases, and with experience, the surgeon can find these at the operating table. Arterial blood gases provide crucial information on the state of plasma Po_2 and Pco_2. A markedly decreased Po_2 throws into question the meaning of the neurological examination; a greatly elevated Pco_2 may lead to increased intracranial pressure. The standard CBC may be useful in cases in which preoperative blood loss has been significant. Pre- and postoperative hemoglobins or hematocrits may help to determine the adequacy of blood replacement during surgery. Urinalysis usually is not helpful, but bloody urine may indicate abdominal or retroperitoneal trauma. Any derangements in blood volume, plasma Po_2, or Pco_2 should be corrected prior to surgery. This can usually be done while the operating room is being prepared. At the same time, blood typing and crossmatching can be done, the patient's head can be shaved, and broad-spectrum antibiotic therapy is started.

The Operation

I have usually used endotracheal anesthesia, but many neurosurgeons in wartime performed virtually all brain debridements under local anesthesia. The site of the scalp or skull wound and the anticipated debridement determine how one positions the patient on the operating table. I prepare the scalp and missile entry wound with soap and another germicidal agent. The skin entry site is then copiously irrigated with saline and debrided back to healthy, bleeding scalp with a separate set of instruments. In performing the scalp debridement, the surgeon should remember that the scalp wound must be closed without tension to avoid any chance of skin breakdown and subsequent wound problems such as cerebral fungus or CSF fistula. With the low-energy civilian bullet, this is usually not a problem. Combat injuries may sustain extensive scalp lacerations requiring significant debridement. Closure of these wounds without any tension may necessitate extensive scalp undermining, sliding scalp flaps, or relaxing incisions. Successful, elegant closure may require some thought.

My treatment of forehead wounds is somewhat different from that of wounds occurring behind the hairline. Once the forehead skin entry wound has been debrided, I turn a standard coronal scalp flap to approach the bony defect. At the conclusion of the operation, the incision is closed and the forehead skin defect is cosmetically repaired to minimize forehead scarring. Skin wounds behind the hairline are debrided and enlarged in an undulating "S" to provide adequate bone exposure. If I feel that I will be able to close the skin incision without sliding flaps and skin grafts, I take pericranium along with scalp, thereby keeping pericranium intact so that it can be quickly excised to serve as a dural graft at the conclusion of the debridement. If, on the other hand, I anticipate a complex scalp closure requiring split-thickness skin grafts on the skull, I leave the pericranium attached to the skull. Skin grafts can be applied to the exposed pericranium.

A bone flap may be fashioned about the skull entrance wound, and the bony defect may be lifted out en bloc being incorporated in the center of the bone flap. This can be expeditiously done with many of the high-speed instruments available today. This very old technique may have some merit in frontal wounds. The bony missile entrance wound incorporated in the bone flap is then debrided so that loose bone and all foreign material are removed. The flap is then soaked in Betadine and replaced. Although this technique for frontal wounds may prevent large, noncosmetic craniectomy defects, it has the distinct disadvantage of possibly inviting infection by replacing potentially contaminated bone. For this reason, I debride most skull wounds by initially placing a single bur hole adjacent to the bone lacuna and perform a craniectomy about the skull wound. In this way, the bony entrance hole is removed in toto, essentially by simply enlarging it. This provides adequate dural exposure. The dura is tacked up to the skull and then opened in a cruciate fashion. I began this over normal dura and work to the dural defect, which is usually adherent to the underlying damaged brain. Careful separation of dura from pia about the cortical wound prevents further damage to the underlying brain. Usually no dural debridement is necessary, but any particularly soiled dura should be removed. Once the leaves of the incised dura have been folded back, the damaged brain clearly comes into view. Damaged pia-arachnoid is circumferentially electrocoagulated about one centimeter back from the missile track and the brain incised about the perimeter of the track. The track is then suctioned clean of all necrotic brain, blood, clot, and particularly foreign bodies including bone chips. Good light, accomplished by a headlight or lighted retractors, is indispensable for facile brain debridement. Once the damaged brain tissue is removed, bleeding invariably stops with appropriate coagulation, and the brain becomes quite relaxed. If the brain fails to relax with the completion of brain debridement, provided there is no anesthetic complications, one should suspect an undiscovered intracranial blood clot. The subdural space should be inspected, first ipsilaterally then contralaterally. In this instance, postdebridement CT scanning may be of value.

Surgeons have long recognized that indriven bone fragments may become colonized with bacteria and, if not removed, may lead to brain infection, usually an abscess. To facilitate removal, one should count the number of indriven bone fragments seen on preoperative roentgenograms and be sure to remove at least the same number of pieces at operation. Noting the position of the fragments on roentgenograms may help the surgeon to locate them at the time of debridement. When the brain debridement is finished, gentle finger palpation along the track may locate additional fragments not found by the sucker or visually observed.

Metallic fragments within the brain are known to be much less infective than bone. If a metallic fragment is seen readily during debridement of the missile track, I remove it. I do not make a protracted search for such fragments because such a search may lead to additional, unnecessary brain damage.

Once the missile track debridement is complete and bleeding is controlled, the dura is closed. The dura about the missile entry point is destroyed by the missile, and for this reason a small pericranial graft is usually necessary to obtain watertight closure. Great care should be taken to ensure that the dural closure *is* watertight to prevent CSF leak and meningitis in the postoperative period.

I do not favor immediate cranioplasty because bullet or fragment wounds are potentially contaminated. Cranioplasty at the time of brain debridement carries with it a substantial risk of postoperative infection and should be deferred for about one year. In Vietnam, where no future cranioplasty would be availble for civilians, I occasionally debrided frontal lobe wounds via a formal craniotomy flap (already described) and thereby prevented an unsightly frontal craniectomy defect. I observed no infections from this technique, but long-term follow-up was impossible.

I close the scalp in two layers with no tension whatsoever. If a sliding flap must be used to create a tensionless closure, some exposed pericranium at a distance from the wound is of little import when compared to incision breakdown directly over the craniectomy site and resultant brain infection. Such suppuration is not only dangerous for the patient, but very time-consuming for the surgeon because of the daily care required until healing is ensured. With the use of antibiotics, I have not found subgaleal wound drains necessary.

If the missile has crossed the midline, one should remember that it may have assumed its final position in the contralateral hemisphere by ricocheting off the inner table of the opposite calvarium. In this case, contralateral cortical vessels may have been lacerated and a contralateral subdural hematoma may be present. This rare occurrence should be appreciated and highly suspect should the brain not relax following customary brain debridement.

During initial debridement, every effort should be made to remove all indriven bone fragments because of their known infective potential. Usually, many more bone fragments are removed than were appreciated on preoperative roentgenograms. It is useful to take postoperative skull films to ascertain that all indriven bone fragments have been removed. If retained bone fragments are seen on postoperative roentgenograms, clinical judgment is important. In my opinion, if many retained bone fragments are seen on the postdebridement films, the initial debridement was manifestly inadequate. In such a case, the brain wound should be redebrided even if the patient is doing well clinically because the risk of future brain infection is too high. For me, the presence of a single, small retained bone fragment indicates a suboptimal but probably adequate initial debridement. I do not recommend brain wound re-exploration in this case if the patient is doing well clinically because the risk of subsequent brain infection from this single fragment is small. Alternatively, the single retained fragment can be removed if it is superficial and easily accessible, but should be left in place if it is deep and in vital areas. Finally, in the case of the single retained bone fragment, if there is the slightest indication of brain infection in the immediate postoperative phase, the missile track should be summarily redebrided and the isolated bone fragment found, removed, and cultured.

SPINAL WOUNDS

Preoperative evaluation of those with spinal wounds naturally requires a brief but thorough neurological examination. Care should be taken to test penile and perianal sensation to ascertain possible sparing of sensory function. Any sensory sparing indicates that the spinal cord is not totally functionally transected.

Opinions vary widely on the surgical treatment of missile wounds to the spine. Often circumstances influence surgical policy. The likelihood of significant return of neurological function is small following missile wounds to the spinal cord. If many casualties with open brain wounds require help, spinal wounds will assume a lower priority and many will not be operated upon. Virtually all would agree that missile wounds to the spine with concomitant CSF leak require surgery to debride the wound, close the dura, and ensure a watertight closure by closing muscle and skin. Other critiera for surgery include the presence of comminuted bone or metallic fragments within the spinal canal. Ideally, surgical debridement removes these fragments and decreases pressure on the spinal cord or cauda equina, optimizing residual neural function. Furthermore, dural lacerations can be closed to minimize the possibility of meningitis. Many surgeons do not operate on individuals with spinal cord wounds caused by small-caliber bullets or shell fragments if there is no CSF leakage, no obvious bony abnormalities, and no missile in the spinal canal.

Cauda equina injuries deserve more aggressive surgical treatment because the potential for recovery of

nerve function is so much greater than that of the spinal cord itself. Surgical debridement with removal of any indriven bone, clot, and metallic fragments is particularly indicated if some residual neurological function remains.

The missile wound which has passed through esophagus, stomach, small or large bowel and then into the spinal canal is particularly dangerous. Bacteria may be carried into the spinal canal along with the missile and may cause a spinal abscess or meningitis. I believe that laminectomy is indicated in such cases. The vertebral and neural wounds should be debrided and any dural rents closed. Muscle should be used to plug the hole from abdomen, chest, or neck into the spinal canal to prevent any bacteria from entering the epidural space. This is particularly important when the missile has passed through the large bowel before entering the spinal canal.

CEREBROSPINAL FLUID FISTULA

RONALD BRISMAN, M.D.

A cerebrospinal fluid (CSF) fistula exists when the spinal fluid is in continuity with the extra-arachnoid space. The spinal fluid may exit through the nose (rhinorrhea), the ear (otorrhea), or the skin. Trauma is the most common cause.

Traumatic CSF rhinorrhea usually results from an injury in the frontal fossa with leakage via the frontal or ethmoid sinuses, usually associated with a tear in the cribriform area. Less commonly, leakage may occur from the sphenoid sinus. Very rarely, paradoxic rhinorrhea may develop from dural tears and petrous bone fractures which extend into the mastoid air cells and middle ear; when the tympanic membrane is intact, the fluid may pass through the eustachian tube into the nasal passages. Sometimes this fluid does not exit from the nose, but stays in the nasopharynx from where it is swallowed. Fractures of the petrous bone, especilly the longitudinal type, may be associated with disruption of the tympanic membrane and traumatic otorrhea.

CLINICAL FEATURES

CSF rhinorrhea occurs in 2 percent of patients hospitalized with head injury. Patients with fractures involving the paranasal air sinuses are much more likely to develop CSF rhinorrhea, which occurs in 25 percent of these cases. The rhinorrhea usually begins within 48 hours of injury and almost always within 3 months. A

longer delay in onset of rhinorrhea is very rare, but it may occur many years after head trauma. In more than half the cases, traumatic rhinorrhea ceases within a week, but it continues for longer than one month in 10 percent of cases. Anosmia is present in many of the cases and aerocele occasionally. Headache is uncommon, and men are affected as often as women. The amount of leakage is usually small unless a fracture occurs in the middle fossa and enters the chiasmatic cistern, or the fistula involves the lateral ventricle, which may communicate with the ethmoid sinus. Traumatic CSF otorrhea stops spontaneously in the vast majority of cases, usually within the first week.

INFECTION

The possibility that bacterial meningitis may develop is one of the main concerns in patients with CSF fistula. The chances of meningitis occurring are increased if the leak persists for more than 7 days or if there is a large herniation of brain into a paranasal sinus. The meningitis that complicates CSF rhinorrhea is most often caused by penumococci. The use of antibiotics prophylactically in patients with traumatic CSF fistula is controversial and has not been shown to reduce significantly the likelihood of infection. There is some risk that patients treated with prophylactic antibiotics may develop infection with resistant organisms. If prophylactic antibiotics are used, they should be in doses high enough to enter the spinal fluid; they should be broad-spectrum drugs such as penicillin and chloramphenicol; and they should not be given for more than 7 days. Patients with CSF fistula must be observed carefully for clinical findings such as headache, fever, nuchal rigidity, or worsening of state of consciousness, which may indicate the onset of bacterial meningitis. If there is any suspicion of bacterial meningitis, a lumbar puncture must be done to check for cells, protein, sugar, Gram stain, and culture. If meningitis is confirmed or strongly suspected, prompt and vigorous treatment with approriate antibiotics must be instituted.

DIAGNOSIS

A CSF fistula is suspected when clear liquid is seen coming out of the nose, ear, or skin overlying the neuraxis; aerocephalus is present; meningitis (especially repeated episodes) is diagnosed; or a fracture is detected in the bone containing a paranasal sinus.

The presence of a CSF fistula is not always obvious. The flow may be sparse or intermittent. Some easily performed clinical tests may help to confirm the existence of CSF fistula. Postural changes may alter the flow in CSF rhinorrhea. When the supine patient moves to an erect position and flexes the neck, an increase in CSF rhinorrhea may be seen because a large paranasal sinus may act as a reservoir which then empties. CSF in the nasopharynx from a temporal bone fracture, dural tear, closed tympanic membrane, and patent eustachian tube may also exit from the nose when the patient bends forward. Occasionally, the performance of a Valsalva maneuver increases the amount of drainage. During the early stages of traumatic CSF fistula, the CSF may be accompanied by bloody fluid. The CSF may be recognized by the halo effect, which is a colorless wet circle surrounding a bloody stain on a pillow case or sheet.

Confirmation that the fluid is CSF requires quantitative glucose determination. If it is greater than 30 mg/dl, it is probably CSF. A much smaller amount of glucose is present in normal lacrimal fluid, but may give a false-positive result if glucose oxidase test paper is used. If a patient has active bacterial meningitis, the glucose concentration is reduced in the CSF and in fluid from a CSF fistula. If there is any doubt, simultaneous glucose determinations should be made of the fistula fluid and CSF obtained from a lumbar puncture.

If there is very little CSF leaking or if it is contaminated with blood, it may be hard to establish it as CSF. An immunofixation technique for identifying the presence of CSF by demonstrating its two electrophoretically separate bands of transferrin may be helpful.

LOCALIZATION

Before a definitive surgical correction of a CSF fistula is carried out, it is important to try to localize the precise point of dural-arachnoid tear, although this may not always be possible. Some clinical parameters are helpful, but not usually conclusive. If there is traumatic CSF rhinorrhea without anosmia, the cribriform plate is unlikely to be the site of the fistula. The nostril from which CSF rhinorrhea exits is usually, but not always, ipsilateral to the dural-bony defect. A fluid level behind the tympanic membrane may suggest the possibility of a temporal bone fracture and paradoxic rhinorrhea. Hearing loss may also raise the suspicion of temporal bone injury.

Skull films are mandatory for any patient who has CSF rhinorrhea or otorrhea. A fracture may be seen, perhaps pneumocephalus or air-fluid level, as in the sphenoid sinus. Air-fluid levels may be detected more easily if the patient is kept supine for at least 30 minutes before roentgenograms are taken. Polytomography is helpful for evaluating a fracture, base of skull, paranasal sinuses, ethmoid, sphenoid, temporal bones, or other suspicious areas. Computerized tomography (CT) scanning is particularly important. First, it should be done without any contrast enhancement. In the acute posttraumatic period there may be other intracranial pathology such as hemorrhage or contusion which can be detected. Aerocephalus or hydrocephalus may be seen. CT scanning should then be done with bone windows to evaluate fractures, paranasal sinuses, and temporal bones. Metrizamide-enhanced CT is of great value in demonstrating extracranial contrast and often the precise location of the CSF fistula.

A number of other diagnostic tests are not routinely used, but may occasionally be helpful in localization. These include intrathecal injection of substances such as radioisotopes, fluorescein, or indigo carmine and examination of egress sites for these markers. Iodinated ^{131}I serum albumin may be injected into the lumbar (or C1-C2) intrathecal space and cotton pledgets in the nose or ear analyzed for radioactivity. Fluorescein is photoluminescent and may be observed under ultraviolet light. Intrathecal indigo carmine may stain the tympanic membrane blue in cases with otorrhea.

TREATMENT

Most patients with CSF rhinorrhea or otorrhea can be managed successfully without surgery. The patient is kept in a semi-Fowler position and is cautioned to avoid coughing or nose-blowing. Stool softeners are used to lessen the likelihood of straining. Instrumentation of the nose (or ear) is minimized, and occlusive dressings of these orifices are avoided.

Facial fractures, which are seen frequently in patients with CSF rhinorrhea, should be treated early after the patient's general condition has stabilized. This improves the ultimate cosmetic result and may lessen the chance of nasopharyngeal infection. Rhinorrhea frequently stops following reduction of facial fractures, but it is uncertain whether there is a causal relationship.

If the leak persists for more than one week, consideration should be given to spinal CSF drainage, either by repeated lumbar punctures or by an externalized lumbar subarachnoid catheter. CSF rhinorrhea that persists for more than 2 weeks should be treated with craniotomy and intradural repair. Earlier surgery is indicated if the brain is herniated into a paranasal sinus or the rhinorrhea is profuse. Immediate operation is indicated for open wounds after the patient's airway has been secured and the hemodynamics stabilized.

Surgical correction of CSF fistula is done with magnifying loops or operating microscope. The dura is repaired, often with temporalis fascia, and the bony defect is packed with muscle, absorbable gelatin sponge, bone wax, or synthetic plastics. Muscle or absorbable gelatin sponge may be held in place and reinforced with biological adhesives. Wire mesh screen (sometimes coated with acrylic) may be used to cover larger bony openings.

Usually the preoperative examination defines the location of the dural defect, but if it does not, surgical exploration should be carried out until the fistula is repaired and the leak stops. If the side of the fistula is known, but not the precise location, exploration should be done, first of the anterior fossa and then, if this is negative, of the ipsilateral middle fossa. If no localization is noted, thorough exploration should be done of both anterior fossae and, if unsuccessful, the middle fossae.

CSF fistulas from the middle fossa may occur through fractures in the greater wing of the sphenoid bone when lateral extension of the sphenoid sinus extends this far. Direct exposure and obliteration are necessary for these leaks. A more medial defect into the sphenoid sinus, as occurs with any empty sella, an unlikely source of traumatic CSF rhinorrhea, could be handled by transsphenoidal packing.

Sometimas CSF fistulas are hard to eradicate, and recurrences after one or more operations are not unusual. Multiple sites of CSF leak may exist in one patient. Discontinuous fractures, which are responsible for more than one-third of basilar fractures causing rhinorrhea or otorrhea in missile wounds of the brain, may add to the difficulty in diagnosis and treatment.

Hydrocephalus may precipitate a CSF fistula and should be considered when the leakage begins after a delay following trauma or when it recurs. Occasionally, hydrocephalus does not become apparent until after the fistula has been repaired. The treatment of persistent CSF fistula in the presence of hydrocephalus requires the surgical treatment of both conditions: the hydrocephalus with a ventriculoperitoneal shunt and the fistula with direct repair. Persistent CSF fistula, which cannot be cured by direct repair including thorough intradural exploration, may sometimes be treated successfully with a lumboperitoneal shunt even though hydrocephalus is not present.

Iatrogenic traumatic CSF fistula may occur following the transsphenoidal approach to the sella, craniotomy through the frontal sinuses, cerebellopontine angle exposure with entry into air cells of the mastoid or internal auditory meatus, or any operation in which the dura is opened, especially if there is hydrocephalus. It is best to prevent these by repairing the dura, packing an opened sinus, flapping pericranium over an exposed frontal sinus, thoroughly applying bone wax to mastoid air cells, carefully approximating wounds in layers, and shunting patients with hydrocephalus. Postoperative CSF leaks from surgical incisions should be closed immediately. Iatrogenic CSF rhinorrhea that persists requires direct dural repair.

INFECTION

INFECTION OF THE SPINE

PERRY BLACK, M.D.
JACK L. Le FROCK, M.D.

Infections of the spine and paravertebral structures are relatively uncommon, the incidence being less than for intracranial infections such as brain abscess. Categorized in terms of the nature of the offending organism, the two large groupings are infections that are pyogenic and those that are granulomatous. Tuberculosis is the most common granulomatous infection, although fungal infections may occasionally occur, notably in immunocompromised patients. Although tuberculosis is under reasonable control in the developed countries, tubercular infection with the complication of spinal involvement remains a serious problem in some parts of the developing world where tuberculosis is still endemic.

In this chapter, spinal infection is addressed in terms of three anatomical sites: spinal epidural abscess, vertebral osteomyelitis, and intervertebral disc-space infection. Not uncommonly, infection may involve the subdural space or the parenchyma of the spinal cord, but these infections are so rare that they will not be discussed here.

SPINAL EPIDURAL ABSCESS

Pathogenesis

Staphylococcus aureus is the causative organism in most cases of spinal epidural abscess; gram-negative bacilli, tubercle bacillus or other organisms are occasionally implicated. The infections are thought to spread to the spine by the hematogenous route, particularly from skin or urinary tract infections. The infection may gain access to the epidural space by direct extension from a local process or as the result of spinal surgery. There is sometimes a recent history of spinal trauma, although its significance is difficult to assess; one possibility is that the trauma may produce a small epidural hematoma which may then become the site of hematogenous seeding of microorganisms.

Spinal epidural infection is usually secondary to vertebral osteomyelitis but may occur independently. The ventral dural sac in the spinal canal is adherent to the vertebral bodies, while the posterior epidural space is nonadherent and contains fat. Consequently, most abscesses accumulate in the posterior epidural space, except in the cervical region where the majority occur in association with cervical vertebral osteomyelitis. The epidural abscess may consist of liquid pus, firm granulation tissue, or a combination of both; this finding appears to be unrelated to the duration of illness. Tuberculous infection is associated with a fibrous reaction and caseation rather than frank pus. Epidural infection tends to spread to involve multiple levels in continuity, usually 3 to 5 vertebral elements.

The major neurologic hazard is that of spinal cord compression by the epidural mass. On occasion, however, there may be significant spinal cord dysfunction with surprisingly little mass effect. Under these circumstances, the epidural infection may produce thrombophlebitis of the spinal epidural veins (Batson's plexus) resulting in spinal cord infarction, clinically recognized as a "transverse myelitis".

Clinical Manifestations

In situations where bacterial seeding of the epidural space is by hematogenous dissemination, early signs of infection may be those of bacteremia, characterized by fever and malaise. If infection originates in a vertebral body, nonspecific complaints such as fever may be associated with back pain and local spinal tenderness. Spinal pain may progress to local nerve-root pain and, if untreated, to spinal cord compression and motor or sensory impairment; bladder and bowel sphincter dysfunction commonly accompany the paraparesis. Localized spinal pain is the most consistent symptom of spinal epidural abscess. Rapidity of progression is variable. With hematogenous spread to the epidural space, progression of symptoms and signs is likely to be rapid (hours to days). Chronic cases, by contrast, are generally associated with vertebral osteomyelitis, in which the spread from the vertebral body may take weeks to months. In children, nonspecific features of fever, irritability, vomiting, and headache may predominate; rigidity of the spine and spinal tenderness may be diagnostic clues.

Diagnostic Procedures

Rapid neurological deterioration, or suspicion of meningitis constitutes an emergency situation and requires urgent diagnositc evaluation. Obtain a white blood cell count and differential to detect leukocytosis. Radiographs of the involved region of the spine may show vertebral osteomyelitis or a paravertebral mass in the thoracic region or expansion of the psoas shadow in the lumbar area. The radiographs, however, may be entirely normal in the presence of a spinal abscess.

Lumbar puncture to rule out meningitis, and myelography to identify spinal cord compression are the two most important diagnostic studies in this situation. It is desirable to perform the lumbar puncture to obtain cerebrospinal fluid (CSF) as part of the myelogram. If the suspected spinal lesion is distant from the lumbar area, perform a lumbar puncture to obtain a specimen of CSF, and then inject the contrast dye for myelography through the same needle. Because the epidural infection may have tracked to the lumbar region, advance the lumbar puncture needle slowly, and remove the stylet frequently to detect epidural pus; if pus is encountered, do not penetrate the dura in order to avoid introducing infection into the subarachnoid space. If the suspected lesion is in the lumbar area or if pus is encountered in the lumbar epidural space, perform the CSF puncture and myelogram by the cervical route.

Examine the CSF by Gram stain, acid fast stain, and India ink stain. Conduct a white blood cell and differential count and assess glucose levels; compare the CSF glucose with the serum glucose level. Culture the CSF for aerobes, anaerobes, fungi, and acid-fast bacilli, and submit the CSF for latex agglutination tests to detect *Cryptococcus*.

In the emergency situation, neither the CT scan of the spine nor a radionuclide bone scan is likely to contribute to rapid diagnosis. However, in the more chronic form of spinal epidural abscess or vertebral osteomyelitis, a bone scan is likely to "light up" infected areas of the spine days to weeks before plain x-ray films of the spine may reveal bony destruction. Depending on its technical resolution, a CT scan may show an epidural collection.

When a paravertebral mass is present, diagnostic needle aspiration under fluoroscopic guidance may be carried out; introduce the needle several centimeters lateral to the midline and direct it obliquely toward the involved vertebral body, taking care to avoid penetrating the dura or the pleura. Aspiration of pus may be of value therapeutically, but, more importantly, the pus may identify the offending organism and permit selection of appropriate antimicrobial therapy.

Treatment

Start systemic antibiotic therapy immediately after obtaining a specimen of the epidural material. Initially select the antibiotics based on the Gram stain results, and subsequently adjust them on the basis of the culture and antibiotic susceptibility findings. Continue antibiotic treatment for 4 to 6 weeks. If there is myelographic evidence of spinal cord compression, carry out urgent spinal decompression. Since most epidural abscesses lie in the posterior part of the epidural space, perform a standard decompressive laminectomy to unroof those segments overlying the area of compression. In the cervical region, the abscess is more likely to be associated with vertebral osteomyelitis, so that an anterior cervical approach is necessary to resect the involved vertebral body and to evacuate the ventral epidural collection. Remove the pus or granulation tissue, and irrigate the epidural space with saline. After closing the wound, the surgeon has the option of placing a tube which serves as a drain and a route for postoperative instillation of antibiotics. A drain, however, is probably not essential if the purulent material has been evacuated and if the patient is given specific high-dose systemic antibiotics, which are likely to penetrate the epidural space without the need for local antibiotic instillation.

The dura is usually an effective barrier against penetration of the subarachnoid space from an overlying epidural abscess. Consequently, although there may be a sterile CSF inflammatory response, meningitis is usually not associated with the abscess. If meningitis is present, the urgency for specific antibiotic therapy is even greater.

The prognosis for survival and for prevention of serious neurologic deficit is good if the purulent collection is removed and vigorous antibiotic therapy is promptly instituted. As a general rule, the longer a neurologic deficit has been present the less likely the prognosis for reversibility of the deficit.

VERTEBRAL OSTEOMYELITIS

Pathogenesis

Infection reaches the vertebral column by direct extension from local infection in the neck, chest, or abdomen or via the spinal epidural veins (Batson's plexus). Another common source is urinary tract infection which may be caused by instrumentation of the urinary tract. Diabetics and drug addicts are at increased risk of vertebral osteomyelitis. *Staphylococcus aureus* is the most common offending organism, but a host of others, including gram-negative bacilli and mycobacteria, may be responsible.

Clinical Manifestations

In children, there is usually an abrupt onset with fever, malaise and back pain, but in adults, the onset is characteristically gradual and the course may extend over weeks to months before the diagnosis is established. Aching pain and localized tenderness in the involved region of the thoracic, lumbar or cervical spine should cause the physician to suspect the diagnosis. Careful palpation of the spine may reveal point tenderness which can be a useful diagnostic clue to the possibility of vertebral osteomyelitis. In adults, low-grade fever is present in about one-half of the cases. In about one-quarter of all cases, there is associated neurologic impairment, secondary to extension of the vertebral infection to the spinal epidural space or as the result of vertebral collapse with cord compression. The neurologic dysfunction can range from mild weakness and sensory loss to paralysis and bowel- and bladder-sphincter disturbance.

Diagnostic Procedures

Peripheral leucocytosis may or may not be present, but the erythrocyte sedimentation rate (ESR) is usually elevated. Plain x-ray films of the spine may be normal in the early stage, but the radionuclide bone scan with technetium or gallium generally lights up the spinal infection. In later stages, plain films show lytic changes in the affected vertebral bodies. In the more chronic stages, some new bone formation occurs, so that there is a combination of osteolytic and osteoblastic changes. Usually, several adjacent vertebral bodies are involved. CT scans or laminograms can be useful adjuncts to detail the vertebral disruption. In tuberculous osteomyelitis, collapse of multiple vertebral elements result in gibbus formation with angulation of the spine. A distinction can be made radiologically between vertebral osteomyelitis and metastasis from a primary neoplasm; when infection is present, the disc space is generally eroded, particularly so in tuberculous infection; by contrast, the disc space is generally preserved in cases of metastatic destruction of the vertebral body.

If a paravertebral abscess is present, evacuation by needle aspiration or open drainage may be required. Needle aspiration or a percutaneous core biopsy of an involved vertebral body may be carried out for histologic verification and for bacteriologic study. If needle aspiration fails to identify the organism, a positive blood culture may serve as the basis for selection of antibiotic therapy. In the presence of a neurologic deficit, myelography will identify the site of spinal cord or nerve root compression. In any event, it is essential to obtain bacteriologic identification of the organism, since this is the key to rational selection of antimicrobial therapy.

Treatment

In the absence of neurologic impairment, treatment is based on the principles of placing the spine at rest and administering parenteral antibiotics for 4 to 6 weeks, based on meticulous susceptibility testing of the offending organism(s). In the cervical region, relative immobilization of the neck can be facilitated by halter traction (up to 5 pounds), which often affords pain relief. Continue bedrest until the acute symptoms subside; then permit the patient to ambulate if there is no evidence of instability; prescribe a spinal brace for support. If there is a question of meningitis in the acute stage, apply the prin-

ciples of management that were discussed previously in connection with spinal epidural abscesses.

In patients with neurologic deficit, carry out surgical decompression of the spinal cord or nerve roots, and provide intraoperative antibiotic coverage. Since the compression is often ventral, an anteriolateral approach to the spine is best. In the cervical region, the standard anterior approach with a longitudinal incision placed along the anterior border of the sternocleidomastoid muscle on one side provides excellent exposure of multiple levels of the lower two-thirds of the cervical spine. In the thoracic region, a costotransversectomy approach affords access to the vertebral bodies as well as to the ventral epidural space. In the lumbar region, access to the vertebral bodies is achieved by a retroperitoneal approach, similar to that used for lumbar sympathectomy; alternatively, a posterior laminectomy approach is usually feasible, since the dural sac containing the cauda equina can be gently retracted medially to expose the posterior aspect of the lumbar vertebral bodies (below the level of the conus medullaris).

When there is spinal instability, bone fusion can be carried out even in the presence of infection, provided that pus and necrotic debris have been removed, and that the patient is placed on appropriate antibiotics. During spinal decompression or fusion, it is desirable to monitor intraoperative spinal cord evoked potentials in order to minimize the risk of trauma to the cord.

In cases of tuberculous osteomyelitis associated with neurologic dysfunction, there are two schools of thought concerning surgical intervention. Spinal immobilization and long-term antimicrobial therapy are usually considered the best approach. On the other hand, there are those who recommend surgical decompression. We are of the opinion that the same principles of surgical decompression should apply to both tuberculous and pyogenic infection. In both situations, meticulous bacteriologic study and selection of appropriate antimicrobial therapy are vital.

As in the case of spinal epidural abscess, the prognosis in vertebral osteomyelitis is generally favorable provided that proper antibiotic management is promptly instituted and that surgical decompression is carried out when there is evidence of cord or nerve root compression.

DISC-SPACE INFECTION

Pathophysiology

Infection of the disc space is a relatively uncommon complication following excision of a herniated disc (usually in the lumbar area). Somewhat more common is the spontaneous development of disc-space infection without prior spinal surgery. The latter form is thought to be produced by the hematogenous spread from an infective source elsewhere in the body, although a specific source often remains undetermined. The spontaneous form of disc-space infection tends to be more common in children than in adults, which has been attributed to the observation that the disc space early in life is well supplied with blood vessels from the adjacent vertebrae and that these vascular channels gradually disappear by the second or third decade. The normal adult disc is relatively avascular, which probably accounts for the lower frequency of blood-borne infection of the disc in adulthood.

Staphylococcus aureus is nearly always the offending organism in children; this bacterium also predominates in adults, but a wide variety of other organisms may be implicated and hence the importance of isolating the organism, especially in adults, before making a decision regarding selection of antibiotic therapy.

Clinical Manifestations

Discitis can affect the intervertebral disc at any level of the spine but is most common in the lumbar region. Children may be affected from approximately 1 year of age through adolescence. There is a higher incidence of discitis in diabetic adolescents. Children commonly present with low-grade fever, irritability, and malaise. If they are able to describe symptoms, back pain is a prominent complaint and paravertebral muscle spasm is a significant finding on examination. Sometimes the child will present with a limp or will refuse to walk, and the spinal origin of the problem may be missed unless the examiner palpates the spine in search of point tenderness and muscle spasm.

In adults with spontaneous discitis, the onset is generally more insidious, extending over weeks to months before the diagnosis is suspected. Patients complain of well localized back pain; if the lesion is in the lumbar spine, there is referred pain down one or both legs or to the hip or groin. As in children, there is localized spinal tenderness, paravertebral muscle spasm, and limitation of spinal motion. Neurologic impairment is unusual in children but is more likely in adults, secondary to an extradural inflammatory reaction with spinal cord or nerve-root compression. In recent years, it has been observed that intravenous drug users appear to be predisposed to discitis.

Postoperative disc-space infection is also difficult to diagnose because patients routinely have back pain and muscle spasm after surgery. However, if the spasm is severe and prolonged (beyond a matter of weeks), consider a diagnosis of disc space infection, despite the absence of any evidence of wound infection.

Diagnostic Procedures

The white blood cells count in children and adults is often normal or only moderately elevated, but the erythrocyte sedimentation rate is almost uniformly elevated. Blood cultures are positive in about one-quarter of patients with pyogenic infection of the disc space; when positive, the blood culture can be used as a guide for antibiotic therapy and can obviate the need to obtain a culture from the affected disc space.

Plain x-ray films of the involved areas of the spine show localized disc-space narrowing as the first radiologic sign, but the films may be normal until several weeks after onset of the symptoms. Narrowing is followed by blurring of the end-plate and irregularity and lytic destruction of the subchondral portion of the vertebral body. In later stages, after many months of healing, there is sclerosis and spontaneous interbody fusion. Laminograms or CT scans are helpful in characterizing the lesion. The most valuable radiologic study is the radionuclide bone scan with technetium or gallium. The bone scan shows a localized area of increased uptake; spot views using the pin-hole collimator provide greater diagnostic detail. The bone scan, however, is of less value in postoperative discitis, since increased uptake is normally expected following disc surgery. Reliance in the diagnosis of postoperative infection is placed on serial plain x-ray films and CT scans.

Perform percutaneous needle aspiration of the affected disc space in an effort to obtain material for culture; this is crucial in order to select appropriate antibiotics, unless the blood culture has been positive. Disc-space culture in children is said to be less vital than in adults, since the organism in children is likely to be *Staphylococcus aureus*. A problem with simple needle aspiration is that the infection is usually not purulent and positive cultures are obtained in no more than one-third of the cases. If no material can be aspirated, inject 1 to 2 ml of saline through the needle and reaspirate the patient. A superior technique which yields positive cultures in about two-thirds of the cases uses the trephine biopsy needle, which can be introduced percutaneously under local or general anesthesia or in open surgical biopsy. Three types of trephine aspiration/biopsy needles are available: the Ackerman, Craig, and Ottolenghi needles. The biopsy/aspiration technique not only provides tissue for histologic examination but also increases the likelihood of obtaining a positive culture. Histologic verification of infection is valuable in patients in whom an organism is not isolated; a further advantage is the occasional finding of an unsuspected tumor. To place the diagnostic procedures in perspective, early isotope bone scan and early biopsy of the affected disc are recommended.

Treatment

The key to management is the administration of parenteral antibiotics for 4 to 6 weeks, basing the selection of antibiotic on blood culture or biopsy/aspirate from the affected disc space. Bedrest is recommended for comfort until the acute symptoms of back pain and spasm subside. Rigid immobilization in a body cast is probably unnecessary. After the initial acute phase, permit the patient to ambulate with a simple spinal support for comfort. Use the sedimentation rate and the plain x-ray films of the spine to indicate resolution of the infection.

Children tend to recover over the course of a few weeks to several months; the course in adults may be more prolonged. In individuals, usually adults, in whom the symptoms persist and the x-ray films fail to show bone healing, open surgical debridement of the disc can be carried out; a spinal fusion might be added at the time of the disc debridement. In the unusual circumstance of neurologic impairment secondary to spinal cord or nerve-root compression, surgical decompression is mandatory unless there are general medical contraindications. In general, the long-term outlook for most patients with disc-space infection is favorable.

PYOGENIC BRAIN ABSCESS

MICHAEL E. CAREY, M.D., M.S.

Pyogenic brain abscess continues to be a medical and neurosurgical problem. Brain abscesses may be grouped and understood according to etiology. Some occur in conjunction with sinus or mastoid infection. From an infected sinus, bacteria reach the brain either by direct invasion through the adjacent bone and dura or by venous spread from the sinus through an emissary vein into the subdural space or brain proper. Likewise, a brain abscess may arise from an area of scalp or skull infection, bacteria entering the brain as from an infected sinus. Whether the site of antecedent infection is sinus, skull, or scalp, the brain abscess in such cases is likely to be in close proximity to the original infected site. Trauma (as a compound comminuted skull fracture) may also lead to the occurrence of a brain abscess; bacteria are implanted in the brain by the instrument creating the trauma or enter the brain later through the breached dura. Naturally, the abscess is in contiguity with the site of trauma. Hematogenous or metastatic brain abscesses occur when bacteria from elsewhere in the body enter the brain by the blood stream. Chronic lung infections, such as bronchiectasis, have been a common initial source of infection, although the skin and mouth also have been frequently implicated as the underlying bacterial source. The direct extension of the middle cerebral artery from the internal carotid plus laminar flow considerations cause most blood-borne bacteria to enter the middle cerebral artery complex. Hence, most hematogenous brain abscesses occur in the distribution of this artery and frequently present, clinically, with hemiparesis or speech and language problems. Individuals with congenital heart disease and right-to-left vascular shunts are particularly prone to hematogenous brain abscess because bacteria normally present intermittently in the blood stream are not filtered out in the lungs. For similar reasons, pulmonary arteriovenous fistulas are associated with the occurrence of brain abscesses. People with right-to-left shunts have high hematocrits and increased blood viscosity. Their blood, therefore, tends to sludge. This capillary sludging may lead to microinfarcts of the brain which can be colonized by bacteria from the blood stream. Only occasionally do brain abscesses occur after meningitis.

Pathologically, a pyogenic brain abscess initially begins as an area of cerebritis, which the brain attempts to wall off by a fibroblastic reaction initiated by surrounding capillaries. Severel weeks are required for significant encapsulation. Outside the fibrous brain abscess wall, a glial reaction occurs. Occasionally by this means the brain's own host-defense mechanisms may successfully contain an abscess. Most often, however, the abscess continues to expand, acting as an acute or subacute space-occupying intracranial lesion. Because the white matter of the brain is less vascular than the gray and less able to wall off an abscess, most brain abscesses expand toward the ventricles as they expand. In the usual untreated case, the abscess within the brain continues to enlarge, and death most often ensues from tentorial herniation and brain stem compression. Sometimes, because of poor encapsulation deep in the white matter, the abscess may burst into the ventricular space and cause ventriculitis, meningitis, and rapid death from these effects.

Busy neurosurgical services in underdeveloped countries may see as many as 20 pyogenic brain abscesses a year. In such circumstances both physicians and surgeons have a high index of suspicion that any intracranial lesion may be an abscess. In the United States and other highly developed countries, even a busy hospital may admit only two to four patients a year with pyogenic brain abscess. Naturally, in these circumstances the probability that any single patient will have a brain abscess is much lower. For this reason, the correct diagnosis may not be ascertained, and as the abscess enlarges during the delay in diagnosis, the patient may undergo fatal neurological decompensation from temporal lobe herniation and brain stem compromise.

Clearly, the key to successful treatment is prompt diagnosis. A careful history, with emphasis on any possible antecedent infection, is important. A chronic lung lesion or chronic osteomyelitis is a particularly ominous antecedent. This being said, it should be noted that up to one-half of all brain abscesses occur without any known prior infection. Neurological signs and symptoms associated with a brain abscess depend on the location and size of the abscess. If the abscess involves a porition of the motor strip, for instance, hemiparesis will ensue; with left temporal or posterior frontal lobe locations, speech and language impairments occur. As the mass enlarges, symptoms of intracranial hypertension appear: headache, nausea, vomiting, papilledema, and lethargy.

The common laboratory aids for the diagnosis of

infection may be unrevealing. In many cases of brain abscess, the peripheral blood WBC count is not elevated or only midly so, with no or minimal shift to the left. Temperature may be normal or only slightly elevated. Surprisingly, an "old" test, the erythrocyte sedimentation rate (ESR), may be elevated with a brain abscess, and frequently this test is the only clue that the intracranial problem is an infection. Unfortunately, in this "modern" era of medicine, the ESR is often omitted from the preliminary work-up of patients with intracranial mass lesions.

Currently, the CT scan is the optimal diagnostic test. When searching for a brain abscess, the brain CT scan should be done with and without contrast. Often a zone of rather regular ring enhancement exists about a brain abscess, with edema lying outside this area. Those practicing in hospitals without a CT scanner should not despair: radionuclide brain scans can localize about 90 percent of all brain abscesses, and even the EEG frequently can identify an area of abnormality caused by a brain abscess. Angiography is an excellent way to diagnose a brain abscess as well because of the mass effect of the abscess and because the angiographic contrast medium sometimes outline part or all of the lesion. Lumbar puncture is unrewarding and dangerous; it should not be performed for the diagnosis of brain abscess. Not only is little diagnostic information provided, but removal of spinal fluid from the lumbar subarachnoid space in the presence of an intracranial space mass and elevated intracranial pressure may cause tentorial herniation and neurological deterioration or death of the patient.

Once an abscess is suspected, high doses of broad-spectrum antibiotics should be started. Most brain abscesses contain staphylococci and streptococci, but gram-negative organisms or mixtures of gram-negative and gram-positive bacteria now often cause many brain abscesses. Anaerobic bacteria are commonly encountered as well; Bacteroides are often associated with temporal lobe abscesses consequent to chronic otitis media. One should tailor initial antibiotic choice to what bacteria one suspects to be causing the brain abscesses. For initial broad-spectrum therapy, I give intravenous penicillin G (12 mega units per day) and chloramphenicol (1 g every 6 hours), but would add metronidazole (15 mg/kg^{-1}) initally followed by 7.5 mg/kg every 6 hours thereafter) when dealing with a mastoid-induced temporal lobe brain abscess because of the high probability of the presence of Bacteroides in the abscess.

In the past I have used preoperative, operative, and postoperative steroids because brain abscesses are often associated with cerebral edema, but currently, the place of steroids in the management of brain abscess is controversial because steroids delay encapsulation and may retard the passage of antibiotic across the blood-brain barrier. Whether they effect edema associated with a brain abscess is not known. These theoretical considerations notwithstanding, if the patient has much edema associated with the abscess perhaps steroids are in order. If the edema is mild and not causing a major mass effect, steroids are better omitted.

The aim of surgical treatment of pyogenic brain abscess has been to get rid of the purulent mass, which acts as a space-occyping intracranial mass. Four methods have been used to achieve this end: drainage, aspiration, excision, and aspiration or drainage followed by excision. Each method has had its proponents, and in the hands of advocates, each method has shown similar results.

Poorly encapsulated abscesses, particularly in the motor or speech areas, might best be considered for aspiration or drainage procedures so that less brain may be damaged. If aspiration is to be done, a bur hole is placed over the abscess and the dura incised in a cruciate fashion. After coagulation of the pia-arachnoid so as to seal off this space, a large needle is inserted into the abscess and pus aspirated. A few milliliters of a local antibiotic such as bacitracin may be inserted into the collapsed abscess cavity and the needle withdrawn. The skin wound is then closed. Collapse and resolution of the abscess may be followed by CT scanning, and aspiration repeated as indicated.

Once pus is obtained from an abscess, I immediately culture it (aerobically and anaerobically). Fungal and tuberculosis cultures should be prepared as well. Naturally, ultimate antibiotic choices will be determined by the culture and sensitivities obtained from the abscess pus. Because of their importance, I prefer to prepare aerobic and anaerobic cultures immediately in the operating room by placing the pus directly in appropriate culture media such as aerobic and anaerobic blood culture bottles. Microaerophilic and anaerobic organisms are quite sensitive to air exposure and may not grow if exposed to the atmosphere. Hence, merely sending the abscess specimen off to the laboratory for subsequent culturing (perhaps hours later) will prove inadequate for obtaining growth of many organisms. Poor culture technique results in many reports of "sterile" abscess and precludes optimal antibiotic selection.

The purulent material should also be smeared for Gram staining because often organisms obtained from the abscess do not grow in culture media, particularly if the patient has had antibiotic therapy prior to surgical treatment. In these cases, Gram stain may provide the only clue to causative bacteria and proper antibiotic selection.

If drainage is to be used, a bur hole is placed over the abscess and the dura opened. The subarachnoid space is sealed with electrocautery, and a pointed brain cannula is directed toward and into the abscess. The character of any capsule can be noted as the cannula perforates it. Pus egressing from the cannula can be aspirated into a syringe. At this point care should be taken so that the surface of the brain is not soiled by the purulent material. Once the abscess has been located and pierced, the cannula should be withdrawn before all the pus has exited and the capsule has collapsed. Insertion of the drainage tube into a collapsed abscess may be difficult. After the metallic brain cannula has been withdrawn, a rubber catheter of proper length is quickly slid down the cannula track into the abscess. It is sutured to the skin so that about 1 cm protrudes beyond skin level. The wound is irrigated particularly thoroughly and the skin wound then closed. The inside of the abscess cavity can be irrigated with antibiotics. After this, dressings are built up around the base of the catheter to prevent direct pressure from being applied to the protruding catheter. This prevents its being driven into the brain further should the patient lie on it. Fluffs are placed over the end of the catheter to catch subsequent abscess drainage. Head dressings are changed daily by the operating surgeon and the abscess irrigated with appropriate antibiotic solution. There is no hurry about removing the catheter within the abscess; it may remain in place for several days to a week or two. Once drainage from the abscess ceases, the draining catheter can be gradually removed. I generally advance the drain about 1 cm per day. I recommend no set size of catheter. Clearly, the inside diameter must be large enough to afford drainage of the pus. If the pus is viscous, drains of larger internal diameter are in order. Care must be taken not to insert either the initial probing cannula or the draining catheter past the abscess and into the ventricular system. This could result in fatal ventriculitis.

Abscess resolution following drainage, as well as following aspiration, can be monitored easily by CT scanning. Both aspiration and drainage are excellent ways of quickly draining large amounts of pus in critically ill patients with increased intracranial pressure. They may be done easily under local anethesia. If not curative, drainage and aspiration may tide the patient over and allow a better preoperative neurological status prior to elective excision. Both drainage and aspiration may fail if the abscess is multiloculated or if adjacent "daughter" abscesses are present. In these instances, neither method drains all the pus and the intracerebral infection continues.

Excision of the abscess via craniotomy is the technique favored by many. It is perhaps most successful in those cases in which host defense mechanisms have allowed some abscess encapsulation to occur, and particularly when the abscess is in a neurologically less critical area of the brain, such as the frontal lobe. If the CT scan demonstrates a multiloculated abscess, excision is mandatory. A formal craniotomy is performed as for any space-occupying intracranial mass. The abscess is located by probing with a brain needle or by direct suction downward to the abscess capsule. Once the abscess has been located, it is gently dissected free of the brain. One endeavors to remove the mass in toto without spilling intracapsular contents, but this is often easier said than done. Soilage of the surrounding brain should be prevented by the placement of cottonoid patties; if any pus spillage does occur, the area should be copiously irrigated with antibiotic-containing solution. Frequently, the abscess mass may be reduced in size and its removal expedited by aspiration of the contained pus.

CT scanning is unsurpassed as a means of following resolution or recurrence of an intracerebral abscess. Following successful treatment, the zone of intracerebral edema resolves and brain distortion disappears. Finally, the area of abscess may be represented by a small hypodense area. One should remember that a pyogenic abscess may recur whatever the initial therapy. Recurrence should be suspected if the patient is not progressing satisfactorily or if the CT scan does not exhibit characteristic resolution.

Particularly if aspiration or drainage is selected as the initial form of therapy and if the CT scan shows persistence of the abscess or if neurological deterioration occurs, the surgeon must be prepared to revise his form of therapy by retapping, redraining, or excising the abscess at any time, day or night. A flexible approach to the problem must be maintained.

Recently, reports of medical cures of brain abscesses have appeared in the literature. This has been made possible mainly by a better understanding of antibiotic selection plus the ability to follow the brain lesion by CT scanning. Impressive cures have been reported of multiple hemispheral abscesses as well as small and deeplying abscesses within the basal ganglia or brain stem. Antibiotic treatment alone is more likely to be successful with abscesses less than 3 cm in diameter. Undoubtedly, medical treatment successes are more likely to be reported than are failures. When conscientiously tried, medical treatment has been successful only about 60 percent of the time. If medical treatment of a brain abscess is contemplated, it should only be undertaken by a specialist in antimicrobial therapy acting in concert with a neurosurgen. Neurological deterioration may occur quickly and without warning, and emergency surgical treatment may be required. Because the mass effect of the abscess is so deadly, it would be inappropriate to consider a drowsy or comatose patient with a large abscess as a candidate for medical therapy.

Multiple reports have shown that the surgical mortality of a brain abscess is directly proportional to the decrease in the patient's level of consciousness at the time of treatment. A decreased level of consciousness reflects brain stem compromise from brain herniation owing to the mass of the abscess and associated edema. The surgical mortality of patients who are alert has ranged from 10 to 20 percent; for those minimally responsive or unresponsive to pain, it has been 60 to 80 percent. Clearly, whatever form of surgical therapy is undertaken, it must be performed when the patient is in a good neurological state. Brain stem integrity at the time of treatment appears much more important to survival than the actual mode of therapy. The literature is replete with recent reports in which simple aspiration(s) has provided as good results as excision.

In the preantibiotic era, pyogenic brain abscess had a 60 to 80 percent mortality. With the advent of penicillin and other antibiotics in the 1940s, plus better diagnostic tools such as angiography and radionuclide scanning, it was hoped that the mortality associated with brain abscesses would fade to insignificance. This, however was not to be. Worldwide, brain abscess mortality ranged from 25 to 40 percent from the late 1940s through the early 1970s. Again, with the development of CT scanning, it was hoped that brain abscess mortality could be drastically reduced. Unfortunately, even with CT scanning, brain abscesses currently have a 15 to 30 percent mortality. One factor contributing to the continued high mortality continues to be delayed recognition of the lesion. Delayed diagnosis provides time for the abscess to increase in size, eventually causing temporal lobe herniation, brain stem hemorrhage, and death. Hematogenous brain abscesses have been particularly difficult to diagnose, especially when no antecedant infection has been evident, and they continue to be associated with a particularly high mortality. Thus, the key to further reduction in brain abscess mortality appears to be timely diagnosis, which can only come from continual clinical awareness of the problem.

Complications of intracerebral brain abscess include specific neurological deficits (e.g., hemiparesis, aphasia, reduced intellectual capacity, and hemianopsia), abscess recurrence, and seizures.

The incidence of seizures following brain abscess is in the neighborhood of 50 to 75 percent. Several years ago excision was believed to be less likely to be associated with seizure occurrence, but this has not proved to be the case. The development of seizures has been shown to be independent of the mode of surgical therapy. The occurrence of seizures after brain abscess has a peak incidence 4 to 5 years after successful treatment, and because of this, I believe that anticonvulsants should be continued for at least 5 years.

GRANULOMATOUS ABSCESS IN THE BRAIN

HUMBERTO J. ORTIZ, M.D., Ph. D.

Most granulomatous brain abscesses are due to infection by fungi. Fungal infections of the nervous system are almost always the result of hematogenous spread from a lesion in the lungs—less commonly from another primary site of infection. The lung infection occurs by inhalation of soil particles, a common habitat for many fungi. The widespread use of antibiotics, corticosteroids, and cytotoxic and antimetabolic drugs has caused an increase in the incidence of fungal infections. The advent of organ transplantation with immunosuppression and the prolongation of life in patients with neoplastic and some metabolic diseases have also increased the number of patients at risk for fungal infections.

A potential fungal etiology must then be considered in the differential diagnosis of a cerebral mass lesion in patients with evidence of lung disease and patients with an immunocompromised status. If the cranial CT scan shows evidence of simultaneous abscess and meningitis or simultaneous abscesses and subdural empyema, fungal disease is also a likely possibility. Preoperatively, skin and serologic tests may be used in some fungal conditions; if active lung disease is present, studies of sputum may yield the diagnosis. Since fungal cultures may take 4 to 8 weeks, special stains such as silver methenamine can help to establish a preliminary diagnosis. Intraoperatively, any abscess whose contents have an unusual coloration or granules should be suspected of being a possible fungus infection, and a specimen should be obtained for special stains and fungal cultures. If, after drainage or excision of a presumed

bacterial abscess, the cultures are negative and the patient persists with fever and other symptoms, fungal infection should also be suspected.

Most fungal diseases generally respond to systemic treatment with amphotericin B and/or 5-fluorocytosine. Newer antifungal agents are under investigation at the present time. The duration of treatment in immunosuppressed patients will have to be longer than for the usual patient.

Fungi may be of two forms: molds, which are composed of tubular elements called hyphae, and yeasts, which have a thick cell wall. Some fungi are dimorphic, that is, they grow as molds in artificial media and as yeasts when seen in tissues. Examples of dimorphic fungi are Histoplasma, Blastomyces, and Sporotrichum.

The actinomycetales (Actinomyces and Nocardia) are more properly classified as bacteria and are sensitive to penicillin and sulfonamides. But since the pathologic changes they induce in the brain are more like those of other fungal diseases, they are included in this section.

The phycomycetes (Rhizopus and Mucor) have a predilection for the diabetic in acidosis. *Mucor* characteristically involves the blood vessels, causing occlusion and infarction.

SPECIFIC DISEASE ENTITIES

Coccidioidomycosis occurs in arid climates like the San Joaquin Valley. The dimorphic fungus *Coccidioides immitis* lives in the soil and is acquired by inhalation. From the lung, spread occurs hematogenously; it usually causes a subacute or chronic meningitis similar to that seen with mycobacteria (tuberculous meningitis). Only rarely does it give rise to a focal granulomatous mass lesion in the brain or cerebellum which simulates a brain tumor. Hydrocephalus secondary to the granulomatous basilar meningitis may require a shunting procedure. Treatment of the meningeal infection with amphotericin B both systemically and intrathecally, is recommended prior to shunting to avoid dissemination of the infection with the shunt. Lytic vertebral lesions, coccidioidal spondylitis, may also occur. In nonendemic areas, skin tests may be useful; in endemic areas, serologic tests are used.

Paracoccidioidomycosis, which is caused by *Paracoccidioides brasiliensis,* occurs mostly in Latin American from Mexico to Argentina. The primary focus of the disease is pulmonary. Neurologic involvement may be either in a meningitic form or a pseudo-tumorous form (paracoccidioidoma). The granuloma is usually single, well circumscribed, and similar to the tuberculoma. Diagnosis usually requires identification of the organisms in tissue. It is treated with amphotericin B or sulfonamides. Surgical treatment of the mass lesion may be necessary.

Cladosporiosis, also known as cerebral chromo-blastomycosis, may be caused by Cladosporium, Hormodendrum, and other groups of pigmented fungi. It occurs predominantly in the tropics, but may occur in temperature zones. Basilar meningitis and/or granulomatous brain abscesses may occur. The cerebral lesions may be darkly pigmented, multilocular, and well encapsulated. Surgical removal is frequently necessary, but 5-fluorocytosine has also been recommended. Its efficacy in the treatment of this entity has not been established. Diagnosis depends on identification of brown septate hyphae in tissues.

Blastomycosis (Gilchrist's disease) is caused by *Blastomyces dermatitidis.* It is most common in the South Central part of the United States. Involvement of the nervous system occurs via the hematogenous route from a primary lung lesion. Infection is contracted by inhalation of soil particles. Meningitis or abscesses may occur; the abscesses may be parenchymal or extradural. The extradural abscesses may occur in the cranial or spinal compartment secondary to bony involvement and extend for many segments; the radiographic changes in this case may mimic those of tuberculosis. The CT scan shows an irregular rim-enhancing lesion that is initially hyperdense without contrast.

There are no serologic or skin tests of value in defining blastomycosis as there are for histoplasmosis, coccidioidomycosis, and cryptococcosis. Ventricular or spinal fluid may be positive on smears, but identification in tissue samples has a higher yield.

Mortality is now less than 15 percent. Of all the systemic mycoses, *B. dermatitidis* is the most sensitive to amphotericin B. Surgical excision may be necessary for mass lesions, but alone may be insufficient therapy. Intravenous amphotericin B to a total dose of 2 g is recommended.

Histoplasmosis in its pulmonary form is the most common mycotic infection in the United States. It is endemic in the Ohio, Central Mississippi, and Saint Lawrence River Valleys. The causative organism is *Histoplasma capsulatum.* Central nervous system involvement is similar to that seen in tuberculosis,

meningitis, miliary granuloma, histoplasmoma (a focal destructive lesion), and bony vertebral abscesses with extradural spinal cord compression.

The CT scan of the focal mass lesion reveals a lesion with ring enhancement. Skin testing may be useful in nonendemic areas; serologic tests may be used in endemic areas. Surgical treatment may be required for mass lesions or in cases of postmeningitis hydrocephalus. It should be followed by amphotericin B administered systemically for at least 10 weeks, but in some cases therapy may need to be prolonged.

The prognosis depends on early diagnosis and treatment. The very young and the very old have the worst prognosis. The coexistence of other infection such as tuberculosis also worsens the prognosis. The mortality rate may be as high as 25 percent with disseminated histoplasmosis.

Phycomycosis (rhinocerebral mucormycosis) is caused mostly by fungi of the *Rhizopus* and *Mucor* genera. It is acquired by inhalation. The disease is most commonly seen in patients with diabetic ketoacidosis and typically consists of nasal and paranasal sinus involvement with orbital cellulitis, followed by evidence of a frontal or temporal lobe mass. Multiple homolateral cranial nerve findings are common and frequently suggest cavernous sinus or orbital fissure syndromes. Because of the tendency of the microorganisms to invade blood vessels, intracranial aneurysms may occur.

Plain roentgenograms of the skull may reveal paranasal sinus involvement. The CT scan shows the orbital and intracranial involvement. If phycomycosis is a consideration, angiography may be justified prior to operative intervention because of the tendency of the infection to involve blood vessels. Biopsy of black necrotic turbinates or nasal mucosa can be examined for the nonseptated branching hyphae with special stains (PAS or silver methenamine) and cultured in Sabouraud's glucose-agar medium.

Corticosteroids should be avoided, since control of the diabetic condition is crucial. Treatment with amphotericin B, given systemically to a cumulative dose of 2 g, is mandatory. Surgical debridment of involved tissue may require combined otorhinologic-ophthalmologic-neurosurgical approaches.

The prognosis depends on control of the diabetic condition, the degree of nervous system damage prior to diagnosis, and the severity of the blood vessel involvement.

Aspergillosis is usually due to infection with the organism *Aspergillus fumigatus.* It may occur in a primary form in a normal patient or in a secondary form in immunocompromised individuals. Primary infection occurs in the lung by inhalation, and central nervous system involvement may follow in the form of meningitis and/or abscess. The abscesses are frequently multiple. Vascular invasion and aneurysm formation also may occur. Most fungal mycotic aneurysms are due to *Aspergillus.* Rarely, extradural spinal cord compression may be the presenting symptom. Diagnosis usually depends on tissue or culture identification of the fungus.

Immunologic tests, when positive, are helpful. Computed tomography may reveal a solid or cystic lesion with ring enhancement and without significant amounts of edema.

Medical treatment with systemic amphotericin B is recommended. Surgical excision of brain or extradural lesions may be necessary.

The prognosis is better in the primary forms, in which the nutritional and immunologic status of the patient is normal.

Petriellidosis is caused by *Petriellidium (Allescheria) boydii.* Central nervous system infection may be in the form of meningitis or brain abscess. Diagnosis depends on morphologic identification of the organism in tissue or culture or on serologic studies with immunodiffusion techniques.

Focal brain lesions should undergo operative debridment. Medical treatment with amphotericin B is recommended, but is unsatisfactory.

Candidiasis (candidosis) is caused by *Candida albicans* and usually is a low-grade meningitis, but cerebral abscesses or granulomas also may occur. The abscesses are frequently microscopic, but large abscesses acting as mass lesions may occur.

Diagnosis usually requires identification of the organism in tissue.

Treatment of these large lesions consists of surgical evacuation and systemic treatment with amphotericin B. 5-fluorocytosine may be required in some cases; occasionally, intrathecal treatment also may be required. Ketoconazole, rifampin, and terconazole also have been recommended.

Candida also shows vascular tropism, as do *Mucor, Aspergillus,* and *Blastomyces*, and may cause occlusion of vessels or aneurysm formation.

Cryptococcosis (torulosis) is the most common mycotic infection affecting the nervous system, and it is caused by the fungus *Cryptococcus neoformans.* Tissue lesions may be gelatinous (mucinous) or granulomatous. In the nervous system the organism may give rise to a chronic meningoencephalitis similar to tuberculosis and/or to a focal intracranial mass lesion (toruloma).

India ink examination of the cerebrospinal fluid or of tissue removed at surgery may provide a rapid diagnosis. Immunologic tests in blood and spinal fluid may be of assistance.

Surgical excision or aspiration of mass lesions should be followed by systemic treatment with amphotericin B; occasionally 5-Fluorocytosine or miconazole may be required.

Cryptococcal meningitis may be followed by communicating hydrocephalus, requiring a shunting procedure.

Actinomycosis is usually caused by *Actinomyces israeli.* Typically, small yellowish granules called sulfur granules are seen: they are composed of a central basophilic area surrounded by radially arranged club-shaped filaments. The organism, which is not really a fungus, but a fungus-like bacterium, responds to penicillin treatment.

Central nervous system actinomycosis is almost always secondary to disease elsewhere in the body. Cerebral abscess is the most common neurologic presentation, but intracranial or intraspinal epidural abscess as well as diffuse meningitis may also occur.

Brain abscess may occur as a single, multiloculated lesion or as multiple lesions. The capsule at the time of diagnosis is usually thick and enhances with intravenous contrast in computerized tomography. Meningitis may occur in association with the brain abscess. Clinically, increased intracranial pressure, with or without focal deficits, is the most common presenting sign. Treatment requires excision if possible or aspiration of the abscess, both followed by 6 weeks of penicillin treatment. Tetracyclines or rifampin may be used in patients allergic to penicillin.

Spinal epidural abscesses usually arise secondary to actinomycotic vertebral osteomyelitis. A "coarse sieve" appearance of the bones has been described radiographically, but the discs are usually spared. Back pain with a cutaneous fistula and progressive paraparesis should suggest actinomycosis. Decompressive laminectomy and antibiotics are the recommended treatment, although antibiotics and steroids have been recommended by some.

The prognosis after treatment is fairly good owing to the response to penicillin treatment.

Nocardiosis is usually caused by *Nocardia asteroides.* This organism is a fungus-like bacterium, not a real fungus, and responds very well to treatment with sulfa drugs.

Involvement of the nervous system is usually secondary to pulmonary disease and is most commonly seen as a brain abscess combined with meningitis. The abscess may be single, but is frequently multiple or multiloculated. The abscess capsule may be thin and not well defined. Computerized tomography scan without contrast shows hypodense lesions, but after contrast shows multiple contiguous ring-like lesions with lucent centers. The clinical picture may combine signs of meningitis with those of focal mass lesions.

Treatment may require excision if possible or aspiration of the abscess followed by prolonged treatment with sulfa drugs (sulfisoxazole or sulfamethoxazole). Blood levels of the drugs may be measured during treatment. Six weeks of treatment after cessation of *Nocardia* activity have been recommended.

The prognosis has improved since the advent of sulfa drugs and CT scanning, but can still be poor in some patients with multiple central nervous system lesions. Immunosuppressed patients should be treated for much longer periods of time.

PARASITIC DISEASE OF THE BRAIN AND SPINAL CORD

HUMBERTO J. ORTIZ, M.D., Ph. D.

Parasitic diseases are very common, particularly in the third world. Human infestation may occur via cutaneous, intestinal, or pulmonary routes—depending on the parasite—with the corresponding primary manifestations of the disease process. The involvement of the nervous system in the parasitosis then occurs via hematogenous dissemination from the primary region of involvement; this hematogenous spread may be arterial or venous. The correct preoperative diagnosis is not difficult in endemic areas or in areas of developed countries with large immigrant populations where the index of suspicion is high. Yet in most regions of the United States, the diagnosis frequently is not made prior to operation.

There are certain situations which should suggest to the physician the possibility of parasitic disease in a patient undergoing diagnostic work-up for a central nervous system lesion. When the suspicion arises, we should inquire about foreign residence or travel or other possible exposure to parasitic sources whether occupational or recreational. Cutaneous or serologic tests are available to help in the diagnosis of some parasitic diseases. The immunosuppressed patient, whether from disease such as AIDS or lymphoproliferative disorder or from the treatment of other conditions with corticosteroids or immunosuppressants, is at a very high risk of acquiring a parasitic disorder if exposed. Patients who present with central nervous system involvement and simultaneous or preexisting pulmonary, gastrointestinal, or hepatic disease should be suspected of having parasitic disease. When peripheral eosinophilia is noted in a routine blood count, parasitic disease should be included in the differential diagnosis. If cerebrospinal fluid is obtained, as for example in patients being investigated for intraspinal lesions, a mononuclear pleocytosis, with or without eosinophilia and an elevated protein content, should suggest the possibility of parasitic disease. On computed tomography of the brain, cystic cerebral mass lesions, with or without adjacent areas of calcification, should raise the possibility of parasitic disease. This is particularly true if CT-guided stereotaxic biopsy is being considered because of the risk of spillage in parasitic cysts. Radiographs of bony lesions, whether spinal or cranial, may show a mixed lytic-blastic pattern in most parasitic diseases involving bone.

In general terms, the treatment of central nervous system parasitic infections requires the correct diagnosis, removal of significant mass lesions, and prolonged systemic treatment with chemotherapeutic agents effective against the specific organism. Newer drugs are being developed, and among the most efective at present seems to be praziquantel (Biltricide). The prognosis depends not only on the effectiveness of the drug, but on the degree of nervous tissue damage that preceded the correct diagnosis and treatment. The nutritional and immunologic status of the patient are also important factors in prognosis. Serial serologic and immunologic tests provide good follow-up regarding the response to treatment and help to determine the correct duration of the treatment.

During surgical procedures on these patients, extreme care must be taken to avoid spillage of the cyst contents on unprotected brain or subarachnoid space since this makes the disease harder to manage. When the specimen is submitted for pathologic examination, the pathologist should be advised that parasitic disease is a possibility to ensure adequate examination of the tissues including serial sections of the cyst wall or contents.

It is hoped that future application of and improvement in public health measures will decrease the incidence of parasitic diseases throughout the world. Present knowledge regarding causation and transmission can make this a reality, but only if government efforts and fiscal resources are applied intensively.

Parasitic diseases that may require neurosurgical intervention include cysticercosis, echinococcosis, schistosomiasis, paragonimiasis, amebiasis, toxoplasmosis, and coenurosis. All of these entities may give rise to cerebral involvement; the first four may, in addition, give rise to spinal involvement.

CYSTICERCOSIS

This is the most common parasitosis affecting the nervous system. The disease is caused by the larval form (*Cysticercus cellulosae*) of the pork tapeworm (*Taenia solium*). In the western hemisphere it is seen most frequently in Mexico and South America. The infection is acquired through the gastrointestinal tract by drinking or eating contaminated food or water. The organisms later reach the nervous system via the hematogenous route. Upon reaching the nervous system, the parasite may localize in the brain parenchyma, the subarachnoid space, the ventricular system (through the choroid plexus), or a combination of these. The presenting symptoms and signs will depend on the predominant localization of the larva. In the case of parenchymal localization, when the parasite dies, an acute inflammatory reaction is unchained which may cause more harm than the larva itself. Edema is frequently present at this time around the parenchymal lesions and can be visualized in cranial computerized tomography. These lesions in the parenchyma may be single or multiple, usually rounded, soft tissue masses or cystic lesions. With time the lesions may calcify, usually becoming sphere-shaped with an eccentric nodular calcification within (the scolex). In cases of meningobasal or intraventricular localization, the predominant pathologic finding and clinical presentation is hydrocephalus; in addition, ventriculitis or ependymitis may be present. Diagnostic studies in these patients may require the direct injection of positive contrast into the ventricular system or subarachnoid spaces for proper visualization of the cysts since the cyst density is similar to that of the cerebrospinal fluid. Asymmetric ventricular enlargement or asymmetric basal cisternal enlargement should always suggest the possibility of a cystic structure in these CSF spaces.

Diagnosis of neurocysticercosis depends on (1) history of exposure in an endemic region, (2) a lesion identified in CT scanning compatible with the disease, and (3) when necessary, tissue obtained at operation. An enzyme-linked immunosorbent test in blood is available, but it is not always positive in the presence of disease. Complement fixation or precipitation assays are supportive but not absolute tests at present.

The treatment of uncomplicated cases consists of praziquantel, 50 mg/kg/day, distributed in three doses daily for a 15-day period. If cerebral edema is present, corticosteroids can be given concurrently (dexamethasone, 4 mg q6h. Treatment may be repeated in 1 or 2 months.

The neurosurgeon may be called to see the patient with neurocysticercosis for one of the following symptom complexes. A patient with a focal neurologic deficit, frequently a progressive hemiparesis commonly associated with a seizure disorder of focal origin, CT scanning may show a solid or, more frequently, a cystic lesion with some peripheral enhancement; the lesions may also be multiple. Multiple lesions, if not associated with a predominant lesion with impending herniation, are best treated with praziquantel and steroids and followed closely with serial CT scans. Large single cystic lesions associated with a decreased level of consciousness or signs of impending herniation are best handled surgically. The preoperative preparation should include steroids. The surgical approach is planned to include use of the CT scan in order to reach the lesion through the most direct route that avoids important cortical areas. Intraoperatively, the lesion can be localized by means of ultrasound or gentle palpation with a blunt cannula. Every attempt should be made to deliver the cyst without rupturing it if this can be done without undue stretching of the cortex. If the cyst has to be ruptured because of its large size, the cortex and subarachnoid space should be protected with cottonoids. The cottonoids are then removed and the cortical surface thoroughly irrigated after cyst delivery. Hydrostatic expulsion may be done by inserting a small rubber catheter alongside the cyst to its deeper surface, followed by gentle irrigation until the cyst is delivered. A Valsalva maneuver performed by the anesthesiologist may also help. The cyst wall should not be grasped with toothed or pointed instruments. A small pipette may be used to provide atraumatic traction on smaller cysts. The cyst is submitted for pathologic examination; typically it contains a single invaginated scolex, which is characterized by four suckers and a double row of hooklets. Treatment with corticosteroids and praziquantel should be given to these patients as soon as the diagnosis is made.

A second group of patients that may come to the neurosurgeon's attention are those presenting with intracranial hypertension without hemispheric findings or with a dementing process. The cranial CT scan separates this group into two subsets: one with pseudotumor (small ventricular system and diffuse parenchymal involvement) and a second subset with hydrocephalus. The former can be treated with praziquantel and steroids. The latter usually needs further diagnostic tests to establish the etiology of the hydrocephalus and indicate the correct treatment. Most patients with hydrocephalus due to neurocysticercosis have either the racemose, basomeningeal cysticercosis or an intraventricular cyst. In the former case, the hydrocephalus is communicating; in the latter, obstructive. A small group may have aqueductal stenosis secondary to ependymitis. The differentiation of these several types frequently can be made on cranial CT scanning, but some difficulty may arise in differentiating fourth ventricular cysts. The initial treatment of these patients may be carried out by a shunting procedure, and if a question of intraventricular cyst arises, a transvalvular contrast injection is done to visualize the ventricular system in radiographs or CT scan. If an intraventricular cyst is identified, surgical removal should be recommended for various reasons. The cyst can cause ventriculitis, become adherent to the cerebral substance, and cause progressive symptoms; it is also less likely that praziquantel or similar agents will cause the disappearance of these intraventricular cysts. The surgical approach depends on the location of the cyst. Transcallosal or transcortical approaches may be used for lateral or third ventricular lesions; suboccipital craniotomy is necessary for fourth ventricular lesions. In addition to the precautions outlined in the management of the supratentorial mass lesion, certain facts should be kept in mind regarding intraventricular cysts. First of all, they are frequently mobile and may migrate, even through the aqueduct. The preoperative CT scan and the operation should be as close in time as possible; in addition, the patient should be scanned in a position as close to the operating room position as possible. The CT scan with intravenous contrast should be examined closely, looking for enhancement in areas of contact between cyst and brain. If present, these areas constitute regions of denser attachment of the cyst capsule and therefore increase the risk attendant in an attempt at total removal.

Some cases of meningobasal cysticercosis may not respond to the initial shunting procedures and praziquantel. In these cases, posterior fossa craniectomy and an attempt at microscopic removal of the multiple cysts in the cisterns of the posterior fossa may be indicated. When dense arachnoiditis is present, it is best not to persist with surgical removal but to depend on the shunt and bony decompression to provide some palliation.

A third and smaller group of patients with neurocysticercosis comes to the attention of the neurosurgeon with a clinical picture of progressive paraparesis. Pathologically the lesion may be intramedullary (hematogenous spread) or, more commonly, leptomeningeal, that is, extramedullary intradural (spread via the cerebro-spinal fluid). The cerebrospinal fluid may show a mononuclear pleocytosis, elevated protein, and eosinophilia (on a Wright's stain). Myelography reveals the location of the lesion, usually thoracic. Praziquantel and steroids may be tried if the block is not complete and the clinical evolution is slow; otherwise, surgical decompression is the treatment of choice, that is, laminectomy and removal of the lesion.

ECHINOCOCCOSIS (HYDATID DISEASE)

The causative organism, *Echinococcus granulosus,* is the larval or hydatid stage of the dog tapeworm (*Taenia echniococcus*). The disease is most common in the sheep- and cattle-raising areas of South America, North Africa, and Australia. It is also seen in South Africa, Central Asia, and Europe. Endemic foci also exist in the lower Mississippi valley, in the sheep-raising areas of the Western United States including the Central Valley of California, and in some Alaskan villages.

The infection is acquired through the gastrointestinal tract by drinking or eating contaminated water or food. The liver and lungs are the primary sites of involvement, but some organisms spread hematogenously to brain and bones. Cerebral hydatid cysts tend to occur in children and young adults in the distribution of the middle cerebral artery and tend to be single, slow-growing, and associated with little or no inflammatory reaction or edema. Children usually present with increased pressure, whereas young adults often have hemispheric focal signs and symptoms. Radiographs may show thinning of the bone overlying the lesion, and CT scanning reveals a well-delimited cystic lesion with CSF-like attentuation and with little, if any, capsular enhancement and no surrounding edema. Vertebral hydatidosis is more common in older adults; the lesions are microvesicular, invasive, and progressive with initial involvement of the centrum and pedicle of the vertebra in the thoracic, lumbar, or sacral areas. Neurologic involvement occurs by compression. Unilocular or multilocular cavitation may be seen on roentgenogram.

Diagnosis of echinococcosis of the nervous system depends on (1) history of exposure in an endemic area, (2) a clinical picture suggestive of nervous system involvement (in endemic areas, a history of chronically increased intracranial pressure and relatively little neurologic deficit), and (3) a positive skin test (Casoni's) and complement-fixation test (Weinberg's). In cases requiring surgical intervention, the parasite or its body parts may be identified in the lesion.

Medical treatment consists of mebendazole (Vermox), 50 to 100 mg/kg/day in three divided doses with meals for a minimum of 3 months. Plasma levels should be 80 ng/ml or higher as measured by radioimmunoassay. This use of mebendazole is not listed in the manufacturer's package insert, nor is the medication approved by the FDA for this use.

The surgical treatment of large cystic cerebral lesions is based on the principles described in the section on neurocysticercosis. When lesions are very large, the cyst wall may be punctured with a small needle and the cyst partially emptied. If spillage of cyst contents occurs, the contaminated area should be irrigated with hypertonic saline solution. Because of their large size and their occurrence in children, a significant problem is the postoperative dead space resulting from the craniocerebral disproportion. Dural plication or reversal of the bone flap is a more physiologic way of dealing with this problem than the use of foreign bodies to obliterate the dead space. Drainage of fluid collections occasionally may be necessary at later dates, as after surgical removal of large supratentorial tumors in children.

In vertebral hydatidosis, decompressive laminectomy is often required; in addition, every effort to remove all the hydatid material should be made to avoid risk of cutaneous fistulas. The operative area should be irrigated with hypertonic saline at the end of the procedure. When preoperative films or CT scans reveal a predominant anterior involvement, a modification of the laminectomy is required: a costotransversectomy approach is preferable to transpleural approaches. Autogenous bone is preferable if fusion is necessary in these cases.

Intraorbital hydatidosis produces unilateral progressive exophthalmos. The lesion is readily visualized on CT scans of the orbit and may be removed by the standard transcranial approach to the orbit.

PARAGONIMIASIS

The disease is caused mainly by the trematode *Paragonimus westermani.* Most of the reported cases have originated in the Far East and Southeast Asia. Man usually acquires the infection by eating uncooked crustaceans. Initial symptoms include hemoptysis due to pulmonary involvement.

Cerebral paragonimiasis frequently presents as a mass lesion with seizures and a progressive neurological deficit. About 50 percent of the patients show calcifications in plain skull radiographs. The CT scan shows single or multiple cystic lesions with associated calcifications. Pathologically, the lesions tend to predominate in the posterior regions of the supratentorial compartment and may be solid granulomas or poorly encapsulated abscesses or cysts.

Diagnosis depends on (1) the history of exposure in an endemic area, (2) a compatible lesion on CT scanning, and (3) positive results of complement fixation tests. This immunologic test is also helpful in following the response to treatment.

Traditional medical treatment consists of bithionol, 40 mg/kg/day on alternate days for 15 doses; frequent hepatic function tests are necessary when this drug is used. Recently, praziquantel has been used in the treatment of paragonimiasis.

Surgical treatment is indicated for large single cystic lesions or solid granulomas complicated by increased intracranial pressure or brain displacements. If the lesions are multiple and disseminated, medical treatment is preferable. On occasion, with longstanding lesions, it may be preferable to evacuate the cyst cavity, leaving the cyst wall in place.

The surgical procedure and precautions are similar to those described in the section on neurocysticercosis.

Spinal paragonimiasis has a predilection for the thoracolumbar area, the usual presentation being a progressive paraparesis from extradural compression. The lesion, in the lower thoracic or lumbar areas, frequently extends for four vertebral segments or more, so that extensive laminectomy for decompression may be necessary. Radiographic changes are nonspecific. Myelography from above and below is useful to define extent of involvement.

All operated patients, cranial or spinal, should receive medical treatment once the diagnosis is established.

SCHISTOSOMIASIS

This group of disease is usually acquired by coming in contact with infected waters. The cercaria, after leaving the snail (intermediate host), may penetrate even the intact skin of man. In the Far East, the organism is usually *Schistosoma japonicum*, whose smaller eggs are more likely to cause cerebral involvement. In North Africa, the organism is *Schistosoma Haematobium*, and in South America and the Antilles, *Schistosoma mansoni*. These latter two generally involve the spinal cord via Batson's plexus of veins. In all schistosomiasis, the adult worms remain in the intestinal or urinary bladder venous systems, and the eggs may go to the nervous system, where granulomas or acute inflammatory lesions may result. The granulomas may act as mass lesions in the brain or spinal cord, causing focal deficits or compression of adjacent tissues.

Diagnosis is based on (1) history of exposure in an endemic region, (2) eggs found in the stool or urine, (3) a clinical presentation compatible with neuroschistosomiasis, and (4) immunologic tests on blood or spinal fluid. Of the last-mentioned, the circumoval precipitin test is the most accurate.

Medical treatment consists of either praziquantel or oxamniquine (Vancil). *Schistosoma mansoni* and *Schistosoma japonicum* can be treated with oxamniquine, 15 mg/kg as a single dose, whereas *Schistosoma haematobium* should be treated with oxaminiquine, 10 mg/kg every other week for three doses. African strains of schistosoma should be treated with oxaminiquine, 15 mg/kg *bid* for 2 days. Corticosteroids help to reduce the inflammatory reaction and edema associated with the lesion.

In the Western Hemisphere, the neurosurgeon sees spinal schistosomiasis more frequently than he sees cerebral schistosomiasis. The most common localization of the spinal schistosomal granuloma is in the conus medullaris. Symptomatology includes bilateral lower extremity pain and weakness with bladder and rectal sphincter involvement. Straight leg-raising test is usually positive; the ankle reflexes are absent while the patellar reflexes are preserved; the rectal sphincter is lax and the bulbocavernous reflex absent. The cerebrospinal fluid shows a mononuclear pleocytosis with 100 to 200 cells/mm^3 and protein elevation to about 150 mg/dl. The myelogram may be normal or show widening of the conus medullaris; occasionally a myelographic block is present. Treatment with corticosteroids and oxaminiquine suffices in most cases. The prognosis is good for return of motor function, but only fair for full return of sphincter function. If a complete myelographic block is present and neurological deterioration is progressing, laminectomy with dural grafting can be of help. Biopsy of the enlarged conus should be avoided if the diagnosis of schistosomiasis is established. Biopsy of whitish granular lesions in the pia-arachnoid of the nerve roots or posterior cord surface may yield the diagnosis.

Cerebral schistosomiasis may present with an acute encephalopathic picture or with a chronic granuloma causing focal deficit and increased intracranial pressure. As mentioned earlier, cerebral invlement is more common with *Schistosoma japonicum* infections, but may occur with the other schistosomes. Cranial CT scan localizes the lesion. If surgery is necessary, preoperative steroids are helpful. Decompression should help to establish the diagnosis, but cerebral damage may be unavoidable in some cases because of the intermingling of normal cerebral tissue with the components of the granuloma.

COENUROSIS

This rare infection is caused by the larval cyst or coenurus of the dog tapeworm *Taenia multiceps*. Unlike a cysticercus, which has a single scolex, a coenurid larva contains a number of scolices. The infection may involve the brain or the spinal cord with multiple small granulomas or with large single or multiple multiloculated cysts. Racemose involvement of the posterior fossa as in cysticercosis may also occur. Children or adults may be affected, and the clinical presentation is usually one of increased intracranial pressure due to the location of the coenurus in the region of the fourth ventricle or basilar cisterns.

Diagnosis depends on (1) history of exposure, (2) compatible clinical findings and diagnostic studies (CT scan), and (3) identification of the parasite on removed tissues. Dozens of scolices, visible as little white spots on the delicate cyst wall, are characteristic.

Surgical treatment follows the principles outlined in the section on cysticercosis, particularly the discussion on fourth ventricle and basilar cistern cysts.

AMEBIASIS

The disease is caused by ingestion of the cystic form of *Entamoeba histolytica*. The gastrointestinal tract and liver are commonly involved. Cerebral involvement may then occur in a stage of extraintestinal or invasive amebiasis. Cerebral lesions often have a thin wall surrounded by significant edema. On CT scan an irregular hypodense area without a well-defined capsule may be seen. The lesions may also be multiple or multiloculated. Children or adults may be affected, and the presenting symptoms are those of a focal supratentorial lesion with increased intracranial pressure.

Diagnosis depends on (1) history of exposure, (2) a suggestive clinical picture or computerized scan, (3) isolation of the ameba from stools or infected tissues, and (4) positive findings on immunologic tests such as indirect hemagglutinating antibody or micro-ELISA techniques.

Medical treatment for cerebral amebiasis should consists of metronidazole, 750 mg *tid* for 10 days. If the organism is resistant, dehydroemetine (can be obtained from CDC, Atlanta), 1 mg/kg (up to 65 mg) per day for 10 days, should be used. If cure has not been obtained, chloroquine phosphate, 500 mg *bid* for 3 days and then 250 mg *bid* for 3 weeks, may be used. Corticosteroids should only be used in extreme cases of focal mass lesion with impending herniation and for a very short period of time because of the risks of secondary bacterial infection in amebic brain abscesses.

Surgical treatment may be necessary in large cystic lesions. When the capsule is not well formed, it may be necessary to just aspirate the contents, protecting as always the surrounding brain against spillage. The pathologist should be advised that ameba are suspected so that immediate warm wet slide preparations can be obtained.

Patients with amebic cerebral abscesses may develop secondary bacterial abscesses in the areas, and antibacterial antibiotics should be given to prevent this possibility.

A search for hepatic abscesses with ultrasound, liver radionuclide scanning, or CT scanning should be carried out in patients with cerebral amebiasis and the appropriate treatment given if such a lesion is found.

TOXOPLASMOSIS

The disease caused by the obligate intracellular parasite, *Toxoplasma gondii*, is one of the most widely distributed protozoan infections. The disease may occur in congenital or acquired forms. The acquired form is seen frequently in adults or children who are immunocompromised because of disease or medications. Toxoplasmosis is the most common cause of focal brain lesions in AIDS patients. The infection is acquired by contamination with cat excreta. Involvement of the nervous system can cause multiple small nodules or large necrotic granular masses. The clinical picture may be subacute or acute, with supratentorial focal deficits being a common manifestation. On cranial CT scan, multiple ring-enhancing or nodule-enhancing lesions that often involve the basal ganglia are characteristic of cerebral toxoplasmosis.

The diagnosis depends on (1) history of exposure, (2) compatible clinical and CT picture, and (3) positive findings on serologic tests. The serologic tests include the Sabin-Feldman dye test and the indirect fluorescent antibody test for IgM. On occasion, brain biopsy or lymph node biopsy for microscopic examination and mouse inoculation is necessary. Electron microscopic examination may be necessary and tissue processed for that eventuality.

Medical treatment in cases of acquired cerebral toxoplasmosis requires at least 4 to 6 weeks; in cases of immunosuppressed patients, it may need to be given longer. Pyrimethamine is given in a loading dose of 2 mg/kg in two doses, followed by 1 mg/kg up to a maximum of 25 mg/day. In addition, sulfadiazine is given in a loading dose of 50 to 75 mg/kg, followed by 75 to 100 mg/kg in four doses. Corticosteroids should be avoided except in dire emergencies.

Surgical treatment may be required in patients with large mass lesions or in patients with small lesions in which a diagnosis cannot be made in any other way. The surgeon must remember to take precautions in patients with AIDS—the same precautions he would take when operating on a patient with hepatitis, for instance. The biopsy has a better possibility of being diagnostic if taken from the periphery and not the center of a necrotic lesion.

SPINAL DISORDERS

CERVICAL FRACTURE

JOSEPH M. PIEPMEIER, M.D.

Cervical spinal cord injury can be a difficult management problem. The complexity of treatment and the need for integration of patient care has created a need for specialized medical facilities that combine the expertise of emergency physicians, neurosurgeons, orthopaedic surgeons, urologists, physiatrists, and specialized nurses. The information in this chapter is based on the experience at the Spinal Cord Injury Center of Yale-New Haven Hospital.

Despite a continuing effort by physicians to identify a therapy that improves the patient's chances for neurologic recovery, no treatment or combination of therapy has emerged that significantly produces better results. It is clear, however, that inappropriate treatment can inhibit expected neurologic recovery or cause further neurologic loss, and failure to anticipate potential complications by recognizing early indications of problems can contribute to prolonged hospitalization and increased disability. Current treatment methods cannot, in general, reverse loss of neurologic function, but can help to prevent many posttrauamatic complications.

EPIDEMIOLOGY OF CERVICAL SPINAL CORD INJURY

Cervical cord injuries occur in patients of any age, but are most common in the 15- to 30-year-old age group. Males outnumber females by a 3:1 ratio. A majority of these injuries result from motor vehicle accidents. Diving injuries are common in young patients, whereas falls are a more frequent cause in the elderly. Injuries sustained during contact sports and penetrating injuries such as gunshot wounds characterize the remainder of cases in most series.

Sixty percent of the cervical spine injuries occur at the C5 and C6 segments; 30 percent at the C4 and C7 segments; and 10 percent above C4. The majority of these injuries result in fracture and dislocation of the spinal column caused by hyperflexion, hyperextension, and axial loading. These forces usually produce a fracture of the vertebral body and disruption and dislocation of the lateral and posterior elements. As a result, there may be both anterior and posterior compression of the spinal cord at the level of injury. Fractures without dislocation occur in 15 percent of the patients as a result of axial loading forces, whereas dislocations without fracture usually occur from hyperextension, hyperflexion, and/or rotational forces in only 5 percent. In 10 to 15 percent of cervical injuries, no detectable fracture or dislocation can be found. This happens most frequently in elderly patients with cervical canal stenosis from spondylosis and osteophytic bars or in the very young, in whom relatively lax ligaments permit dislocation and spontaneous reduction, resulting in a cord injury without a demonstrable radiographic evidence of spinal column injury.

At the time of the initial neurological examination, approximately 50 percent of the patients demonstrate a complete loss of motor and sensory function below the level of injury. Although the total loss of function does not imply anatomic transection, it always indicates a very severe injury. Preservation of some motor and/or sensory function that is of no practical use to the patient can be detected in one-third of the patients. Retained useful motor and sensory function can be found on the initial examination in 15 to 20 percent. The ability to perform a complete and detailed neurological examination is extremely important because rational treatment plans and realistic prognoses are influenced by the degree of spinal cord injury detected on the initial examination.

PATIENT EVALUATION

Any patient who experiences trauma above the shoulders is at risk of sustaining a cervical spine injury. Injured patients with an altered level of consciousness from suspected head injury or alcohol also should be managed as if a cervical spine injury is present until proven otherwise. Bilateral loss of motor and/or sensory function is diagnostic of cord trauma, but clues such as neck pain, abnormal or difficult respiration, vasomotor instability, bradycardia, hypotension, or cardiac arrhythmia in the young should serve as a warning that a cervical spinal cord injury may be present. These latter findings can result from the loss of accessory respiratory muscle and sympathetic nerve function.

A detailed neurological examination is mandatory

and should include testing of individual muscle groups in all four extremities with a grading of the amount of muscle strength present. Muscle strength should be recorded as no contraction, contraction without movement, non-antigravity movement, antigravity movement, movement against resistance, or normal strength. Sensory testing should include an evaluation of pin sensation, touch, and pressure sensation over every dermatome from C2 to S5. Vibratory and position sense should be tested in the toes, ankles, knees, hips, fingers, wrist, elbows, and shoulders. Both the presence and the quality of sensation should be noted. Deep tendon reflexes at the ankles, knees, biceps, triceps, and brachioradialis should be tested and recorded as normal, increased, decreased, or absent. Abdominal, cremasteric, and anal response reflexes, as well as the presence or absence of Babinski sign and rectal sphincter tone, should complete the examination. The results of this examination should not be trusted to memory, but should be recorded and compared with subsequent examinations. Detailed examination forms are useful in providing a permanent record for the patient's hospital chart. They also serve as a reminder of the components of a complete examination.

The topographic arrangement of fibers in the corticospinal and lateral spinothalamic tracts are arranged so that the sacral efferent and afferent fibers are in the most lateral position of the lateral funiculus. Consequently, an expanding traumatic gray matter hemorrhage and/or white matter edema that does not involve the entire cross-sectional area of the cord may preserve these fibers, and rectal sphincter tone and perianal sensation may be the only evidence of an incomplete injury (sacral sparing). Since there is a significant difference in the neurological prognosis when sacral sparing is present as compared to a complete lesion, this portion of the examination should not be omitted. Deep pain or pressure sensation in anterior tibial or Achilles tendon areas may also denote incompleteness of the lesion.

Cervical cord injuries usually are considered to cause paresis and sensory loss in all four extremities, but it should be remembered that any pattern of weakness and/or numbness may occur. Specifically, unilateral weakness with contralateral pin sensation loss (Brown-Sequard syndrome) or weakness and numbness in the upper extremities with retained strength and sensation in the legs (central cord syndrome) are also evidence of a spinal cord injury. Therefore, depending on the severity of injury and the region of the cord involved, various neurological deficits can result.

HIGH CERVICAL INJURIES

Injuries to the high cervical cord (C1 to C4) are life-threatening because of loss of phrenic nerve function (C3 to C5) and respiratory arrest. Severe injuries in this area usually result in death unless the victim receives immediate respiratory support. Airway management is treacherous since head movement can produce addi-

tional cord injury. Either nasotracheal intubation or cricothyroidotomy is the safest method for obtaining respiratory control in a patient with an unstable fracture. These patients may also become hypotensive and bradycardic as well as hypoxic and require rapid resuscitation by means of airway control, respiratory support, intravascular volume support and, when necessary, atropine and vasopressor administration.

A burst fracture of the ring of C1 (Jefferson's fracture) usually results from an axial loading force to the head. This fracture is best demonstrated radiographically on an open-mouth view that reveals lateral displacement of the articulating facets of C1. This fracture is considered stable and usually heals with proper external immobilization.

Odontoid fractures are also best seen on an open-mouth radiographic view or a lateral cervical spine film. In many cases, fractures that extend through the tip of the ondontoid (type 1) or through the base of the odontoid (type 2) do not fuse properly since the vascular supply to the odontoid has been disrupted. If the fracture line extends through the body of the C2 vertebra (type 3), fusion is more likely to occur with proper immobilization.

A hangman's fracture results in the displacement of C2 on C3 with an associated fracture of the pedicles of C2. This injury usually results from hyperextension of the head. Fractures of C1, the odontoid, and C2 do not often produce severe neurologic deficits unless there has been gross displacement; then they are usually fatal.

LOW CERVICAL INJURIES

The most frequent cervical injuries occur at C5 and C6 with fracture and dislocation. Because the maximal amount of normal cervical spine flexion and extension occur at these levels, they are more susceptible to displacement. Although the preservation of cord function is extremely important, the return of root function in the lower cervical spine is also significant and can make the difference between a functional and a useless upper extremity. Therefore, reconstitution of an obstructed neuroforamen should be considered even when the chances for a return of cord function are very poor.

Initial patient management should include securing an airway, evaluation of the respiratory status, and respiratory support when needed. The loss of sympathetic activity can result in hypotension and bradycardia. Intravascular volume replacement and prevention of venous pooling in the legs by means of Ace wraps or Mast trousers serve to elevate the blood pressure sufficiently in most patients. Failure to maintain a normal blood pressure is an indication for the use of vasopressors. Bradycardia does not require treatment unless it causes further hypotension. Atropine is effective in increasing the heart rate in these patients. Although most spinal cord injured patients receive steroids during their hospitalization, there is no clear evidence that this medication significantly improves the rate of neurological recovery.

RADIOGRAPHIC EVALUATION

The initial roentgenogram in any severely traumatized patient suspected of a cervical spine injury should be a view of the lateral cervical spine. This film is inadequate unless it clearly shows all seven vertebral segments. Specialized views (Swimmer's view) or tomograms may be necessary in patients with short necks or muscular shoulders. Although most injuries are associated with a fracture and/or dislocation, a clear spinal column abnormality may not be present. Soft tissue swelling between the vertebral column and the tracheal air shadow may be the only radiographic evidence of a cervical injury. Additional views are then necessary to complete the radiographic evaluation of the spine. High resolution CT scanning with coronal and sagittal reconstruction provides the best evaluation of cervical injuries. This technology has replaced the need for most myelograms. Small doses of intrathecal contrast (metrizamide) by a C1–C2 puncture enhances the resolution of intraspinal details. Routine myelography is occasionally used with air, Pantopaque, or metrizamide, and the resolution can be enhanced by polytomography.

CT scans and roentgenograms should be examined closely for areas of fracture and dislocation, to evaluate the dimensions of the spinal canal, and to assess the degree of instability. Frequently, repeat films are necessary to monitor the area of injury and are mandatory if the patient suffers further neurological deterioration.

PATIENT MANAGEMENT

Every patient with a suspected injury of the cervical spine should be immobilized initially on a firm surface in a cervical collar or by sandbags to prevent neck motion. Once the injury has been confirmed by the neurological examination and x-ray studies, skeletal traction should be applied, preferably with Gardner-Wells or similar skull tongs. Garnder-Wells tongs can be inserted into the skull under local anesthesia without necessitating an incision. The spring-loaded mechanism in the tongs permits a safe insertion without penetration of the inner table of the skull. In order to exert a direct axial force of traction, the tongs should be inserted in a line just above the tip of the mastoid processes. Reduction of dislocations are then attempted by adding weights to the traction. An initial weight of 5 to 10 pounds is preferred, and weights are added in 5-pound increments. This procedure is best performed in the x-ray department so that after every addition of weight, the neurological examination and lateral spine films can be repeated. Constant monitoring is necessary to evaluate the patient for any increase in neurological deficit, increase in dislocation, or distraction. Should these events occur, the weight should be immediately reduced. Muscle spasms can inhibit reduction of a dislocation and can be treated with intravenous diazepam. Weights should be added until a maximum of 50 pounds is reached. Although additional weight may be helpful in completing a reduction, it should be used with extreme caution.

After successful reduction of dislocations or reconstitution of a normal canal diameter, further diagnostic studies (myelogram, CT) can be performed to evaluate any soft tissue (disc, hematoma) cord compression. If dislocations cannot be reduced by this method, an open reduction may be necessary. Surgical decisions are based on the patient's neurological status, the severity of other traumatic injuries, and the evidence of continued cord compression. If a surgical decompression is performed, the procedure should be planned to include an internal fixation and fusion. Continued cord compression in patients with incomplete cord injuries is considered to be an indication for emergency decompression and fusion. In patients with complete cord injuries, emergency surgery has not been demonstrated to be of any significant benefit. Approximately 60 percent of our patients with cervical injuries undergo spinal surgery during their hospitalization. The majority of these procedures are performed for spinal stabilization to permit early patient mobilization.

Additional patient management techniques are directed toward preventing further complications and optimizing the chances for neurological recovery. The most frequent causes of mortality in the acute phase of patient care are respiratory complications, including pneumonia, atelectasis, aspiration, respiratory failure, and respiratory arrest. Vigorous pulmonary toilet and frequent blood gas monitoring are routine in the care of these patients. The loss of accessory respiratory muscles and abdominal distention lead to further pulmonary compromise in the recumbent patient. By elevating the head of the bed, maintaining a clean tracheobronchial tree with endotracheal suctioning, and keeping gastric distention controlled, one can prevent most pulmonary complications. Spinal cord injured patients can become fatigued, and resultant hypoxia and hypercarbia may necessitate intubation and respiratory assistance with a controlled ventilator. Patients with high cervical injuries are particularly susceptible to such respiratory failure and need close monitoring for respiratory distress. Early intubation can prevent further deterioration and respiratory arrest.

Cardiovascular instability, hypotension, bradycardia, and irregular cardiac rhythms are common during the initial 2 to 3 weeks following cervical injury. This instability is caused by the loss of sympathetic activity, relative parasympathetic hyperactivity, and peripheral venous pooling. Hypoxia can cause significant drops in pulse rate in patients requiring controlled ventilation owing to a loss of the pulmonary inflation reflex. This severe bradycardia can be prevented by pretreating patients with oxygen or atropine prior to disconnecting the ventilator for endotracheal suctioning. Various cardiac rhythm irregularities frequently occur during the acute postinjury period and do not usually require pharmacologic intervention. However, intensive care unit personnel should be instructed in the management of atrial and ventricular ectopy, bradycardia, and common arrhythmias. Volume replacement and vasopressors are useful in treating hypotension. It is not unusual to observe a neurological deficit increase with hypotension and improve when the blood pressure is elevated, presumably reflecting changes in spinal cord blood flow.

Bladder and bowel evacuation often require assistance. The urinary bladder can be managed initially by constant drainage, but within 12 to 24 hours it should be emptied by sterile intermittent catheterization at a frequency required to keep the residual volume less than 500 cc. Within the first week, bowel evacuation should be regulated to a daily movement stimulated by a suppository or low saline enema. A standard regimen of treatment is most effective in preventing obstruction and distention.

Venous thrombosis is always a risk in plegic and recumbent patients. Low-dose (5000 units) subcutaneous heparin administered twice daily helps to prevent deep vein thrombosis and lowers the risk of pulmonary embolism. Antiembolic stockings also assist the venous return to the heart from immobile legs.

Skin integrity must be observed frequently, and early signs of redness and desquamation are a warning of impending skin breakdown. In order to prevent decubitus ulcers, the patient's position should be changed every 2 to 3 hours. Soft padding around bony prominences protects the skin throughout the patient's hospitalization.

Physical therapy is started as soon as the patient is hemodynamically stable. Active and passive range of motion as well as exercises for weakened muscles help to prevent further skin breakdown, loss of range of motion, and contractures.

RESULTS OF TREATMENT

The amount of neurologic recovery following cervical spinal cord trauma depends on the severity of trauma initially sustained by the cord. Because of this fact, the initial neurological examination should be complete and detailed in order to make rational treatment plans. The benefit of surgical decompression in the management of these injuries remains unclear. Surgical decompression has not been demonstrated to improve the neurologic recovery in patients who sustain a complete and immediate total loss of spinal cord function. Although emergency decompression may be performed on patients with incomplete lesions and radiographic evidence of continued spinal cord compression, the benefit of surgery in these patients has not been proved. However, early decompression and fusion does permit early mobilization and probably contribute to shorter hospitalization and fewer complications.

Of the patients who demonstrate no preserved cord function immediately following injury, only 5 percent regain functional use of their legs. If there is no improvement in function within 24 hours, the incidence of functional recovery drops to less than 1 percent. These recovery rates probably indicate that some of the initial examinations were unreliable because of patient intoxication, head injury, or hypotension and that some function was missed on examination. It should be noted that a return of function does not mean that the patients have no disability. Most patients with "functional" recoveries can ambulate only with braces and walking aids. The recovery rate in patients with even minimally preserved motor or sensory function immediately following injury is significantly better. Approximately 50 percent of these patients regain the ability to ambulate within one year. Patients with preserved useful motor and sensory function immediately following injury have a 90 percent chance of ambulating. Deterioration of neurological functional status occurs in less than 5 percent of the patients. Despite the fact that the current treatment methods for acute cervical cord trauma have been ineffective in significantly improving neurological recovery, inadequate treatment can result in further loss of neurological function or prevent expected recovery. Meticulous care of the patient can prevent many of the common complications and reduce the incidence and severity of subsequent disability. After the patient is discharged from the hospital, it is imperative that adequate follow-up evaluations by neurosurgeons, orthopaedic surgeons, urologists, and physical therapists continue. The cooperative effort of these specialists improves patient care and increases the patient's chances of returning to society.

THORACIC FRACTURE

PAUL C. McAFEE, M.D.
THOMAS B. DUCKER, M.D., F.A.C.S.

The acute management of thoracic fractures and fracture-dislocations provides many challenges for both the orthopaedic surgeon and the neurosurgeon. The initial considerations involve resuscitative efforts to save the patient's life, (to preserve neurological function) and to maximize stability. The initial resuscitative efforts consist of insertion of intravenous catheters, restoration of adequate blood pressure, and prevention of spinal shock. A Foley catheter is usually inserted in patients with neurogenic bladders to preserve detrusor muscle function. In addition, patients need careful monitoring of respiratory function because of possible intercostal muscle paralysis. A nasogastric tube is routinely inserted to prevent abdominal distention from an ileus. A full radiologic evaluation and physical examination should be performed to rule out concomitant fractures of the cervical or lumbar spine; multiple spinal injuries are more common than was once believed. Finally, cimetidine should be given routinely to reduce the high incidence of stress ulcers. The administration of steroids is controversial and probably of no benefit in thoracic or other spinal injuries. While several animal studies suggest that the immediate administration of steroids improves the chances of subsequent neurological recovery in certain injuries, the incidence of stress gastrointestinal ulcer is as high as 25 percent in the clinical population to which steroids had been administered. The incidence of stress ulcers in patients who had not been given steroids was less than 5 percent.

When a patient presents with thoracic fractures the patient should be evaluated for (1) continued spinal cord compression which interferes with neurological recovery, and (2) possible instability of the spine.

EVALUATION FOR POSSIBLE SPINAL CANAL DECOMPRESSION TO OPTIMIZE THE ENVIRONMENT FOR NEUROLOGICAL RECOVERY

In patients with incomplete spinal cord injury, the possibility of neurological recovery depends on the amount of trauma at the time of initial injury as well as the potential for removal of bone or disc fragments which compress the spinal cord. Generally, in patients with unstable burst fractures or any injury that causes comminution of the vertebral body, the cause of spinal cord compromise is anterior, and the current revolution in surgical spinal techniques has resulted in various operative techniques to decompress the spinal cord through *anterior* approaches. In nearly every case of upper thoracic spine fracture (T1 to T3), this involves a costotransversectomy-type approach. From T4 to T11, the anterior procedure of choice is a thoracotomy because the transthoracic approach provides the best visualization of anterior compression. At the T12 level and below, the anterior decompressive approach is an extrapleural retroperitoneal decompression. Through these anterior approaches, direct visualization of the segmental arteries and veins is provided, and they can be carefully clamped in the anterior portion of the vertebrae. With each of these approaches, the cause of neurological deficit can be visualized directly, and the disc or bone fragments that are compromising the spinal canal can be removed under direct vision. After corpus or disc is removed, an anterior fusion utilizing iliac crest bone graft is performed to prevent further instability. This allows for optimal neurological recovery.

Several large series of patients followed for 2 years or longer after anterior decompression have shown that approximately 80 percent of patients who present with incomplete spinal cord injuries can recover at least one grade of motor function following anterior decompression. Bohlman in Cleveland, Larson in Milwaukee, and large series here in Maryland at the University of Maryland and Johns Hopkins have shown that approximately one-third of patients who have such severe neurological deficits as to be nonambulatory eventually regain enough motor function to walk without aid following anterior decompression. Therefore, the primary goal of therapy in patients with thoracic fractures, after the acute resuscitative measures are performed, is to evaluate the patient for possible spinal canal decompression. The radiographic method of choice is metrizamide CT myelography. With high-resolution, fourth-generation CT myelography, it is possible to directly visualize the spinal cord as well as any encroaching bony fragments. Anteroposterior and lateral tomography is not currently utilized if plain CT and CT myelography are available. We currently use a C1-C2 puncture and insertion of intrathecal contrast. Both CT and myelography can be obtained without need of turning the patient from side to side or to the prone position. Even in patients with extremely unstable injuries, after plain radiographs are obtained, CT myelography is performed as expeditiously as possible.

ASSESSMENT OF SPINAL STABILITY (NONOPERATIVE TREATMENT VERSUS INTERNAL STABILIZATION)

In the evaluation of spinal stability, the primary radiographic modalities for study of the thoracic spine are AP and lateral plane radiographs and high-resolution computed tomography; a contrast study such as myelography is not actually necessary. The greatest current advance in the orthopaedic management and determination of spinal stability after traumatic fractures is the development of the "three column theory". Francis Denis defined three columns in the thoracolumbar spine. The anterior column comprised three structures: the anterior longitudinal ligament, the anterior portion of the vertebral body, and the anterior portion of the anulus fibrosus. The middle osteoligamentous column comprises the posterior longitudinal ligament, the posterior aspect of the vertebral body, and the posterior aspect of the anulus fibrosus. The third longitudinal column of spinal stability comprises the posterior elements such as the posterior facet joints and facet joint capsules, the ligamentum flavum, the interspinous ligaments, and the posterior aspect of the neural arch.

There are six main categories of injury based on the mechanism of injury of the middle osteoligamentous column.

1. The *wedge compression fracture* is defined as compressive failure of the anterior column, secondary to an axial load. There is no posterior ligamentous injury and no failure of the middle osteoligamentous column. The wedge compression fracture is therefore a stable injury and requires internal fixation only if it occurs high in the thoracic spine (T1-T4). Wedge compression fractures occurring at two or more vertebral levels in the upper thoracic spine can cause progressive cervicothoracic kyphosis and can therefore cause secondary spinal cord compression. Multiple adjacent wedge compression fractures should therefore be stabilized with Harrington compression rods.

2. A *stable burst fracture* is defined as failure of the anterior and middle longitudinal columns, secondary to an axial load. Because by definition there is no disruption of the posterior elements, these are stable injuries and do not normally require interior fixation. These fractures can be managed successfully with a thoracolumbar sacral orthosis (TLSO). Most stable burst fractures heal without subsequent deformity, without causing progressive pain, and are not associated with progressive neurological deficit—provided the patient is maintained in a TLSO for a 3- to 6-month period. The duration of immobilization for TLSO is determined by the radiographic appearance.

3. The *unstable burst fracture* is an injury with compressive axial failure of the anterior and middle column which also involves complete disruption of the posterior elements. These are extremely unstable injuries and require internal fixation to prevent further compression of the spine. As the vertebral bodies compress, owing to axial load, the bone fragments from the vertebral bodies are retroposed against the neural structures. Therefore, as soon as a patient with an unstable burst fracture is medically acceptable for consideration of an operative procedure, internal fixation by means of Harrington distraction rods is indicated. The current "state of the art" technique uses Drummond buttons with Harrington distraction rods. This is a method of stabilizing unstable burst fractures that does not require the passing of wires or instrumentation devices into the spinal canal. This is an excellent fixation method and allows the patient to be mobile out of bed without wearing an external orthosis. In addition, with more rapid mobilization of the patient, there is a lower incidence of

pulmonary embolism, respiratory infections, urinary tract infections, and problems due to heterotopic ossification.

4. A *Chance fracture* is by definition a stable injury. There is distraction of the posterior and middle columns. This is a very characteristic injury which occurs only in the upper lumbar and the lower thoracic areas, usually secondary to a seat-belt injury. It is of interest to note that the application of the seat-belt in a motor vehicle accident causes a distraction force to be transmitted to the posterior aspect of the thoracic spinal column. As the patient flexes forward over the restraint of the seat-belt, the posterior aspect of the spine is pulled apart. Therefore, these injuries can usually be managed with a body cast or well-molded orthosis which hyperextends the spine. This brings the posterior elements of the spine back together. Because Chance fractures are injuries through bone, excellent long-term results and healing are the normal result. If the posterior part of the thoracic spine fails by ligamentous disruption, this generally results in an unstable injury. However, with Chance fractures, the posterior aspect of the thoracic spine fails by fracture, resulting in a stable situation after conservative treatment.

5. A *flexion-distraction injury* is the most serious injury to involve ligamentous disruption of the posterior elements. A flexion force applied to the thoracic spine usually results in a facet subluxation or dislocation. The anterior aspect of the vertebral bodies are crushed, whereas the posterior aspect of the thoracic elements are spread apart. This injury requires posterior internal fixation with Harrington compression instrumentation. This injury is also associated with more severe neurological deficits than the Chance fracture.

6. A *translation injury* is defined as any injury of the thoracic spine which results from a shearing failure of the middle osteoligamentous middle column. Holdsworth originally described this injury and termed it a "slice" fracture. This is the most unstable of all thoracic spinal injuries, and it is associated with the highest incidence of paraplegia and complete neurological deficits. There is basically a complete loss in continuity of the patient's spinal canal, and ligamentous discontinuity from one vetebral level to the next. The treatment of these injuries is directed toward more rapid mobilization and earlier rehabilitation of the paraplegic patient. Therefore these injuries are usually treated with Luque segmental spinal instrumentation (SSI). Luque segmental spinal instrumentation has revolutionized the treatment of these injuries because it permits patients with complete paraplegia to be out of bed, using a wheelchair, within 4 days of surgical stabilization. The Luque SSI method allows for unequaled stability of the thoracic spine and is

the method of choice in stabilizing thoracic injuries associated with complete paraplegia. The main drawback in the technique occurs when it is used in patients with preserved neurological function. The technique necessitates passage of 18-gauge wires underneath the lamina. Therefore, if a patient has intact neurological function, there is a theoretical risk of iatrogenic neurological deficit. In patients with severe translation injuries who have preserved neurological function (i.e., incomplete neurological deficits), a modified method of segmental instrumentation which does not necessitate passing wires into the spinal canal is appropriate. Drummond wires secure the bases of the spinous processes, thus allowing the stabilization of multiple segments of thoracic posterior elements without placing the already compromised spinal cord in jeopardy.

CONCLUSION

Generally speaking, the more translational displacement or distraction a given injury has, the more unstable it is. It is usually appropriate to perform the anterior decompression of neural tissue first except with severe ligamentous disruption (distraction or translational injuries). With compression injuries and burst fractures, primary anterior decompression is indicated. However, distraction or translational injuries are traditionally treated in two stages: first, by posterior stabilization, and second, by anterior decompression. There is no sense in performing an anterior corpectomy and strut grafting if the spine can shift out of alignment and displace the bone grafts.

With current treatment protocols, the instability of the injury and the incomplete neurologic deficit are managed simultaneously. It is possible to perform anterior spinal canal decompression simultaneously with posterior spinal instrumentation. Other one-stage techniques for stabilizing an unstable injury and decompressing the spinal cord involve a transthoracic corpectomy followed by application of an anterior spinal plate. At the present time, however, long-term follow-ups of large numbers of patients are not available, but our early results are encouraging.

FRACTURE OF THE LUMBAR SPINE

EDWARD L. SELJESKOG, M.D., Ph.D.

When considering management of lumbar spine fractures, priority is given to identification of the injury. Often, the victim of a lumbar spine injury has coexisting intra-abdominal, retroperitoneal, or pelvic injuries, which often signficantly overshadow the spinal problem. All too often, the diagnosis of a spinal injury is made retrospectively, after neurological loss is identified following stabilization and treatment of the coexisting and preeminent life-threatening problems. To avoid a pitfall of this sort, clinical suspicion is the watchword; appropriate follow-up with clinical and radiographic assessment is required.

Once a lumbar spine fracture is identified, two major issues need to be addressed: an assessment of the stability of the injury and an evaluation of the patient's neurological status (which indirectly assesses a possible need for spinal decompression).

When considering spinal decompression, a standard neurological evaluation of sensory and motor function and reflex activity in the lower extremities is standard, with particular reference identifying radicular neuro-

logical loss, since many thoracolumbar and lumbar spine injuries have evidence of changes involving only one or several nerve roots of the cauda equina. Of more importance is an assessment of spinal cord conus function, particularly in spinal injuries at the level of the conus, at the thoracolumbar junction, or in injuries which involve the first lumbar vertebra. This requires an evaluation of perineal sensation, gluteal motor activity, rectal sphincter tone, and the presence of an anal-wink reflex. Often in these thoracolumbar injuries, alterations in the latter two tests are the only identifiable abnormalities. The major point to be emphasized in the neurological assessment of the thoracolumbar and lumbar fracture patient is that the neurological changes may be incomplete and minimal, quite a different picture than that presented by the more cephalad spinal injury which involves the thoracic or cervical regions, where the spinal-cord injury and resultant neurological change is all too often profound.

The second major point to be considered in the evaluation of lumbar spine injury is stability of the fracture or injury. This requires a very thorough radiographic evaluation, including tomography and CT scanning. Instability is often apparent, particularly in cases of major fractures that involve the vertebral body, such as the axial loading burst or lateral-rotational types of injuries. In these injuries, there is usually evident fracture comminution and angulation, and in the more severe situations, actual subluxation or translation of vertebral elements. In the less complicated injuries, tomography and CT scanning are helpful in identifying the degree of bony comminution within the fractured elements. CT scanning is particularly helpful to identify fractures of the posterior elements, which are poorly visualized through the use of more standard radiographic techniques.

Following this initial radiographic evaluation, one should have gained an overall sense of the severity of the bony injury, and more importantly, an impression of its stability. In the event that the injury is a stable fracture (which is often the case with the simpler wedge-compression types of injury) without significant fracture of the posterior elements, management is simplified; the injury is often best treated with bedrest and if required, cast or brace immobilization. The latter permits early ambulation, once the patient's general condition has stabilized.

In contrast are those injuries which cause suspicion of or show evidence of instability, as is often the case in the more severely comminuted burst, lateral-rotational, or translational types of fractures. These may involve disruption of posterior elements and some degree of subluxation or translation of vertebral elements. As one might anticipate, many of these patients have neurological impairment, manifested by either conus or cauda equina dysfunction. In unstable situations of this sort, one must address the need for decompression, but should also consider fracture reduction and stabilization. Stabilization is usually best accomplished operatively, since there does not appear to be much place for closed fracture reduction or manipulation. This is particularly important in patients with significant intraspinal bone and for those with neurological dysfunction. Operative fracture reduction is most expeditiously accomplished from a posterior approach, utilizing the Harrington rod technique. This technique affords the opportunity to anatomically reduce the fracture under direct visualization and concomitantly achieve a reasonable degree of early stability. Depending on the degree of initial instability and the achieved level of operative stability, early mobilization frequently requires the additional use of a polypropylene jacket until solid bony healing has occurred. In order to permit long-term bony stability, one needs to carry out a concomitant bony fusion of the lateral masses and facets at the level of the surgery, usually with the so-called rod long-fuse short technique at the time of the Harrington rod procedure. In severe types of injury, particularly those at the thoracolumbar junction where there are present considerable flexion-extension forces stressing the fusion site, jeopardizing fracture healing, stability, and anatomic reduction, external body jacket immobilizatin is usually required, frequently for periods up to 6 to 9 months. In the absence of neurological loss, this type of operative intervention for stabilization can be carried out electively once the patient's acute medical and surgical problems have stabilized.

In addition to a decision regarding the need to achieve fracture reduction and stabilization, the need for early decompression of neural elements within the spinal canal must be assessed. This decision is based on the initial and complete neurological examination, as well as the initial radiographic assessment. Identification of intraspinal bone fragments is imperative, either on plain x-ray films, tomography, or CT scanning, since their removal can certainly enhance the potential for neurological recovery. Retained bone fragments within the spinal canal and compression of roots of the cauda equina often prevent or impair neurological return. It should be emphasized that the potential for recovery of neurological loss within the cauda equina is significant, even though the initial neurological impairment may be major in degree. Even severe injuries with paraplegia and those involving the thoracolumbar junction carry with them the potential for neurological improvement, especially in the extremities. The recovery of function related to the conus in these injuries is, of course, often a different matter, and incontinence and impotence are frequent long-term consequences of this injury. Nevertheless, every opportunity for recovery should be afforded these compromised neural elements, and complete assessment of the injury with an aggressive plan of decompression is reasonable and justifiable.

In patients with minimal evidence of bony change within the spinal canal, as judged by tomography and/or CT scanning, and where the patient is neurologically normal, there is little need for myelography or the introduction of contrast material into the spinal fluid for visualization of the conus, nerve roots, and dural sac. On the other hand, in the equivocal situation, where one cannot be certain regarding the degree of compromise of the spinal canal, metrizamide myelography, with concomitant CT scanning often helps to clarify the situation. This is particularly the case where there is questionable neurological dysfunction. It is surprising in situations of this sort how often one identifies major soft tissue change within the spinal canal which was not evident on standard tomography or nonCSF enhanced CT scanning. In the patient with definite evidence of neurological loss, involving the conus or single or multiple nerve roots, metrizamide myelography and CT studies are also helpful in identifying any coexisting soft tissue elements or disc material within the spinal canal, in addition to any already visualized bone.

Once one has identified spinal canal compromise, a need for decompression exists, especially in view of the potential for neurological recovery. Minimal intraspinal changes in a neurologically normal patient can be treated expectantly. On the other hand, removal of major elements within the spinal canal, even if they are not involved in neurological loss, should be strongly considered, since there is long-term potential for further encroachment on the spinal canal if post-traumatic bony spurs, kyphosis, or arthritic changes develop in the future.

After identifying the need for decompression, one must consider whether the procedure is best accomplished via an anterior, or posterior, or posterolateral approach. This decision rests in part on the location of the intraspinal bony or soft tissue change. If the mass lies entirely ventral to the dural sac and has relatively intact posterior elements, decompression is best accomplished via an anterior approach, either transthoracically in the case of thoracolumbar or first lumbar vertebral injuries, or retroperitoneally in the case of fractures involving the mid and lower lumbar spine. If the degree of bony decompression is sufficiently significant to require a partial vertebrectomy, one must always consider an anterior strut fusion, utilizing a rib graft. This is a particularly useful technique at the thoracolumbar junction where one can occasionally, even at this lower thoracic level, utilize a vascularized rib pedicle graft.

If, however, a combination of anterior spinal canal compromise and major disruption of posterior elements is involved, the patient will require spinal stabilization in addition to decompression. In this situation, stabilization is most easily accomplished posteriorly, utilizing a Harrington rod technique. One should then consider approaching the decompression of the spinal canal posterolaterally, while at the same time accomplishing the stabilization/Harrington rod procedure. Removal of posterior elements and particularly pedicles or facet joints may further destabilize the spine. One must be ever mindful, however, of the need for adequacy of the decompressive procedure; good visualization of the intraspinal canal, particularly when the bony or disc fragments lie ventral to the dural sac is imperative. Limited removal of these already unstable posterior elements, unilaterally or bilaterally, has minimal effect on stability but aids in the decompression and, more importantly, its verification. Often, in situations of this sort, the spinal decompression has been incomplete, and a second procedure is required. It is better to sacrifice some minor degree of stability in these injuries in order to be assured of the completeness of the decompression.

In summary, the initial assessment of lumbar and thoracolumbar injuries requires a complete radiographic and neurological assessment of the patient. In the event that a problem of instability is identified, operative intervention for stabilization is usually the preferred form of management in an attempt to facilitate solid bony healing and early stability, but more particularly to permit early ambulation and rehabilitation. This, of course, has to be considered within the context of the patient's general medical and surgical condition. For the most part, stabilization is best and most easily accomplished via a posterior approach using the Harrington rod technique. This generally achieves the goals of stability and has reasonably good long-term results, achieving solid fracture healing with a minimum of pseudoarthrosis or deformity complications.

In contrast, anterior stabilization, although it has some advantages, usually requires more prolonged external immobilization until solid intervertebral healing

has been achieved. The anterior fusion technique is most often indicated when a patient requires a major anterior decompression involving a partial vertebrectomy.

When considering the need for decompression, radiographic confirmation of any significant degree of spinal canal compromise is usually an indicator for decompressive surgery, particularly if the patient has any suggestive evidence of neurological impairment. Aggressive and complete decompression is especially important in the lumbar spine, where the potential for neurological recovery is decidedly brighter. Even when a patient is neurologically normal, one can make a very reasonable argument for a decompressive procedure, should the compromise of the spinal canal prove to be significant. Metrizamide myelography, coupled with CT scanning has proven to be a very valuable adjunct when making this surgical decision.

The best avenue for decompression is dictated by the circumstances of the individual case. Where the major impingement on the dural sac is purely ventral, with relatively stable posterior elements, an anterior approach is usually the procedure of choice. In contrast, where there is major spinal disruption, with compromise both anteriorly and posteriorly, with a coexisting need for early spinal stabilization, the problem of decompression is often best addressed via a posterior approach, decompressing the spinal canal posterolaterally through the pedicle and approaching the dural sac laterally. Occasionally this will require a bilateral approach which sacrifices some degree of spinal stability in order to enhance and be assured of the adequacy of decompression. In most situations of this sort, which require either a unilateral or bilateral posterolateral approach, Harrington rod fusion is required to provide additional early stability of the fractured area.

Finally, it should be noted that as a matter of routine, postoperative evaluation of these surgical cases, including tomography and more particularly, spinal CT scanning, is prudent in order to be absolutely assured of the completeness of decompression and to be confident that there is no persisting neural compression to impair neurological recovery. Additionally, of course, these patients will require long-term follow-up with appropriate x-ray studies to assure maintenance of fracture reduction, and ultimately, solid bony healing. With the use of these principles and techniques, one can be confident that the patient has been provided an optimal milieu for neurological recovery. With this sort of approach, many cases with initial serious neurological impairment can ultimately demonstrate a rather surprising degree of neurological recovery, even to the point of relatively independent ambulation.

ACHONDROPLASIA: NEURORADIOLOGICAL INVESTIGATION AND SURGICAL MANAGEMENT OF CRANIOCERVICAL JUNCTION AND PAN-SPINAL STENOSIS

J. A. WINFIELD, M.D., Ph.D.
HENRY WANG, M.D.

Achondroplasia is the most common form of congenital bony dysplasia and constitutes the major cause of dwarfism. Although there is an autosomal dominant Mendelian penetrance, approximately 75 percent of achondroplasts are new spontaneous mutations. With the exception of their short stature, these pleasant individuals are normal in every other respect with normal intelligence and a near-normal life expectancy.

Although the defects are not fully understood, membranous bone formation appears to be normal or mildly hyperplastic, with hypoplasia of chondral bone formation. This disparity in bone growth results in typical facial and skull features. There is midfacial hypoplasia which can contribute to respiratory difficulties, basal synostosis that leads to constriction of the foramen magnum, and a large head circumference, consistently above the 97 percentile at birth. Long-bone and vertebral-column growth is also affected; longitudinal bone growth from epiphyseal centers is hypoplastic and transverse growth from periosteal contribution remains normal. These growth characteristics lead to shortened ribs which may cause restrictive lung disease, foreshortened and stocky extremities, and pan-spinal stenosis.

In both the normal individual and the achondroplast, vertebral-body growth occurs from a single epiphyseal center, and neural arch growth from two epiphyseal centers. In the achondroplast, this results in poor longitudinal growth of the vertebral body with a 1:1 ratio of disc to vertebral body height in adults and short pedicles which are of normal thickness due to the periosteal growth. In the newborn, the interpedicular distance is already narrowed and there is further narrowing of this distance as one descends to the sacrum. This is in marked contrast to the normal spine where the interpedicular distance increases as one descends to the sacrum. In summary, these abnormal growth characteristics lead to specific anatomical bony abnormalities which include: (1) constriction at the level of the foramen magnum, (2) 40 percent reduction in the interpedicular distance throughout the spinal column, (3) short, but normal thickness pedicles, and (4) diminished diameter of the nerve-root foramina. Further neurologic compromise can arise from the presence of marked abnormal curvatures of the spine including: (1) hyperlordosis of the lumbar area (70% of adults), (2) long kyphosis at the thoracolumbar junction occurring over extended segments, (3) less commonly, a sharp angulated gibbus occurring over a single wedged vertebra, (4) kyphoscoliosis (30% of adults).

Until recently, most neurological complaints in adult achondroplasts were attributed to thoracolumbar stenosis. Occasional patients underwent suboccipital decompressions and staged pan-spinal canal decompression. A rare teenager may present with symptoms of neural claudication and require a decompressive procedure. There is now substantial evidence that, in infants, cervicomedullary compression secondary to foramen magnum stenosis may be responsible for apnea, sudden death, persistent delayed motor development, and multiparesis. In children under the age of 5 years, we have not found stenosis of the spinal canal to be the cause of neurological abnormalities in the extremities, and in this age group we have directed our attention to the craniocervical junction. Since these children are predisposed to primary respiratory abnormalities caused by midfacial hypoplasia and restrictive chest-lung disease, multidisciplinary evaluation is essential to rule out non-neurogenic causes for the respiratory abnormalities before cervicomedullary compression is considered as the etiology. To date, we have studied 27 children in conjunction with Dr. S. Reed in the Department of Pediatric Genetics. Neural compression causing respiratory problems was considered a major factor in 10 of the 27 children. Three of these 10 children were neurologically normal and had only respiratory difficulties. The other 7 children had multiparesis, delayed motor development, and hyperreflexia with clonus, as well as respiratory difficulties.

In the adult achondroplast the clinical presentations vary but are usually secondary to thoracolumbar stenosis. Symptoms of back pain, intermittent sciatica, paresthesias, and difficulties with bowel and bladder may be antecedent, beginning during childhood or in the teens. Occasionally, patients may present with acute sciatica and a foot drop, in which case an acute disc herniation should be suspected. More commonly, symptoms of classic neural claudication are described by the patient. On neurological examination, one usually finds a mixed upper and lower motor-neuron pattern of weakness with absent reflexes in one lower extremity and a downgoing toe, compared with hyperreflexia, clonus, and a Babinski in the other leg. Sensory levels at the spinal levels T8 to T12 are also common.

Following admission and careful detailed neurological examination, we feel that multiple studies are essential in planning surgical intervention and should in general include: (1) complete spinal and skull base plane x-ray films, (2) cystometrograms, (3) pulmonary function studies, (4) electromyography nerve conduction test, (5) spinal cord evoked potentials.

The neuroradiologic techniques used in the evaluation of achondroplastic patients with compressive spinal disorders includes myelography, computerized tomography (CT), and magnetic resonance imaging (MRI), either performed singly or in concert.

For myelography, low-concentration, small-volume, nonionic, water-soluble x-ray contrast (e.g., metrizamide 190 mg I/ml of 4 ml to 8 ml) is used, and a CT scan of the spine is performed as soon as possible following myelography. The patient should be kept in the upright position while waiting for CT scanning. For 6 hours following myelography keep the patient sitting upright or elevate the head at least 30° and provide adequate hydration. Since all of these patients have a congenitally narrowed spinal canal and a very small subarachnoid space, the route of choice for spinal needle insertion is a lateral C1-C2 puncture for all patients over 10 years of age. For patients under 10 years of age who show no symptoms of lumbar stenosis, myelography should be performed using an oblique lumbar needle approach at the L2 or L3. Only a 25-gauge spinal needle should be used in order to minimize damage to dura and nervous tissue, and to prevent a CSF leak.

Plain CT (without intrathecal metrizamide) does not provide clear delineation of the individual structures and compartments within the spinal canal because of the small subarachnoid space, except in the craniocervical junction. However, following intrathecal contrast, CT enables one to visualize the severity and extent of the spinal-cord compression along the entire neuraxis and also allows one to discern the thecal sac and its surround distal to the apparent complete block on plain myelogram.

In the evaluation of the craniocervical junction, plain CT or metrizamide CT cisternogram provides adequate diagnostic information. In young achondroplasts with cervicomedullary compression, when metrizamide cisternogram is warranted, 3 ml to 4 ml or 100 mg I/ml concentration metrizamide is instilled intrathecally via a lumbar puncture (without fluoroscopy) in the CT scanner room; by positioning the patient, the contrast is gravitated toward the craniocervical junction and axial CT sections are obtained immediately. The entire examination is done with the patient either under general anesthesia or heavily sedated at the discretion of the anesthesiologist. (We usually take advantage of this anesthetized state to perform preoperative evoked potentials either following anesthetic induction or following myelography before anesthesia reversal). Thin axial CT sections (4 mm slice thickness, 4 mm table increment) of the area of interest are obtained. Using the multiplanar reformation computer software program, coronal, sagittal, and oblique images can be generated. Linear area and volume measurement can also be accurately performed.

Although MRI provides good delineation of bone, subarachnoid space, and nervous tissue of the spine, scarcity of MR scanners, cost, and lengthy time of the examinations still make this modality impractical for most patient workups.

Once the entire neuraxis has been assessed neuroradiographically, the clinical picture, neurological examination, and other diagnostic studies need to be carefully collated, since multiple defects without clinical symptoms may be present on diagnostic myelographic and CT studies. All patients are placed on steroids prior to radiologic studies and are continued on steroids through the postoperative period.

Regardless of age, several anesthetic considerations are important. Venous access is, in general, poor and all patients require placement of a central line, which further facilitates postoperative fluid management. Because of midfacial hypoplasia, intubation can be extremely difficult, and awake fiberoptic nasal intubation is often performed in adults. As a general rule, all patients are left intubated for several hours postoperatively in order to prevent unnecessary reintubation and its complications. Intraoperative evoked potentials are used in all achondroplastic infants who require suboccipital decompression and, whenever possible, in all other decompressive procedures on adult achondroplasts.

Suboccipital decompression in the infant is performed in the prone position. The child is carefully positioned over chest rolls and the head fixed with a padded horseshoe ring. Due to the well known problems with CSF dynamics, these infants are placed on Diamox preoperatively (75 mg/kg/day in 3 divided doses), and a right frontal ventricular drain may be placed. Extracranial ventricular drainage is used for several days postoperatively to allow for wound healing and to prevent the development of a pseudomeningocele.

A midline incision is made from the inion posteriorly to the spinous process of C4 or C5. Standard subperiosteal dissection of the paraspinous muscles is performed with removal of the muscle from the arch of C1 and spinous process and lamina of C2. No space will exist between the posterior lip of the foramen magnum (which will be hyperplastic) and the arch of C1. Great care should be taken with the subperiosteal removal of muscle for the arch of C1, since the vertebral artery is often in an abnormal position, lying more medial than expected or exiting the foramen transversarium between C1 and C2 and passing over the arch of C1. The posterior arch of C1 can then be removed, using the high-speed drill. Occasionally, because of the hyperplasia of the occipital bone, the suboccipital bone must be removed with the high-speed drill before the arch C1 can be removed. Once the suboccipital bone and arch of C1 are removed, one usually finds a persistent "napkin ring" dural structure. Duroplasty represents a formidable task in the infant with persistent circular and occipital sinuses. The dura is opened in the midline beginning just above the cephalic level of C2. When the dural level at the suboccipital region is reached, the dura is further opened in the midline between consecutively placed pairs of wet clips. The suboccipital portion of the dural opening only needs to extend in the cephalic direction for 1 to $1\frac{1}{2}$ cm. At the midpoint of the dural incision, the dura is then retracted posteriorly and stitched to the muscle laterally, creating a diamond-shaped dural defect. The dural defect is then patched with fascia lata or a periosteal graft and is sutured in place with a running suture. Paraspinous muscles are then closed in "multiple" layers and the skin is closed using a running stitch. Postoperative management is routine except that the ventricular drain is left in place for several days. One of the 10 children who underwent suboccipital decompression required placement of a permanent ventriculoperitoneal shunt after developing communicating hydrocephalus. Short-term follow-up to date has been extremely rewarding with resolution of respiratory problems, acceleration in acquiring motor milestones, and substantial improvement or complete resolution of multiparesis.

Surgical management of thoracolumbar stenosis in the adult achondroplast represents a most technically challenging spinal procedure. When a conus syndrome predominates the clinical picture, we generally perform a T8 to S1 decompressive laminectomy. Despite great surgical care, venous blood loss may be substantial, and adequate blood products should be available preoperatively. Because of prominent thoracolumbar kyphosis and hyperlordotic lumbosacral curvature, great care must be taken when positioning the patient in the prone position. Use of commercially available spinal frames is not recommended as these frames may cause "bowstringing" of the cauda equina with reduction of the naturally acquired thoracolumbar curvature. Baseline spinal-cord evoked potentials should be performed before and after placing the patient in the prone position. A midline incision is made after injecting lidocane and epinephrine into the paraspinal muscle, and a standard subperiosteal dissection is performed. The spinous processes are then removed using a large rongeur. Often, overgrowth of the facets will virtually obliterate the space lateral to the spinous process. Next, the initial laminectomy is performed using a high-speed drill. At no time should a Kerrison punch be used. The dura is extremely thin and the ligamentum flavum hypertrophied and often scarred down to the dura. Great care must therefore be taken to prevent large dural tears when removing the ligament. If a tear occurs, it must be repaired using an interposed fat graft. Due to the marked decrease in size of the neural canal, unrepaired dural tears will invariably result in extrusion of segments of the cauda equina with nerve entrapment and severe postoperative pain. Often multiple unilateral facetectomies will be required to adequately decompress the conus and cauda equina. Despite multilevel facetectomies, stability is usually not a problem, although we advise patients to wear a thoraco lumbar spine brace postoperatively. Once the midline laminectomy is completed, further lateral extension and foramenotomies can be performed using the high-speed drill and micro Kerrison punches. The L5–S1 area represents a particularly dangerous area to decompress but decompression into the sacrum is essential. The neural canal is extremely stenotic at this level and the dural sac rises posteriorly to enter the sacrum. A large fat graft is placed over the entire exposed thecal sac and standard muscle closure is performed.

For the acute disc herniation syndrome, we recommend a complete laminectomy prior to exploration of the disc space. The surgical principles and operative techniques for cervical and upper thoracic laminectomies are identical to the lumbar surgery. The head is generally held with the Gardner-Wells head holder. The majority of the bone work is performed using the high-speed drill.

The overall surgical results in the literature are mixed, with only prevention of further neurologic progression and often some worsening of neurologic symptoms postoperatively. With careful attention to anatomical relationships, steroid use, careful attention to patient positioning at surgery, judicious surgical technique, and use of the high-speed drill, we have obtained gratifying results, often with complete return of bladder function and motor strength in patients who presented with several months of bladder dysfunction and significant motor weakness. Long tract findings often persist, but remain stable.

BASILAR IMPRESSION, PLATYBASIA, OS ODONTOIDEUM, AND FRACTURE OF THE ODONTOID PROCESS

JULIAN T. HOFF, M.D.

While basilar impression, platybasia, os odontoideum, and fracture of the odontoid process are distinct entities, they have clinical, diagnostic, and therapeutic similarities that warrant discussion of them as a group in this chapter.

DEFINITIONS

Platybasia. This is a descriptive term for the appearance of the base of the skull on a lateral plain skull radiograph. The normal angle between a line drawn tangentially along the floor of the frontal fossa and a line parallel to the clivus is about 145 degrees. If that angle is more obtuse than 145 degrees, then platybasis exists. Platybasis, per se, is asymptomatic.

Basilar Impression. Basilar impression is protrusion of the upper cervical spine into the base of the skull at the foramen magnum. It may be congenital in origin or it may be acquired. This displacement of the skull downward on the upper cervical spine has been likened to a "pumpkin on a stick". It develops in Paget's disease typically, but also occurs in other illnesses affecting bone such as osteomalacia, rickets, and osteogenesis imperfecta. Congenital anomalies associated with basilar impression include occipitalization of the atlas and spina bifida of C1.

Os Odontoideum. The normal odontoid process develops embryologically from separate osseous centers. Failure of fusion of the odontoid process to the body of C2 occurs occasionally and results in a separated odontoid process from body of C2. This condition is known as os odontoideum. Signs and symptoms may be absent. The anomaly may mimic a nonunion fracture of the odontoid process. Os odontoideum and a malunited fracture of the odontoid may be clinically and radiographically indistinguishable. Some authors believe that trauma is the underlying cause of os odontoideum and that it is almost always a result of fracture nonunion.

Fracture of the Odontoid Process. Fracture of the odontoid process results from acute trauma to the head and neck. The fracture may occur at various points along the peg-like structure. Usually the fracture occurs in the midportion of the odontoid. Less often the fracture involves only the tip, or the fracture occurs at the base and extends into the body of C2 itself. The odontoid is seldom dislocated significantly because it is attached to several strong ligaments. In general, fractures of the odontoid heal well, particularly those at the midportion or at the base of the process. Occasionally nonunion develops as well as instability of the C1-C2 interspace.

CLINICAL PRESENTATION

Basilar impression, os odontoideum, and fracture of the odontoid process may all affect the musculoskeletal system and central nervous system. Compression and distortion of nerve roots in the suboccipital region and in the posterior aspect of the neck cause local pain. Pain often radiates over the occipital scalp because the second cervical dorsal nerve root is compressed at its root foramen or because of excessive motion in the intervertebral joint. Nerve root compression in this area does not cause detectable motor function loss, but sensory loss can sometimes be recognized. Occasionally brain stem signs develop, particularly if basilar impression is present or if the odontoid process that is either free or fractured compresses the upper cervical cord or lower brain stem. Hypoglossal nerve paresis, nystagmus, dysphagia, vertigo, and weakness of the sternocleidomastoid and trapezius muscles may appear.

Compression of the spinal cord is the most ominous clinical sign of these bony lesions. Long tract signs including hyperreflexia in all four extremities, weakness, spasticity, ankle clonus, and extensor plantar responses are typical. Sensory loss may be diffuse, with or without a detectable sensory level.

Occasionally congenital anomalies of the cervical spine, including os odontoideum and basilar impression, are associated with other anomalies in the cervical area. A short neck with webbed trapezius muscles suggests the presence of Klippel-Feil syndrome. Spasmodic torticollis may also occur.

Subjective complaints, in addition to headache, include fainting episodes, particularly on turning the head or flexing the neck; dizziness; and diplopia. Sometimes Lhermitte's sign, the phenomenon associated with paresthesias in the legs and back produced by flexion or extension of the neck, is experienced by the patient when the cervical cord is compressed or stretched.

Acquired lesions of C1 and C2, not associated with fracture, develop in patients with Down's syndrome and in those with rheumatoid arthritis. In both conditions, the upper cervical spine may become unstable as ligaments lose their tensile strength. Progressive subluxation of C1 on C2 then develops. Cord signs and symptoms and neck pain appear in a manner similar to that occurring with os odontoideum and fracture of the odontoid process.

NATURAL HISTORY

The patient with platybasia alone, a radiographic finding, has no specific signs or symptoms and no sequelae because of the abnormal shape of the base of the skull. Patients with basilar impression, on the other hand, develop progressive difficulty at the foramen magnum level because of progressive invagination of the cervical spine into the foramen. Uncontrolled metabolic bone disease accounts for the progressive deformity. Long tract signs including spasticity, clonus, and weakness are typical. Similar clinical changes develop in patients with os odontoideum and fracture of the odontoid process. Some patients have little or no difficulty despite the presence of basilar impression, judged radiographically, or odontoid fracture.

If nonunion of a fractured odontoid process develops, arthritic change is accelerated. Neck rotation is then limited progressively. Pain is often present, particularly at the base of the skull.

DIAGNOSTIC CHOICES

Plain films of the cervical area and skull are the initial radiographic step. Typically, platybasia is recognized because of the angulation between the frontal fossa and the clivus. If the angle is greater than 145 degrees, platybasia is said to be present.

Basilar impression is noted classically on plain films by two measurement techniques. The first is the position of the odontoid process in relation to Chamberlain's line as shown on a lateral skull film. The line is drawn on the lateral film between the hard palate and the posterior rim of the foramen magnum. If the odontoid process lies above that line, basilar impression is said to occur. The second line is Fischgold's bimastoid line. A line is drawn between the mastoid tips on an AP view of the skull. The line should lie above the odontoid process. If the odontoid process protrudes above Fischgold's line, basilar impression is diagnosed.

Plain radiographs of the cervical area may detect

an os odontoideum, particularly on a lateral or open-mouth AP view. Fracture of the odontoid is also seen best on these projections. Open-mouth AP views of the upper cervical spine are essential in order to visualize the intervertebral area between C1 and C2, as well as the base of the skull.

Plain films may be augmented by tomographic views of the area. AP and lateral projections demonstrate the integrity of the odontoid process in clear detail, as well as its relationship to the foramen magnum anteriorly and posteriorly.

Flexion/extension views may be used if stability of the spine in the cervicomedullary area is questionable. These views are done with either plain film or with tomographic techniques. The relationship of the space between the odontoid process and the anterior portion of the atlas is an essential observation. That gap should not exceed 2 to 3 mm in the adult. In children under 5 years of age, the normal interval may be up to 5 mm because of the relative flexibility of the ligaments investing the odontoid process and holding it against the atlas.

Flexion/extension views should not be obtained when the patient is anesthetized or comatose. Because this maneuver is potentially harmful to the patient, it should be done when he or she is awake and able to gauge the safe limits of flexion and extension subjectively.

Cervical myelography with water-contrast medium is an important diagnostic tool, provided there is question of compression of the cervical cord and roots. This technique, coupled with CT scanning in the transverse dimension, can give precise anatomic detail in the area. Sagittal reconstruction of the CT scans can add further to bony features of the area of interest. The relationships of the foramen magnum, the odontoid process, and adjacent structures are clearly shown by these tests.

Other diagnostic techniques that are sometimes useful include somatosensory evoked potentials for function of the cord to augment the clinical neurological examination and electromyography of the neck muscles if a question of root compression exists. These techniques are rarely needed.

TREATMENT CHOICES

Basilar Impression. If the spinal cord is compressed and clinical signs are related to that level of compression, decompression is essential. In the case of basilar impression, the primary problem is that of the bony structures anterior to the spinal cord and medulla. Secondary compression of the cord and medulla may develop posteriorly from the intact rim of the foramen magnum. Surgery by the transoral route to remove the anterior rim of the foramen magnum, the invaginated anterior ring of the atlas, and the malpositioned odontoid process is often effective. Posterior decompression, on the other hand, is also effective in some cases provided angulation of the cervicomedullary junction is not acute

so that the decompression procedure damages the underlying cord and stability is provided by the anterior bony structures. The posterior procedure is done most often because complications are fewer.

Os Odontoideum. Treatment is focused on relief of signs and symptoms. Immobilization of a hypermobile joint is an obvious first step. If immobilization is achieved, pain subsides and long tract signs and symptoms may abate. A simple cervical collar can sometimes be effective alone, particularly if stability is relatively good and diagnostic studies show no significant compression of the spinal cord.

Posterior fusion, incorporating C1 and C2 at the minimum, but preferably C1, C2, and C3, is also effective. This procedure serves to immobilize the rim of C1 around the unattached os odontoideum so that it can no longer intermittently compress the cord anteriorly during flexion and extension of the neck. The os should be aligned prior to fusion by skeletal traction. An anterior operation by the transoral route may be employed to remove the os as an alternative form of treatment. The anterior procedure may be accompanied by a fusion anteriorly between C1 and C2 at the same time or posteriorly with bone graft from C1, C2, and C3 at a later time. Wire fixation is done posteriorly to enhance the fusion in the early weeks after operation.

Fracture of the Odontoid Process. Most fractures of the odontoid process heal if the region is immobilized for several months. Initial reduction of the fracture and immobilization are best accomplished with skeletal traction applied to the skull with the neck in neutral position. When alignment is good, external or internal immobilization is carried out.

External immobilization for 3 to 6 months results in a healed fracture in 85 percent of cases. The external devices available consist of (1) continuous traction and bed rest on a Stryker frame or (2) a halo-jacket apparatus and early ambulation of the patient. The halo-jacket device is preferred today because prolonged bed rest is avoided and rehabilitation can be started early.

Internal immobilization is provided by wire fixation of the intact laminae and bony fusion of C1 and C2 posteriorly at the minimum, and commonly of C1, C2, and C3 inclusive. Early stability results in 95 percent of cases. In addition, an external metallic frame is avoided, prolonged hospitalization is unnecessary, and bony union occurs with a high degree of probability.

The choice of treatment depends on the clinical setting and whether or not neurological signs are present. Most physicians today stress early rehabilitation and ambulation of the patient as basic goals, and they choose the treatment options that allow these goals to be reached.

The basic principle of treatment in each of the conditions described in this chapter is to decompress neural structures and stabilize the involved spine and skull. If the primary compression is anterior, anterior decompression is logical and preferable. If compression is posterior, the posterior approach is better. If the compression is both anterior and posterior, posterior compression and fusion are generally indicated because complications are less frequent.

COMPLICATIONS OF TREATMENT

Complications of the posterior route include increased neurological deficit, infection, and cord compression by either the fusion mass itself or from a postoperative hematoma. If a complication arises early, emergency decompression is indicated. In the case of anterior operations, infection is a higher risk and bony fusion is less predictable. In addition, compression of the upper cervical cord may develop during extraction of an os odontoideum, while decompressing the anterior rim of the foramen magnum, or when removing the fractured odontoid process itself.

OUTCOME

Surgery for basilar impression, os odontoideum, and fracture of the odontoid is effective to reduce pain and stabilize neurological disability. If neurological deficits develop secondary to cervicomedullary compression, an accurate diagnosis and early appropriate treatment are essential because clinical outcome depends on the severity of disability existing prior to treatment. Because the consequences of unrelieved cord compression at a high cervical level are so serious, precise and carefully planned management is vital.

NEUROLOGICAL DEFICIT COMPLICATING SCOLIOSIS

SHELLEY N. CHOU, M.D., Ph.D.

Patients with spinal deformities such as scoliosis, kyphosis, kyphoscoliosis, and lordosis are usually seen by orthopaedic surgeons. Neurosurgeons do not, as a rule, see such patients as primary consulting physicians. When a neurosurgeon is consulted regarding such a case, it is usually under one or more of the following conditions:

Group I.   To evaluate neurological deficit due to the spinal deformity and/or rule out intraspinal disease processes such as spinal cord tumors.
Group II.   To assess potential neurological risks of surgical or nonsurgical management to correct the spinal deformity.
Group III. To manage cases in which either nonsurgical or surgical procedures have precipitated neurological complications.

In this chapter, plans of management for the aforementioned conditions and steps toward resolving the problems will be conceptually outlined. There will be no detailed description regarding surgical techniques.

General principles in the management plan deal with information collection (i.e., history taking), clinical objective clarification (i.e., physical and neurological examination), and finally diagnostic procedural confirmation by a variety of imaging techniques.

For groups I and II, information regarding pain, whether radicular pain or myelopathic/dysesthetic pain, provides some indication whether the pain is due to nerve root irritation or compression and, if so, at what approximate level. On the other hand, the myelopathic pain, often less descriptive for lack of words to communicate, has more of a "burning" or "itching" quality. Progression of the pain indicates progression of the disease process. Pain that becomes more severe with change in posture implies spinal loading, which may mean instability of the spinal deformity.

Other symptoms, such as muscular weakness or stiffness of lower extremities, a feeling of numbness, and, in more advanced cases, urinary bladder symptoms and sexual or bowel problems may be present. In most cases symptoms develop insidiously over many years. Occasionally acute symptoms may be precipitated by trauma.

It is important to remember that symptoms of spinal cord compression due to idiopathic or congenital spinal deformity manifest themselves when the patient is at the so-called "growing spurt" period, that is, in the teens. When the thoracic spine, particularly from T3 to T8, is involved, there is far more risk of neurological compromise. Additionally, of the variety of spinal deformities, kyphoscoliosis appears to be the major culprit causing spinal cord compression, kyphosis the next, and scoliosis the least.

Spinal deformity also may be associated with a spinal cord tumor, usually of the intramedullary variety. Rarely, a herniated intervertebral disc may cause marked scoliosis, which may be the presenting symptom instead of radicular pain due to the disc lesion.

The examiner should pay special attention to both the spinal deformity itself and associated findings of cutaneous abnormalities, such as a hair patch over the spine and stigmata of neurofibromatosis. The so-called bending test is a simple one to perform. In this test the patient is simply asked to bend forward to touch the floor with both hands. The patient with congenital or idiopathic spinal deformity would bend down and back up without deviating to either side. The patient with a spinal deformity and a spinal cord tumor would deviate to one side. The reason for this difference is not known.

Obviously a full neurological examination should be performed. Findings of spasticity, hyperreflexia, and sensory deficit should be noted. The examination should always include a rectal examination to test the sphincter tone, that is, sphincter voluntary contraction and sensation.

Radiologic examination of such patients should include x-ray films of the entire spine, in both the erect and the supine position. These views demonstrate not only the deformity, but also whether the deformity is exaggerated with loading (i.e., erect position). In patients with kyphosis, the apex may be rigid or flexible which may have import regarding options and risks of therapy. In a patient with a rigid apex traction using increasing weights will not only be unfruitful but also risky in potentially producing neurological deficits. One should also look for scalloping of the vertebral bodies, pedicular erosion, spina bifida, and signs of diastematomyelia. Such findings, except the last, increase the possibility that an associated spinal cord tumor is present.

Contrast studies such as large volume myelograms have been used successfully to exclude intrinsic spinal cord disease. Now that MRI is available, this new technology will become the procedure of choice.

This overall assessment should both rule out intraspinal lesions and provide information to assess risks involved in nonoperative or operative corrections of the spinal deformity. It should be emphasized that the indication for surgical decompression of spinal cord compression due to spinal deformity is progressive myelopathy. The surgical approach should be an anterior decompression followed by a fusion. For a lesser degree of angulation involving limited vertebral segments, the Capner procedure, which is an extrapleural approach, may be used. For more extensive deformity, the transthoracic, sometimes combined with the retroperitoneal, approach is the procedure of choice.

In group III patients, the neurosurgeon is dealing with neurological complications of nonsurgical or surgical management.

The nonsurgical neurological complications result from skeletal traction (either too much or applied too quickly). Generally, the orthopaedic surgeon uses halo-femoral traction for these patients with flexible (nonrigid) spinal deformities. The weights applied depend on the patient's size and body weight. The intent is to reduce the deformity as much as possible nonsurgically, then to perform a spinal fusion to stabilize the spine. If this traction is too forceful or is enforced too quickly, certain neural elements would also be adversely distracted, thus producing a variety of neurological deficits. Such deficits can be cranial nerve palsies VI, IX, and X—in that order;

peripheral nerve palsies, the brachial plexus, peroneal nerve; sympathetic trunk traction in the neck to cause Horner's syndrome; and finally spinal cord distraction. When any or several of these complications occur, it is imperative to discontinue the traction to allow the deficits to recover; fortunately, most of them do recover if detected early. The traction then can again be applied, but obviously more deliberately and carefully to achieve the desirable reduction. It should be obvious that these patients under traction should be neurologically monitored.

The most-feared complication is postoperative paraplegia. The majority are due to overdistraction by instrumentation, as with the Harrington rods. A certain number of such complications may be due to direct injury of the spinal cord by a surgical manipulation. The intraoperative "wake up" test described by Vauzelle et al is helpful in avoiding such tragedies. The test consists of letting the patient "wake up" during surgery after the instrumentations are fixed to see whether the patient's leg movements are still intact. It sounds almost primitive, but most patients have no recollection of this experience. Whether spinal cord evoked potential monitoring can unfailingly replace this test is still not known at present.

The patient who becomes paraplegic on awakening from surgery should be immediately returned to the operating room to have the instruments removed. Time is of the utmost importance. A 3- to 4-hour delay may result in permanent paraplegia. Unless there is direct pressure on the spinal cord by broken bone, a dislocated hook, or hematoma, laminectomy is not indicated.

It should be emphasized that when the neurosurgeon is called to evaluate such a patient, there is little time available. Information should be collected quickly and concisely and decision making should be prompt. The situation usually is made difficult by the fact that the patient is just beginning to come out of anesthesia and cannot cooperate with the examiner. The patient is usually in extreme pain. Movement of the legs and urination may be difficult, not on the basis of neurological compromise, but on the basis of pain. The neurosurgeon should perform the examination carefully and expeditiously. A rectal examination is very important to test the sphincter tone and the sphincteric contraction. If the preponderance of the neurological function of the lower extremities and the sphincters is intact, neurological function of the lower extremities and the sphincters is intact, a period of careful monitoring is indicated. In my experience most of these patients improve functionally in time. However, if the neurological function deteriorates during this period of observation, the patient should be returned to the operating room for removal of the instruments.

SPINAL METASTASIS WITH AND WITHOUT NEUROLOGICAL DEFICIT

JOSEPH H. GALICICH, M.D.

Metastatic disease of the spine is a common and often disabling complication of cancer. It may occur with virtually any malignancy, but its incidence among the various types of cancer differs widely. Spinal metastases have been reported to be present in as many as 70 percent of patients who die from breast cancer. Other cancers that commonly metastasize to the spine are those of prostate, lung, and the hematopoietic system. In approximately 10 percent of patients, the site of origin of the primary tumor cannot be identified.

Pain, the hallmark of spinal metastasis, is almost always the first symptom and may become the most debilitating aspect of the patient's disease. Spinal-cord compression, the most feared consequence of metastasis to this site, occurs in approximately 5 percent of cancer patients who die from their disease. If unsuccessfully treated, the resulting immobility not only is psychologically devastating but also influences survival. Increased susceptibility to intercurrent infection, logistical problems in obtaining care, and waning enthusiasm for vigorous treatment by the paraplegic cancer patient and his or her physicians, all undoubtedly contribute to a decreased survival time.

Although prevention of intractable pain and incapacitating neurological deficit in patients with spinal metastasis is not always possible even with the best of efforts, it is facilitated by early diagnosis and prompt, individualized treatment. Aside from an understanding of the biological behavior of the particular tumor type and its anticipated response to various modes of therapy, rational treatment planning depends upon the general and neurological condition of the patient and a precise knowledge of the extent of the disease in the spine. Much of the uncertainty regarding treatment of spinal metastasis, especially when accompanied by spinal-cord compression, has been generated by results of retrospective studies in which a single method of treatment, either radiation therapy or laminectomy has been employed without regard to important variables, such as radiosensitivity of the tumor, the presence of structural deformity that contributes to cord compression, and the position of the tumor in the epidural space. In patients undergoing surgery, it is often unclear how much of the tumor was removed.

PATHOLOGICAL ANATOMY

The majority of spinal metastases are blood-borne and represent growth of tumor emboli that have lodged in the highly vascularized cancellous bone. Their distribution corresponds well in both the transverse and axial planes to the bulk of this target, with a preponderance located in the body as compared to the arch of the vertebra, and in the thoracic vertebrae as opposed to other regions of the spine. As a corollary to the disposition of such bony metastasis, invasion of the spinal canal by the neoplasm, a secondary event, most commonly occurs anteriorly and is often associated with collapse of the involved vertebral body. Asymmetric origin or growth of the metastasis in a vertebral body and the relatively firm barrier imposed by the posterior longitudinal ligament overlying the middle third of the body accounts for many of the tumors which occupy the anterolateral aspect of the spinal canal. A less frequent but nevertheless significant mode of involvement of the spine is direct extension from primary or metastatic paravertebral neoplasms. Such invasion of the spine is particularly common in cancer of the lung, especially those tumors that originate in the superior sulcus. Aside from destruction of adjacent bone, tumors located lateral to the spine may invade the spinal canal through the foramina. Occasionally, in tumors such as neuroblastoma, this occurs without invasion of the surrounding bone. A small number of secondary tumors that occupy the epidural space present without evidence of bone destruction or migration through foramina. These presumably arise from metastasis directly to the epidural contents. Penetration of the dura by metastatic neoplasm is infrequent. In metastatic disease, intradural tumors usually represent nodular tumor growth in the subarachnoid space, secondary to carcinomatous meningitis or blood-borne intramedullary metastases. Both are uncommon but must be considered in the differential diagnosis of patients with known cancer who illustrate cord and root dysfunction.

The pathological anatomy of spinal-cord compression by metastatic tumor is usually considerably more complex than that encountered in patients with the common benign neoplasms. The differences are due to the more rapid growth of the metastatic tumors, their location in the epidural space, the tendency to involve multiple sites, and the associated destruction of bone. Prior to producing neurological deficit, metastatic tumors have often filled the available space in the spinal canal over many segments far removed from their point of origin. A small increment in the size of the mass, by tumor growth or swelling secondary to infarction, or stasis in the epidural veins, may then produce rapid compression of the spinal cord over a large area. Compression may also be precipitated by a sudden focal narrowing of the spinal canal caused by pathological fracture of one or more vertebral bodies. In this common situation, extrusion of bone or disc into the canal, angulation of the spine, and epidural tumor may all contribute to the compressive force.

DIAGNOSIS

In patients known to have active cancer or in those previously treated for cancers with a predilection for bony metastases, such as breast and prostrate cancer, persistent neck or back pain should be regarded as evidence of spinal metastasis until proven otherwise. The importance of pain, long recognized as an almost universal premonitory symptom of spinal-cord compression, cannot be overemphasized. The one variable shown to be important in almost all clinical series that have evaluated results of treatment of spinal-cord compression caused by metastatic disease is timing of therapy in relation to the severity of neurological deficit. All too often the neurosurgeon is asked to treat an irretrievably paraplegic patient whose back pain, passed off as a sprain, has been present weeks or months before the onset of weakness. The patient as well as the physician should be educated about the value of this important warning signal.

At onset, the pain is usually intermittent, is often precipitated by movement or jarring of the spine as when bending or coughing and is frequently relieved by bedrest; it is almost always well localized to the site of involvement. Radicular pain with or without chronic localized spinal pain, when caused by spinal metastasis, indicates invasion of the epidural space, a paravertebral tumor, or pathological fracture. Severe, unrelenting localized pain of sudden onset is often associated with a compression fracture of the vertebral body.

On examination, localized tenderness is often present when the involved area is palpated or percussed. In advanced tumors of the spine, a paraspinal mass or a gibbus may be evident. In patients with spine metastasis, a negative neurological examination does not rule out significant epidural tumor. Patients without long tract signs who are subsequently shown on myelography to have a high-grade or complete block are not rare.

In patients without neurological deficit, plain x-ray films of the suspected portion of the spine and an isotope bone scan should first be carried out. The latter is usually the more sensitive in detecting early bone disease, and even if bone destruction in the area under suspicion is evident on plain x-ray films, bone scan is useful to determine the existence of occult disease elsewhere in the spine as well as in long bones and skull. Unless obviously at the very end stage of their disease, almost all patients with newly discovered spinal metastases, who do not have major neurological deficit, should also have myelography. A possible exception is the patient in whom the CT scan confirms the presence of metastasis in the vertebral body well away from the spinal canal. Any patient with a paravertebral tumor should have myelograhy prior to treatment, even when there is no demonstrable destruction of the adjacent spine.

In patients who have signs of spinal cord or cauda equina compression, an x-ray study of the entire spine should be done and promptly followed by myelography. If a complete block is encountered, definition of the upper limit of the tumor should be made by instilling radiopaque medium from above C1-C2 puncture. Pantopaque, if left in the subarachnoid space, usually permits gross assessment of the efficacy of treatment of compression without subsequent spinal puncture.

Removal of spinal fluid caudal to a complete subarachnoid block can precipitate rapid progression of spinal cord damage. In patients with obvious evidence of cord compression, 1 to 2 ml of Pantopaque should be instilled without removal of CSF, to determine if a complete block is present. If a complete block is encountered, this amount is usually sufficient to define the lower limits of the tumor. If the block is incomplete to Pantopaque, additional medium can then be injected. Except in the rare case of carcinomatous meningitis which mimics cauda equina compression in which meylography is not diagnostic, examination of the CSF is of little clinical value.

Whenever possible, CT scanning of the involved area should be performed prior to contemplated surgery to determine the presence and extent of bone destruction and paravertebral tumor. In patients who are to have vertebral body resection, sagittal tomography is useful to determine spinal alignment and protrusion of bone into the spinal canal and to assess the integrity of vertebral bodies immediately above and below those to be removed. Nuclear magnetic resonance scanning will almost undoubtedly replace most of these diagnostic procedures; in sagittal section it can simultaneously demonstrate fractures and angulation of the spine, bony and epidural tumor, distortion of the spinal cord, and paravertebral disease.

In patients who are candidates for surgery, results of more rigorous radiologic and laboratory tests may be important in decision making. These include: spinal angiography for tumors known to be highly vascular (i.e., thyroid and renal cell carcinoma) isotope or CT scanning of the liver; and pulmonary function testing in patients who have undergone major lung resection, have pulmonary metastasis, or have been treated with pneumotoxic chemotherapy. A history of recent treatment with drugs known to suppress bone marrow should obviously be taken into account.

TREATMENT

Therapeutic Goals

The armamentarium available for treating spinal metastasis includes chemotherapy, corticosteroids, radiation therapy, and surgery, either alone or in various combinations. Unfortunately, therapeutic options, especially surgical options, are often limited by the extent of the general and spinal disease. Many patients who harbor spinal metastases, whether or not they are accompanied by neurological deficit, have widespread rapidly progressing cancer. When predicted survival is less than six months, the aim of treatment must be palliation by the means least likely to interfere with the patient's remaining life span.

More aggressive therapy, especially of a single spinal metastasis, may be warranted for patients who are in good general health, including patients who are in the early stages of their disease or those known to have indolent tumors, either by the nature of the histology (e.g., follicular cancer of the thyroid) or by the course of their disease.

In addition, there is a small but extremely important group of patients for whom the therapeutic sights should be set higher. These include patients with: tumors in which potentially curative therapy exists, even in the face of metastatic disease such as some lymphomas and germ-cell tumors; apparently solitary spinal metastasis (the primary tumor has been removed and there is no other known metastasis); and primary paravertebral tumors with invasion of the adjacent spine, but without evidence of blood-borne metastasis.

Chemotherapy and Corticosteroids

At present, treatment of spinal metastasis with anti-cancer drugs is generally reserved for patients without significant epidural disease. These drugs are used routinely as initial therapy in patients who have neoplasms that are known to be highly sensitive to specific chemotherapeutic regimens, such as germ-cell tumors, small-cell carcinoma of the lung, lymphoma, multiple myeloma, neuroblastoma, and some sarcomas (e.g., malignant fibrous histiocytoma and osteogenic sarcoma). Supplemental radiation therapy is often given following initial stabilization of these diseases. Other patients for whom initial treatment with chemotherapy may be considered, especially when there are metastases to other sites, are those with tumors (such as breast and non-small-cell lung cancer) in which there is a substantial response rate. If there is no improvement, radiation therapy is indicated. Hormonal therapy for patients with receptor-positive breast carcinoma may be of considerable therapeutic value and may be helpful in controlling pain in patients with prostate cancer. Preoperative chemotherapy has proven to be of benefit to some patients with large paravertebral sarcomas.

Corticosteroids have proven to be oncolytic in some cases of Hodgkins and nonHodgkins lymphoma. They have been used successfully to relieve spinal-cord compression in a few patients with these tumors who cannot receive further radiation therapy and who are not candidates for surgery. Corticosteroids also afford significant pain relief to many patients with spinal metastases from every type of cancer, who have failed other treatment. The major value of corticosteroids, however, is in the treatment of spinal-cord compression. In high doses, they often reverse moderate neurological deficit and usually forestall major deficit long enough to permit adequate evaluation prior to major spinal surgery. The use of corticosteroids in patients undergoing radiation therapy, reduces the risk of swelling of the tumor and in many instances allows time for reduction in the size of the epidural tumor to take place, without further damage to neural tissue.

Radiation Therapy

Radiotherapy is presently the mainstay of treatment for spinal metastases. For patients with little or no epidu-ral disease who have radiosensitive tumors, it often provides palliation for long periods and may afford significant relief of pain for those with relatively radioresistant neoplasms. For patients with spinal-cord compression who are also potential candidates for surgery, the sensitivity of the tumor to radiation is crucial when selecting the initial mode of therapy. In exquisitely sensitive tumors such as some lymphomas, adequate decompression may be achieved within 24 to 48 hours after starting radiation. However, reduction in volume of epidural mass in patients with tumors usually considered to be quite radiosensitive (e.g., breast and prostate cancer) may not begin for a week or more after therapy is initiated. In the case of tumors that are only moderately sensitive, such as most non-small-cell carcinomas of the lung, this period may be as long as 4 to 6 weeks. It is the concomitant use of corticosteroids and not the radiation therapy itself that is responsible for the rapid stabilization or improvement in neurological signs that may be seen in these patients. Furthermore, treatment with corticosteroids must be continued throughout the course of radiation therapy, and the decision for tapering should be made on the basis of myelographic assessment. Radiation therapy or treatment of spinal-cord compression secondary to resistant tumors (e.g., melanoma and carcinoma of the kidney and colon) is usually futile and, when combined with the prolonged use of corticosteroids, only complicates any subsequent attempt at surgical decompression.

Surgery

Relatively few patients with spinal metastases are candidates for surgery. Patients without neurological deficit who may benefit from surgery are principally those with pathological fracture of one or more vertebral bodies that produce intractable pain or potentially dangerous instability. Fracture dislocations of the cervical spine should first be reduced and stabilized with a halo jacket. Internal fixation can then be accomplished. With C1-C2 dislocation, most commonly seen in breast carcinoma, posterior fusion with wire and acrylic followed by radiation therapy, is usually indicated. When a vertebral body or several contiguous bodies have largely been replaced by tumor and the adjacent vertebrae are intact, removal of the tumor-involved bone and vertebral stabilization with pins and acrylic is usually the procedure of choice. In vertebral body replacement that involves the cervicothoracic and the thoracolumbar junctions, it is often judicious to provide additional stabilization by posterior fusion as well. Bone is used for fusion only in patients with very indolent tumors, in whom there is a long life expectancy and radiation therapy is not required.

In isolated paravertebral neoplasms without epidural extension, optimal treatment consists of gross total removal of all tumor, including adjacent tumor-infiltrated bone, *en bloc* if possible, followed by radiation therapy. Much higher doses of radiation than could otherwise be tolerated can be delivered locally by means of brachytherapy. Catheters are positioned over the tumor bed at surgery and are brought out through separate skin incisions. Radiation sources are inserted postoperatively and removed with the catheters when the designated dose has been achieved. If such neoplasms are associated with epidural tumor, this should be thoroughly removed as well, and the brachytherapy should be supplemented by external radiation to the spinal canal.

In patients with spinal-cord compression, considerable improvement in the results of surgery over those previously reported can be achieved not only by earlier diagnosis, but also by better patient selection, tailoring of the approach to the anatomical problem, and attention to stabilization of the spine. Patients who are prime candidates for surgery are those whose life expectancy exceeds six months, who have a single compressive site, have not received radiation therapy to the area, and have minimal signs of cord compression. If such a patient has a very radio-sensitive tumor and no structural abnormalities that contribute to the compression, radiotherapy might be considered as an alternative. However, if the tumor is of a type known to be radioresistant, or if there is considerable local destruction or instability of the spine, surgery should be the obvious choice. Because, with the possible exception of a few tumors known to be highly radio-sensitive, mechanical removal of mass is the only rapid method of decompression, surgery is also indicated in patients with severe but retrievable neurological deficit, especially when it is preceded by a rapid downhill course.

The goal of surgery is to remove all mass, bone as well as tumor, that is compressing the spinal cord and to provide adequate stabilization. Laminectomy is necessary for tumors lying dorsal to the spinal cord and for laterally placed tumors that extend for considerable distances. Laminectomy or hemilaminectomy can be combined with removal of the adjacent facets and pedicles to gain access to anterolateral tumors when the vertebral body is intact. Such a posterolateral approach is often facilitated by the fact that the facets, transverse processes, and pedicles have been replaced by tumor. Metastatic tumors situated anterior to the spinal cord are almost invariably associated with replacement of all, or a major portion, of the vertebral body with tumor. Vertebral body resection usually permits removal of all epidural tumor, but occasionally must be combined with removal of portions of the vertebral arch to gain access to epidural extensions of tumor.

Adequate stabilization is usually provided by replacement of the vertebral bodies with acrylic, reinforced and held in position by two or three stout Steinman pins which span the intervening space and are inserted into the intact vertebral bodies above and below. In the posterior and posterolateral approaches, additional stabilization is usually not required when the corresponding vertebral bodies are intact. However, if they are not, stabilization can be provided by the use of Harrington rods.

Unfortunately, total removal of metastatic tumors of the spine, especially when they involve the epidural space, is rarely achieved by any surgical approach, even when done with the utmost care. For patients who are candidates for either surgery or radiation therapy, surgery followed by radiation therapy would therefore appear to be the most rational form of treatment.

THORACIC SPINAL CORD TUMOR (MENINGIOMA AND NEUROFIBROMA)

FREDERICK A. SIMEONE, M.D.

Meningiomas and neurofibromas are predominant among the benign tumors that compress the spinal cord of adults. Their distribution among the different levels of the spine is relatively proportional, and consequently these tumors occur in the thoracic region more often than in the cervical, lumbar, or sacral divisions of the spine.

These tumors are the neurologist's or neurosurgeon's delight because they can be removed easily, and frequently a grateful patient ultimately reports complete neurological recovery. On the other hand, they frequently mystify the physician who sees the patient early in the course of the illness. These tumors are rarely diagnosed by the primary physician because they are uncommon and the index of suspicion is low. Furthermore, they can masquerade as other, more common conditions. For instance, several patients have undergone gallbladder surgery because the neurofibroma compressed the seventh or eighth thoracic nerve root on the right. Nerve root compression at the third to fifth thoracic nerve roots on the left can launch extensive investigation of angina pectoris. Diabetic patients who develop nerve root compression secondary to these tumors are usually treated for neuropathy. In older patients with these intraspinal tumors and concurrent cervical disc generation, the latter is usually implicated for the myelopathy until a myelogram reveals the culprit. The list goes on.

It is not that these tumors are "great masqueraders". They do occur insidiously, grow slowly, and produce soft, progressive neurological signs and symptoms. As mentioned, some compress thoracic nerve roots and produce chest or abdominal pain. Others grow between nerve roots and only a slowly progressive sensory or motor myelopathy evolves.

Certain distinctions between these tumors and other types of neoplasm which can affect the spinal cord are worthy of mention. Anatomically, neurofibromas and meningiomas are classified as intradural extramedullary tumors. Together they represent most of the tumors seen in this location. The remaining two anatomic sites are extradural (principally tumors that metastasize to the spine and surrounding structures) and intramedullary (primarily tumors that originate from glial cells within the substance of the spinal cord). There are some clinical differentiations which are worth mentioning. In extradural tumors, axial pain is the principal symptom. Tumors that metastasize to the spine usually grow rapidly and produce local pain. On the other hand, intramedullary tumors generally progress slowly and are not associated with local somatic pain. Intradural extramedullary tumors such as neurofibromas and meningiomas generally grow slowly and cause pain if they happen to compress a nearby thoracic nerve root. The development of symptoms does not occur in a pattern that lends itself easily to clinical recognition. The neurological deficit occurs insidiously, whereas with extradural tumors, full-blown myelopathy can develop in a matter of days after the pain is originally perceived. On the other hand, intramedullary tumors are frequently heralded by a peculiar painless numbness which affects the extremities and is not ordinarily associated with local pain.

Over half the spinal tumors seen by a neurosurgeon are of the extradural type, principally metastatic. Of the remaining half, approximately seventy percent are of the intradural and extramedullary type, the majority of which are neurofibromas and meningiomas.

Meningiomas grow from cells of the arachnoid coverings of the spinal cord. They attach themselves early to the inner surface of the dura for blood supply. Neurofibromas grow up in the sheath of a nerve root, usually the dorsal division, and consequently are more likely than meningiomas to produce early pain and numbness. Approximately 80 percent of meningiomas and 40 percent of neurofibromas occur in the thoracic region.

There may be no evidence of either of these type of tumors on plain radiographs. Neurofibromas, because they may grow peripherally on a nerve root, can widen the intervertebral foramina. In the process they may also erode a vertebral pedicle. Foraminal widening and pedicle erosion may be subtle and difficult to determine except in retrospect. However, tumors that have grown large may present in this manner radiographically. When these tumors reach significant proportion, they grow out through the intervertebral foramen and produce a separate extension which will lie in a paraspinal location within or outside the chest cavity. Spine radiographs may show this outpouching. Neurofibromas that have an intraspinal part, with a constriction at the foramen, and then a large outpouching are frequently called "dumbbell" tumors because of their bilobed appearance. Meningiomas rarely erode pedicles or destroy the vertebral architecture. However, longstanding meningiomas may calcify and produce a typical ovoid appearance

within the spinal cord. The study of choice is complete myelography. Recent photographs of meningiomas and neurofibromas in the thoracic region have been generated by magnetic resonance imaging. This technique promises to be an excellent way to visualize the entire spinal canal without the risks and discomfort of myelography, and in future years MRI is likely to replace myelography. Excellent images of meningiomas and neurofibromas have been made with conventional computed tomography, with and without the injection of contrast material in the subarachnoid space. Because the thoracic spine is so long, however, CT scanning is rarely the first study undertaken to diagnose these lesions. They are usually picked on myelography, and then a CT scan is performed through the appropriate levels of myelographic defect.

The myelogram itself can be somewhat diagnostic. Because of their intradural and extramedullary location, the tumors are clearly outlined by the contrast material. They often produce a lima bean-shaped filling defect outlined by myelographic contrast material. Other diagnostic studies are rarely of value in the diagnosis of intraspinal neurofibromas and meningiomas. Electromyography has little role. Although the protein determination of the spinal fluid usually is high, because of the propensity of these tumors to produce complete block prior to their recognition, attention to protein levels is usually a result of historic conditioning.

The role of accurate preoperative radiographic studies cannot be overestimated. The precise location of the tumor within the spinal canal and its relationship, whether anterior, lateral, or posterior, to the spinal cord must be accurately assessed. This is because entirely different operative approaches from the conventional laminectomy are required when the tumor lies anterior to the thoracic spinal cord.

To best summarize the clinical syndrome, a typical thoracic meningioma patient's history and examination will encapsulate the following salient features:

The patient is commonly a middle-aged female. The incidence is three times greater in women and most common in the fifth to seventh decades. She may describe local thoracic pain that radiates to the anterior chest or abdomen. This pain quite typically is worse at night and frequently awakens her from sleep. The pain may be aggravated during the day by motion, coughing, or sneezing. At the time she seeks medical attention she may have few if any neurological findings. More likely, however, she will complain of a vague difficulty with gait. Lower extremity parasthesias are frequent, and these may be quite asymmetrical. She may be unsteady on her feet, unable to climb stairs easily, and weakness can progress so that a cane or walker is required. Bladder difficulty, consisting primarily of urgency and incontinence, is frequent.

Neurological examination shows increased reflexes in the lower extremities, unilateral or bilateral extensor plantar responses, and a sensory level to pinprick and temperature. The sensory level may be quite nonsymmetrical and is higher on the side opposite the weaker lower extremity. On rare occasion there is a band of decreased sensation which results when the tumor compresses a specific thoracic nerve root.

The clinical history is similar for neurofibromas except that they are not found predominantly in women, and they are scattered over a broader age group. Neurofibromas may occur in the teens and any decade thereafter. The index of suspicion for neurofibromas should be increased if the patient has evidence of von Recklinghausen's disease or a previous history of other neuroma removal (such as acoustic neuroma or subcutaneous neuromas). Neurofibromas are more likely to give nerve root signs early in their course. Rarely, a low thoracic neurofibroma or meningioma compresses the conus medullaris of the spinal cord below the innervation to the knees and feet. Consequently, the patient may have neither extensor plantar responses nor hyperreflexia. In these individuals, bladder symptoms are more frequent. However, a lower motor neuron clinical picture can result from a T12 neurofibroma or meningioma.

SURGICAL CORRECTION

The operative procedure must be carefully planned. If the operation is delicately executed, not only is the condition arrested, but spontaneous improvement in most of the neurological signs is the rule rather than the exception. Even patients who have advanced neurological compression secondary to these benign tumors should undergo surgical correction.

The contrast studies are carefully inspected. If the tumor is posterior or lateral to the cord, the back is marked under fluoroscopic control so that the tumor can be precisely located at the time of laminectomy. After the dura is opened, the operating microscope is brought into use. For ordinary meningiomas and intradural neurofibromas, the tumor can be easily separated from the surrounding structures without manipulaton of the spinal cord in any way. A large laterally placed tumor should be "debulked" before it is removed to prevent undue compression of the spinal cord during final delivery of the tumor capsule. Neurofibromas that grow on a nerve root may be traced to an intradural location, and an additional "dumbbell" may be found in the intervertebral foramen itself and require extension of the operative procedure into the posterior mediastinum and paraspinal area. These operations are safely performed, however, and complete excision is usually possible.

The most difficult patients are those whose meningioma or neurofibroma lies directly anterior to thoracic spinal cord. Manipulation of the thoracic spinal cord is particularly dangerous for the following reasons:

1. The thoracic spinal cord is generally avascular in comparison to the cervical and lumbar portions. Blood supply to the thoracic cord is a more or less "watershed" configuration, with the major areas of arterial input coming from above and below. Manip-

ulation of this relativey ischemic spinal cord may produce an intramedullary infarction.

2. The relationship between the diameter of the spinal cord and the diameter of the spinal canal is closer in the thoracic area than elsewhere in the spine. The spinal canal becomes narrow and there is simply no way to retract the spinal cord in order to effect tumor removal. The normal spinal cord is usually pressed up against the lamina, and consequently laminectomy over the cord cannot be safely performed.

For menigiomas that lie entirely anterior to the thoracic spinal cord a costotransversectomy approach is recommended. In this operation, the spine is visualized from the side after removal of one or two adjacent ribs. The surgeon can gain access to the spinal canal by removing the appropriate pedicles and incising the dura laterally while the lung is being retracted. With microsurgical instrumentation, the tumor is gradually teased from its location anterior to the spinal cord. The surgeon's view is a lateral one. With the microscope he can look to the side of the spinal cord and underneath it, bringing the tumor into view without actually manipulating the spinal cord structures. This is a tedious operative procedure, but the results are good. For anteriorly placed tumors, this operation is much safer, despite its more formidable nature, than conventional laminectomy. In rare instances it is not possible to completely remove a neurofibroma or a meningioma. The portion of meningioma that is attached to the dura can be cauterized, and thus the recurrence rate may be reduced.

After these tumors are surgically excised, the spinal cord is significantly deviated because of the chronic localized pressure. As healing develops, however, the spinal cord gradually resumes its configuration and lost function is restored. The patient may have to wait several months before ultimate recovery is realized.

If, for some technical reason, the tumor cannot be totally excised, radiation therapy might be considered. With patience and meticulous attention to detail, virtually all of these tumors should be excised at the primary operation. Reoperative surgery and radiation therapy are complicated and should be avoided. Localized x-ray treatment has been advised in patients who have had incomplete resections. It appears, however, that an already compromised spinal cord is susceptible to radiation necrosis and repeat surgery is difficult after radiation. Consequently the surgeon must strive to perform a complete removal at the time the tumor is discovered and should be both gentle and aggressive in his desire to effect a surgical cure.

Postoperative complications are relatively infrequent. Meticulous dural closure prevents spinal fluid leak after surgery. Most patients notice some immediate improvement in gait and bladder function. This is related principally to the duration of their symptoms, with patients having a shorter history experiencing more immediate relief. Early ambulation is encouraged in combination with physical therapy and reassurance.

Patients who are no weaker after surgery generally describe a progressive improvement in gait, which can continue for a period of several months after surgery. The ending is almost invariably happy.

In summary, thoracic neurofibromas and meningiomas should be considered in any patient who has a slow and relatively painless paraparesis which develops gradually over a period of several months. This is likely to be associated with increased reflexes in the lower extremities, extensor plantar response, and a sensory level. If radiographic studies fail to reveal a distinct bone lesion, complete myelography should be considered. During the study, the myelographer must be prepared, if one of these tumors is discovered, to reposition the patient to determine its extent. After adequate films in all planes are taken, an accurate scratch mark on the back will assist the surgeon in finding the tumor at the time of operation. Consultation with the surgeon at the time of the myelography is encouraged so that additional views may be taken and postmyelograhy deterioration can be monitored.

If, at the time of the myelography, the patient has a complete block, little if any spinal fluid should be withdrawn. This patient should be checked frequently in the immediate postmyelogram interval. If signs of neurological deterioration after the myelogram are observed, high-dose steroids and mannitol therapy should be considered. If these are ineffective in a relatively short time, the patient may be subjected to emergency surgery or spinal cord decompression. Although deterioration after myelography can happen, it is relatively rare, and good results can be expected with prompt medical or surgical decompression.

CAUDA EQUINA EPENDYMOMA

ROBERT M. CROWELL, M.D.

Primary intraspinal neoplasms are rarely intrinsic to the spinal cord. These tumors are generally low-grade with regard to their invasive potential and may extend over many segments of the spinal cord. Many such tumors have a well-defined cleavage plane with adjacent gliotic tissue in the spinal cord. When tumors undergo surgery in early stages, before severe neurological deficit has developed, a gratifying recovery and useful existence may be anticipated. Since many of these lesions are benign, long-term cure may be achieved when total removal is accomplished.

Intramedullary tumors occur in both adults and children. Virtually every type of tumor seen in the brain can occur in the spinal cord; nonetheless astrocytomas are most commonly cervical and thoracic in location, ependymomas are much more frequent in the caudal regions of the spinal cord owing to their prevalence in the conus medullaris and filum terminale. Ependymomas often have a distinct cleavage plane between the tumor and the cord tissue. These lesions are usually soft and solid with a pseudocapsule. They are not usually very vascular, and areas of necrosis may be encountered. Other tumors that may be encountered in this area include teratoma, dermoid, epidermoid, oligodendroglioma, hemangioblastoma, malignant tumors, and lymphomas. Ependymomas of the cord itself produce a fusiform enlargement with no indication of their presence on the surface other than an occasional dilated vein at the caudal end of the tumor. Ependymomas in the conus or filum terminale region frequently grow in exophytic fashion from an intramedullary locus, into the caudate equina, displacing and not infrequently adhering to nerve roots. Because of the expanding nature of such ependymomas, expansion of the osseous spinal canal may develop. Intramedullary tumors receive a blood supply from perforating branches of the anterior spinal and other nutrient arteries.

PRESENTATION

It is remarkable how large tumors in the spinal canal may grow with minimal symptomatology. At last, however, at a critical phase of tumor expansion, the spinal cord can no longer compensate, and deterioration in neurological function develops. Persistent pain involving the dorsal root dermatome in the area of the tumor is often the initial complaint associated with intramedullary tumor. There may or may not be progressive sensory disturbance with dysethesias and even posterior column dysfunction. Sacral sparing may or may not be present with intramedullary neoplasm. In some cases, lower motor neuron symptoms and signs develop in relation to the myotomes of the tumor. Well-defined central cord syndromes, as seen in syringomyelia, are often lacking in cases of intramedullary neoplasm. Symptoms are usually bilateral, but occasionally may be confined to a single extremity. Symptoms are generally progressive with remissions and exacerbations. The duration of symptoms is usually measured in years, although occasionally a case may present with a history of less than 6 months. Consistent with involvement of lumbar and sacral roots, cauda equina ependymomas often present with sensory and motor disturbance in the lower limbs as well as sphincteric incontinence. The degree of neurological deficit is variable, from mild deficit to virtual paraplegia; however, with increasing utilization of new diagnostic technique, cases with relatively mild symptomatology are now presenting with greater frequency to the neurological surgeon for evaluation and management.

EVALUATION

Plain lumbosacral spine films may show widening of the spinal canal in the upper lumbar zone, but the absence of this sign does not exclude the diagnosis. Heretofore, the radiologic confirmation of cauda equina ependymoma has hinged on myelography. In former times, Pantopaque was the contrast medium of choice. Pantopaque myelography was used to demonstrate a fusiform swelling of the spinal cord in the region of the tumor. Generally, a complete block has not been present. Since the introduction of water-soluble dyes (Amipaque), these agents are preferred for the demonstration of intramedullary lesions. When the diagnosis is suspected, the dye should be inserted via a low lumbar puncture (L4–L5 or L5–S1), in order to avoid puncture at the site of the lesion. When there is a complete block, an additional increment of dye should be instilled by a C1–C2 puncture. In rare cases, a differential diagnosis of vascular malformation or syringomyelia may indicate a need for additional studies such as spinal angiography. CT scanning of the spinal canal after the instillation of water-soluble contrast medium permits the identification of upper and lower margins of the lesion as well as the exclusion of a syrinx.

Other diagnostic methods, such as routine computed tomography or polytomography, have not been of practical use in the diagnosis of these tumors. Somatosensory evoked responses may be obtained preoperatively to assist with intraoperative monitoring of root function. Evaluation of bladder function with urologic consultation and cystometrogram is useful as a preoperative baseline. Magnetic resonance imaging offers promise as a tool to demonstrate the lesion without myelography.

SURGICAL MANAGEMENT

A surgeon exploring the spinal cord for a suspected intramedullary neoplasm should make every effort to remove the tumor since inspection, decompression, or subtotal removal creates complicated problems for subsequent surgical efforts at removal. Total removal produces the best results, and the best opportunity for total removal is at the initial surgical procedure.

Under general anesthesia, the patient is placed in the prone position. A standard decompressive laminectomy is performed over the area of the tumor. The facet joints, especially in a child, should be avoided to preclude postoperative spinal instability. The exposure should extend one segment above and below the level of the demonstrated neoplasm. The dura is then carefully opened, and great care is utilized to avoid hemorrhage since this could compromise identification of critical intradural landmarks. After the dura is opened, the operating microscope is wheeled into play at magnifications up to 40μ. The stereoscopic observer tube is utilized

to permit active participation by an assistant. Initially the surgeon must be sure that there is not an anterior extramedullary lesion splaying the cord and the nerve roots. In the case of ependymoma, the extra-axial portion of the lesion is removed initially to afford wide decompression and visualization of roots. Only then is attention directed to the lesion entering the spinal cord itself. Attention is initially directed toward removal of nonadherent tumor, with a view toward enabling clearer visualization and surgical manipulation of such tumor as may be adherent or densely incorporated into conus and roots. If a myelotomy is required, this is done in axial fashion in an effort to preserve as much vasculature as possible. In such a case, 6–0 sutures are placed through the pial margin of the myelotomy on either side in order to provide gentle retraction. The operating microscope and microsurgical instruments, particularly the bipolar cautery and fine dissectors, are used to develop a plane around the margin of the tumor. However, this is done only after its interior is debulked. This procedure may be carried out with the neurosurgical operating laser or the ultrasonic aspirating device, depending on the size and location of the tumor. With the laser, it is possible to remove literally one cell layer at a time; this precise technique does not mechanically interfere with the local neural tissues. The surgeon works primarily on the tumor and not on the spinal cord or nerve roots. Using fine forceps, it may be possible to gently tease the lesion away from the neural elements. In this setting, fine bipolar cautery is used to coagulate adhesions which have been cut with microscissors. In this way the lesion is gently removed from the surrounding neural elements. Blunt dissection is generally avoided. The operative field must be kept scrupulously dry to maintain visualization of the tumor plane. No attempt is made to remove cyst wall because this is not part of the lesion. If there is any question about total removal, small biopsies for frozen sections may be obtained. During surgery, continuous somatosensory evoked responses obtained by stimulation of the posterior tibial nerves and recorded over the scalp may be used to gauge the delicacy of surgery and the maintenance of neurological function. In addition, with a bladder catheter in place, arrangements may be made for intraoperative cistometrography; a nerve root is stimulated to identify the presence of S2, S3, or S4 with elevation in intracystic pressure.

After total removal of the lesion, the dura is closed primarily. Only rarely, when there has been prior surgery and/or radiotherapy, is there intense scarring necessitating reconstruction of the dura with a graft.

The results of surgery in a number of series have been gratifying. In the modern neurosurgical era, increased neurological deficit in this group of patients should be rare, and marked neurological improvement may be noted in some. Patients with mild to moderate neurological deficit often return to normal activity regardless of tumor size. Long-term follow-up has shown a low recurrence rate in cases of total removal of verified ependymoma. The effects of radiation on these tumors has been difficult to gauge. In some instances, beneficial effects have been reported, but a high percentage of histologically unverified tumors clouds the interpretation of such reports. There is little objective follow-up evidence of reduction in tumor size after radiation. Moreover, radiation therapy makes subsequent surgical intervention extremely difficult and is therefore not recommended as a primary approach. Should a patient show recurrence at a later time, reoperation would appear reasonable, with postoperative radiation if excision is incomplete. Only rarely has neurological deterioration been documented in patients after such surgical

intervention. This may be due to a postoperative hematoma, in which case immediate re-exploration would be warranted.

Occasionally, radicular pain in the distribution of nerve roots affected by the tumor has been a postoperative problem. This pain has a dysesthetic burning character, sometimes extremely difficult to control, but has been uncommon in cases in which the conus medullaris was not involved.

SPINAL CORD ASTROCYTOMA OF CHILDHOOD

FRED J. EPSTEIN, M.D.
JEFFREY H. WISOFF, M.D.

Intramedullary spinal cord astrocytoma is a relatively uncommon neoplasm accounting for only 4 percent of central nervous tumors of childhood. Over the past 4 years, we have operted on 100 young patients with very extensive astrocytomas, many of which involved the entire length of the spinal cord. This unusual series has provided us a unique opportunity to study the biology of the tumor and its response to conventional surgical and radiation therapy, and to develop a surgical technique that permits gross total resection of the neoplasms.

NEURODIAGNOSTIC STUDIES

Plain spine roentgenograms frequently demonstrated some degree of scoliosis, varying from mild to severe, and a widened canal often extending from the cervical to the lower thoracic or lumbar levels. Erosion and flattening of pedicles and scalloping of vertebral bodies were a common finding and invariably corresponded to the segments of the spinal cord that were spanned by solid tumor as compared to diffuse widening of the spinal canal, which was usually secondary to associated cysts. Since "holocord" widening is common, it is essential that lumbar myelography be combined with a C1-C2 puncture if a complete subarachnoid block is present. Postmyelography CT scan is routinely performed to help delineate the degree of cord widening. In addition, we routinely perform a delayed CT scan 24 hours after the myelogram to document delayed appearance of intrathecal contrast material within the cyst cavity. Occasionally intravenous contrast has supplemented the spinal CT scan and demonstrated an enhancing neoplasm.

In patients who have had previous laminectomy, real-time ultrasound is performed over the laminectomy defect and has been extremely helpful in delineating the extent of solid tumor versus associated cyst. Since large rostral and caudal cysts are frequently associated with a relatively focal solid tumor of six to ten segments, laminectomy need only be carried out over the region of solid tumor.

SURGICAL TECHNIQUE

The first patients on which we operated for what was presumed to be a holocord neoplasm, a total laminectomy was carried out from C2 to L1. We subsequently recognized that much of the cord widening was secondary to associated rostral and caudal cysts whose walls were non-neoplastic. Therefore it was only necessary to perform a limited laminectomy over the solid component of the neoplasm, as documented by our neurodiagnostic studies.

After the laminectomy is performed, the wound is filled with saline to allow intraoperative ultrasound. With the transducer set at a frequency of 7.5 MHz, the head of the probe (previously covered with a sterile sheath) is gently immersed without touching the dura. The area of solid tumor is localized as well as associated cysts. Intratumoral cysts are small and eccentrically located and have irregular margins. In contrast, the sonographic appearance of the non-neoplastic rostral and caudal cysts is smooth-walled, large, and centrally located.

The dura is opened in the routine fashion over the entire extent of solid tumor as documented by ultrasound. An attempt is made to identify the anatomic midline of the spinal cord; however, the anatomy is often unclear and surface landmarks may be distorted. Careful inspection of the cord surface may identify subpial tumor. Utilizing the operating microscope and the carbon dioxide laser on low wattage (6 to 8 watts), a midline myelotomy is performed. Myelotomy must extend over the entire length of the tumor. The rostral and caudal margins of the tumor sometimes are demarcated by smooth white-walled cyst containing xanthochromic fluid.

Pial traction sutures (6–0) are placed and facilitate tumor exposure, obviating retraction of normal cord. Attenuated white matter overlying the tumor is removed with either the laser or microdissectors and fine suction. Utilizing the cavitron ultrasonic surgical aspirator (CUSA) tumor removal is initiated at either the rostral or caudal pole of the solid tumor. The excision proceeds from within the center of the tumor laterally and anteriorly until a glial-tumor interface is identified. Small remaining fragments of tumor are vaporized with the carbon dioxide laser. In all of our patients, a gross total removal of the tumor with exposure of rostral and caudal cysts (when present) was accomplished. In patients who did not have the cystic dilatations of the spinal cord, a glial-tumor interface was obtained at both poles of the neoplasm. The dural was closed primarily in all patients unless it had been left open at a previous procedure. In these cases, a dural patch was utilized.

Somatosensory evoked potentials are monitored throughout the majority of the operative procedures. Although in some cases there were improvements in the wave form, I am not able to document that this had any clinical relevance. At present, this type of monitoring is desirable in terms of accumulating information, but whether it will prove a mandatory adjunct to spinal cord surgery remains to be seen.

DISCUSSION

Holocord astrocytoma forms a large subgroup (60%) among the spinal cord astrocytomas and, in our series, was a more common occurrence than the more limited neoplasm. Although this has been described in occasional case reports, the prevalence has not been previously recognized as a result of the earlier tendency not to carry out complete neurodiagnostic studies when a complete intramedullary block was observed on myelography.

There are a number of important observations that are clearly relevant in terms of understanding the biology of this group of neoplasms as well as recommending proper surgical management. It has been a consistent observation that the solid component of the astrocytoma is often not so extensive as myelography alone suggests, and indeed the actual location of the neoplasm may be in those segments of the spinal cord that correspond to neurological dysfunction. Demonstration of the rostral and caudal cysts by delayed metrizamide CT scan and ultrasonography is helpful. The lack of significant neurological dysfunction relating to the spinal segment that is distended with fluid is probably directly related to the anatomic location of the cyst within the center of the cord, as compared to the solid component of the neoplasm, which is relatively more diffuse. It is only necessary to expose and extirpate the solid portion of the neoplasm and drain the cysts in order to obtain a satisfactory surgical result. Therefore, a limited laminectomy over the solid portion of the neoplasm is sufficient. The extent of the laminectomy is defined by the combination

of neurological deficit, eroded pedicles, scalloped vertebral bodies, and area of maximal spinal cord widening on plain films and myelography and confirmed intraoperatively with ultrasound.

The presence of cysts that are similar in appearance to those associated with the cystic astrocytomas of the cerebellum suggests that these neoplasms are congenital tumors that had their inception during gestation. The fluid produced by the tumor extends up and down the spinal cord in the region of least resistance, that is, the central canal. We believe that the presence of a widened spinal cord from the cervicomedullary junction to the conus, which is associated with a relatively slowly evolving neurological deficit, is indicative of a very slow growing and perhaps even hamartomatous type of lesion which has a good long-term prognosis and should be treated aggressively. The rare malignant astrocytoma in this population presents with a different clinical picture: the neurological deficits develop rapidly and the prognosis parallels that of glioblastomas elsewhere in the central nervous system.

Benign astrocytomas are often firm, contain calcium deposits, and have no obvious cleavage plane to delineate them from normal neural tissue. The traditional surgical technique of suction and blunt dissection is relatively inefficient and may cause considerable traction on normal adjacent structures, accounting for the high incidence of neurological deficit in older series. The use of the cavitron ultrasonic surgical aspirator (CUSA) and the surgical laser have been indispensable surgical adjuncts in the radical resection of these tumors. The CUSA and the surgical laser permit fragmentation, emulsification, vaporization, and aspiration of the firmest tissue without any movement of adjacent normal spinal cord.

In most cases of holocord tumor, the initial complaint is a weak arm or a mildly weak leg and associated pain somewhere along the spinal axis. The signs and symptoms are consistently relatively minor when compared to the apparently diffuse nature of the pathologic process. It is perfectly understandable why a neurosurgeon, faced with this clinical dilemma, has been most concerned about inflicting a greater neurological deficit as a result of extensive dissection within a rather well-functioning spinal cord. This rationale has been used for a temporizing surgical approach consisting of a limited laminectomy and biopsy and relying on radiation therapy to control tumor growth. Unfortunately, the natural history of these tumors with radiation therapy is slow deterioration and eventual neurological disability.

The outcome following radical resection of these tumors is directly related to the preoperative neurological status. Although a transient increase in weakness or sensory loss was sometimes seen in the immediate postoperative period, only one patient had a significant permanent increase in neurological deficit following operation. Patients with paraparesis or quadriparesis who were ambulatory before surgery had stabilization of their deterioration and usually had neurological and functional improvement over several weeks. The group with severe deficits preoperatively rarely made any significant improvement, although their downhill course abated.

There is no evidence that radiation will cure benign astrocytomas of the spinal cord, and there is abundant evidence that it has a deleterious effect on the immature, developing nervous system. Spinal cord astrocytomas should be recognized as excisable lesions, and radiation therapy should be reserved for possible adjunctive use if there is a recurrence. At that time, it might be employed following a second radical surgical resection.

Children who have undergone extensive laminec-tomy and, in addition, have denervation of the paraver-tebral muscles from tumor as well as operative muscle retraction are likely to develop severe spinal deformities as they pass through periods of rapid growth. They must be treated with body braces, worn during waking hours, for several years after surgery. Close collaboration with a pediatric orthopaedic surgeon experienced with kyphos-coliosis is helpful in managing these patients. Utilizing this regimen, we have had very few patients who have required Harrington rods and fusion for progressive deformity.

SYRINGOMYELIA

NOEL B. TULIPAN, M.D.

The term syringomyelia encompasses a variety of anatomic abnormalities whose common feature is a cavi-tary lesion of the spinal cord not associated with tumor. In the strictest sense, syringomyelia is an enlargement of the central canal of the spinal cord that leads to compres-sion of the fiber tracts and neurons adjacent to the canal. It is postulated that this enlargement results from a developmental obstruction of the outflow of CSF from the 4th ventricle. In its commonest form, this obstruction is associated with an Arnold-Chiari Type I malforma-tion in which the cerebellar tonsils protrude beyond the foramen magnum into the spinal canal. In theory, CSF obstruction leads to pulsatile pressure waves secondary to arterial and venous variations that are transmitted to the central canal. These continual pulsations lead to progressive enlargement of the central canal which occa-sionally ruptures into the substance of the cord. This theory, however, remains unproven. Similar cavitary lesions that lead to similar clinical syndromes may occur in the absence of either an Arnold-Chiari malformation or any obvious ventricular outlet obstruction. For example, syrinx has been associated with other cranio-spinal abnormalities, including Klippel-Feil syndrome, occipitalization of the atlas, and basilar impression. In addition, a history of cervical trauma with or without associated cervical arachnoiditis can be associated with anatomic abnormalities and syndromes that are indis-tinguishable from classic syringomyelia.

SIGNS AND SYMPTOMS

Syringomyelia tends to present later in life, but can occur at any age. The neurological literature describes a classic clinical triad of amyotrophy, especially in the distal upper extremities, hyporeflexia of the upper extremities with hyperreflexia in the lower extremities, and dissociated sensory loss in a cape-like distribution over the cervical dermatomes. These deficits can be explained on an anatomic basis by considering the effects of an expanding mass lesion at the center of the spinal cord. Disruption of the decussating fibers of the spino-thalamic tract leads to a decrease in the sense of pain and temperature, but the fibers of the posterior columns that carry light touch and proprioception are relatively spared. As the cavity enlarges, it encroaches upon the anterior horns and leads to destruction of motor neurons and the muscles that they innervate. Compression of the corticospinal tracts causes spasticity in the lower extrem-ities. Of note is the fact that the descending spinal tract of the trigeminal nerve may also be involved with resultant sensory abnormalities in the face that may initially lead one to suspect an intracranial lesion. Despite the empha-sis in textbooks on this triad, the majority of patients with syringomyelia present with incomplete or unrelated syndromes. Other presenting signs and symptoms include pain, headache, diplopia, and bowel and bladder dys-function.

DIAGNOSIS

Until recently, the definitive diagnosis of syringo-myelia was extremely difficult. Myelography with pan-topaque, the procedure of choice, was used not only to define the cord, but also to outline the cerebellar tonsils which were often displaced inferiorly. Myelography, however, has been replaced by high-resolution com-puted tomography (CT) scanning after subarachnoid injection of metrizamide. It has been found that contrast tends to pool in the syrinx cavity after delays of up to 24 hours. Therefore, the contrast is injected into the lumbar theca; then the cervical cord is scanned at intervals of from 8 to 24 hours. The syrinx cavity appears as a hyperdense core at the center of an otherwise hypodense spinal cord. More recently, the widespread acceptance of the nuclear magnetic resonance (NMR) scanner as a diagnostic tool has led to an interest in its use in diagnos-ing spinal cord pathology. Although the NMR scanner may often resolve the problem of contrast pooling in the syrinx cavity, the author is aware of several false-negative scans. The utility of NMR in the diagnosis of syringo-myelia, therefore, remains unproven.

TREATMENT

Syringomyelia is treated surgically, but controversy remains as to which of the many available procedures is superior. It is generally accepted that syringomyelia associated with an Arnold-Chiari malformation is best treated by decompression of the malformation. A suboccipital craniectomy is performed, and the upper cervical laminae are removed as necessary. Arachnoidal adhesions around the tonsils and roof of the 4th ventricle are removed, and the tonsils are often partially amputated. The dura is then either patched to provide additional room or left open altogether. It has been proposed that a small plug of muscle or other foreign body be placed at the obex to prevent access of CSF to the central canal. Others argue that simple decompression of the 4th ventricle is sufficient. In the absence of an obvious anatomic abnormality, most neurosurgeons opt to attack the syrinx directly. A dorsal incision is made in the cord, either over its thinnest portion or at the level of the dorsal root entry zone where a minimal additional deficit will be incurred. Opinion varies as to whether a silastic tube or wick should be placed within the cavity and brought out into the subarachnoid space. A recent report described a series of patients treated by syringoperitoneal shunting; a small T-tube was placed within the syrinx cavity and was connected to standard peritoneal shunt tubing. The authors reported results that were similar to other reported series in which more conventional surgical therapy was used. Other surgical possibilities include syringo-pleural shunt, terminal ventriculostomy (in which the caudal end of the central canal which is located in the filum terminale is opened into the subarachnoid space), or a combination of posterior fossa decompression and syringostomy. None of these procedures has proven to be significantly superior to another.

Because syringomyelia is a disease with multiple etiologies, treatment must be individually tailored to each afflicted patient.

SPINAL ARTERIOVENOUS MALFORMATION

LEONARD I. MALIS, M.D.

These rare but devastating lesions present with pain in the back or legs which is intermittent for many years. It may resemble claudication, but is not relieved when the patient lies down. The diagnosis is virtually never made during this period. Eventually weakness begins, and then the course is much more rapid, with the average untreated patient becoming paraplegic within 3 years. About 15 percent begin with a sudden stabbing back pain due to spinal subarachnoid hemorrhage. A few begin with a sudden permanent paraplegia, the result of arterial occlusion and necrotizing myelitis. The principle that all progressive neurological disease requires neuroradiologic confirmation of the diagnosis, regardless of how basically typical the neurological picture may be of some degenerative disease, can lead to earlier diagnosis while therapy is still feasible. Metrizamide myelography regularly diagnoses these lesions. The tortuous vascular pattern, with either a long dorsal worm-like configuration or the multiple loops of a vascular nidus, perhaps with a long drain, are quite characteristic.

Improved technology in selective spinal angiography has now made it a virtual requisite in the planning of management. I prefer the highest possible resolution, using stereo magnification films at each pedicle level that provides filling for the lesion. Although digital intravenous angiography can demonstrate the lesions and digital enhanced arterial study may show the pedicles, I have not been willing to operate with the resolution available on these studies.

Some years ago, the failure rate of spinal arterial angiography was still quite high, and we often explored without having filled the lesion, on the basis of the myelographic study alone. I believe the development of the high-resolution angiograms with the combination of rapid early films and films going onward for 20 or more seconds has markedly improved our surgical results.

The lesions occur as a number of types. The most common is the long dorsal lesion, which runs on the posterior surface of the thoracic cord and tends to have a number of major arterial pedicles coming in with the dorsal roots. This system frequently has many tiny connections to the paired dorsal lateral spinal arteries, but nevertheless is a separate circulatory system from the cord. This is the most common lesion, probably occurring in 75 percent of all cases. The next most frequent lesion is a nidus lesion, with one or several major feeders within a few segments usually sharing their flow with the supply to the anterior spinal artery. While the dorsal lateral arterial chain is fed by an arterial pedicle at virtually every dorsal nerve root, the anterior spinal artery is a series of downward tapering vessels coming from ventral arterial pedicles, from two to seven in total number. The artery of the lumbar enlargement, the artery of Adamkiewicz, is defined as the largest pedicle in this area, and its occlusion should regularly produce paraplegia. However, a major shunt to a malformation will have enlarged to meet the malformation's need and may be the largest artery, although not the artery of Adamkiewicz. Occlusion may not have the hazard that would otherwise accompany ligation of the major pedicle of the anterior spinal artery, but there is no certain way of determining this in advance although high-resolution angiography can be of great help in defining the nature of the cord circulation.

Cervical lesions are virtually all intramedullary with multiple large feeders coming in with the roots as well as a comblike network of small arteries coursing posteriorly up the midline raphe from the anterior spinal artery.

Still another small group of lesions is situated at the *foramen magnum* and gets its supply from the two vertebral artery branches which would normally join to form the anterior spinal artery. The flow in the uppermost portion of the anterior spinal artery is often reversed, supplied from the lower root branches and running upward to drain into the malformation.

Some lesions have an epidural shunt and venous drainage, which may be intra-arachnoid or may be entirely epidural. These tend to have multiple veins and feeders within the paravertebral muscles as well.

Finally, the *juvenile malformations* are huge, high-flow, terrifying lesions sometimes associated with other anomalies. These are the malformations that have an audible bruit, sometimes so loud that it can be heard just standing near the bedside.

THERAPY

The untreated outcome is so unfavorable that I believe that active intervention should be undertaken as soon as the diagnosis is made. I do not consider conservative or expectant care to be a reasonable option unless the patient already has catastrophic damage to cord function such as results from the occlusive process that is part of some of these lesions. Even then, this is not a therapeutic option, it is simply an acceptance of the inability to treat. The actual decision that has to be made regarding the patient who still has function is whether embolization or surgical excision is the procedure of choice.

Embolic occlusion of arterial pedicles frequently produces temporary improvement only to have the lesion rapidly pick up a new collateral flow to supply its demands. When embolization is carried out, it should be done in such a manner as to actually occlude the entirety of the lesion while preserving the normal circulation of the cord. This requires demonstration of all the shunts and the use of materials that will enter the lesion yet stay within it. A remarkable degree of skill of the interventional neuroradiologist is a prerequisite. An armamentarium of balloon catheters, which may be manipulated to restrict the flow in one direction while another catheter is used to inject another vessel, may well be required. Partial embolization may require surgical intervention to complete the process. Occasionally a large malformation expands sufficiently after embolization to require urgent surgical decompression.

Complete surgical resection of the malformation remains, in my opinion, the treatment of choice for most of these lesions. A previously operated lesion often has adhesions and scarring sufficient to make the microsurgical dissection unreasonable, and embolization, if it can be achieved, would be recommended. Nidus lesions where the vascular pattern is such that the anterior spinal circulation can be protected may be selected for primary treatment by embolization.

All patients are operated on under endotracheal general anesthesia, with controlled respiration, using fentanyl and curare. The intraoperative antibiotic regimen of intravenous vancomycin and intramuscular tobramycin is routine, with no preoperative or postoperative antibiotic. Hypotension is maintained at 70 mean with intravenous nitroprusside. I no longer record spinal evoked potentials during the surgical procedure, since they have appeared misleading in both directions. I carry out virtually all of the resections with the patient in the 45-degree prone oblique position. This allows freer respiratory movement to the abdomen and thorax without venous compression. Spinal movement with respiration is minimized so that the operative field is kept in the focal plane of the microscope. The position is comfortable for the surgeon, who can sit looking downward at a 45-degree angle without bending over the patient. Adequate support of the surgeon's forearms is achieved with a special padded narrow Mayo table, draped and appropriately positioned. After the laminectomy, (always carried to the full width between the pedicles) and the dural opening, the arachnoid attachments of the vascular loops are separated by sharp dissection. The malformation, if extramedullary, is progressively isolated from the cord. I tend to preserve vascular pedicles throughout the dissection and isolation of the loops of the malformation since following backward to the arterial pedicle will demonstrate when branches supply the cord rather than the malformation.

The use of bipolar coagulation under saline, usually at power levels of 25 or so, is to me an absolute essential in keeping this part of the dissection bloodless and in shrinking large vessels to more manageable proportions to permit their separation and dissection. The older spark gap bipolar coagulators began each burst of current with a high voltage onset spike. My new solid state bipolar coagulator eliminates this spike so that perforation and sticking, as well as charring, have been greatly reduced. Nevertheless, forceps must be kept scrupulously clean and polished, and the use of constant irrigation is required.

I have not observed any of these lesions to have a single shunt. They are quite analogous to the intracranial AV malformations. If a portion of the malformation is left intact it picks up additional circulation and, like the intracranial AV malformations, is demonstrable as a recurrent lesion. However, just as in intracranial malformations, the feeding artery and the draining vein belong to the patient's vascular system. A feeding artery must therefore be protected except for the area that goes directly into the malformation and the venous drainage left with the patient from the point where it no longer has a shunt going into it. Sedimentation of the red cells from the serum in the venous drain can regularly be seen past the point of final shunting. This demonstration of cessation of the venous flow indicates that it is not necessary to pursue the resection for further segments. The intramedullary portions may be followed in through the raphe, progressively reduced in size with the bipolar coagulator to provide the room needed for the dissection. Multiple dentate ligament sections can make rotation of the cord feasible to reach the ventral midline from either side; 6–0 traction sutures placed in the dentate ligaments can provide the support to maintain the cord rotation and so facilitate the ventral dissection. Routine dural closure and layer closure of the wound is done. Postoperative angiographic study is done when there appears to be a significant possibility of incomplete resection. I have done a series of postoperative myelograms after a 1- to 2-month interval in patients in whom I felt there had been complete resection of the lesions. In no case in this group was residual lesion present, and so I now accept my surgical judgment if I am certain of complete removal.

My personal series now amounts to 58 patients operated on since 1967. Complete obliteration of the malformation was achieved in 52 cases. There was one death, due to a massive pulmonary embolus. Four patients unable to walk preoperatively remained unable to walk postoperatively. Four patients still able to walk preoperatively were made much worse postoperatively and could no longer walk. There was slight or modest improvement in four patients and marked improvement or virtually complete recovery in 45. Considering the poor prognosis without interference in the natural course of the illness, the ability to achieve good neurological outcomes in 80 percent of the patients appears to me to be well worth the risk of precipitating the impending paralysis in 7 percent. Nevertheless, patients who are rendered paraplegic by the surgical procedure—regardless of the odds, the natural course of the disease, and the informed consent—in our present litigious society are likely to bring suit. The patient's personality type may indeed be a major factor in deciding whether the surgeon can accept the risk of the procedure.

CERVICAL DISC HERNIATION

CHARLES A. FAGER, M.D.

Symptomatic cervical disc herniation is uncommon and probably accounts for no more than 15 percent of all herniated discs, of which the largest number occur in the lower lumbar spine. This is understandable because cervical intervertebral discs are smaller than lumbar discs and are subjected to far less stress on weight-bearing than that imposed on their lumbar counterparts.

Yet the natural history of their development is remarkably analogous. Degenerative disc disease involves primarily the three lowermost lumbar intervertebral discs, the levels bearing the greatest burden of spinal strain, shearing stresses, and compression forces and those at which most lumbar discs herniate. In identical manner, reflecting the similar wear and tear of almost perpetual neck motion, the lowermost cervical discs degenerate, and at these levels (C5–C6 and C6–C7), disc herniation is most likely to occur. Vulnerability likewise exists at the two adjacent although less busy segments, C4–C5 and C7–T1.

Degenerative narrowing of these cervical disc spaces occurs usually with aging, is probably also related to activity, and is not in itself symptomatic. Under rare circumstances it seems to develop rapidly, is mysteriously independent of rheumatoid disease, facet arthropathy, or other spondylotic change, and may actually produce pain and stiffness in the neck. This is the exception rather than the rule. In patients with neck pain and headache, such radiologic findings alone are often thought to be the cause, or cervical disc herniation is even believed to exist because of the presence of degenerative narrowing seen by radiography. "Pinched nerve" is frequently used as an explanation of muscular neck or shoulder pain in athletes or after minor injury to the neck when the nerve root is actually not compressed at all. As a result, radiologic degenerative changes commonly seen are usually not responsible for symptomatic neck pain.

Many patients with herniated cervical disc, however, exhibit degenerative changes of disc spaces; in others, a perfectly normal cervical spine is seen radiographically with no clue to suggest degenerative disc disease. Likewise, several types of lesion may compress lower cervical nerve roots and cause symptoms, such as a so-called soft ruptured disc or hard osteophyte (spur), the end result of degenerative change and chronic disc protrusion. The most common finding, however, is that of a disc fragment that has extruded through the early semi-hard shell of surrounding degenerative change, an evolutionary stage between pathologic changes at acute and chronic ends of the spectrum.

SYMPTOMS AND SIGNS

The cardinal symptom of cervical disc herniation is pain in the arm, and the diagnosis is easily made by history and physical examination alone. The onset is abrupt, the patient commonly awaking in the morning with pain that is usually pronounced in the shoulder blade, although extending from the back of the lower neck and radiating across, around, or over the shoulder into one arm. The pain may travel to the radial or ulnar forearm or wrist, but it usually stops at the elbow. With C5 nerve root compression (C4–C5 disc herniation), pain usually radiates to the upper arm only. The patient soon becomes aware of some degree of neck stiffness and notices that movement of the neck, invariably extension, produces flashes of severe pain. Activities that require looking upward and raising the chin, as men do in shaving, become an ordeal. Many patients soon learn to keep the head flexed.

The pain is attended commonly by paresthesias when the herniated disc compresses C6 nerve root (C5–C6 disc), C7 nerve root (C6–C7 disc), or C8 nerve root (C7–T1 disc). These sensations, unlike the pain, are described as tingling or electric, at times are accompanied by numbness, and extend to the fingers in a fairly characteristic pattern. Thus paresthesias of C6 root are felt in thumb and index finger; of the C7 root in index, middle, and fourth fingers; and of C8 root in fourth and fifth fingers. As might be expected, tingling of C6 root typically radiates along the radial aspect of the forearm and that of C8 root on the ulnar side. Overlapping of sensory root function exists, however, and a rigid anatomic distribution cannot be presumed in every patient. For example, some patients with C7 nerve root compression complain of thumb paresthesias. In addition to the pain and sensory symptoms, the patient often is also aware of some weakness in arm or hand.

These are the typical presenting complaints in more than 90 percent of patients with herniated disc, and they are often described as symptoms of monoradiculopathy. The fact that the disc frequently herniates during the night suggests probable weakness or attenuation of the posterior longitudinal ligament and disc degeneration. A fragment of disc extrudes laterally where the ligament tends to be weak while neck muscles are relaxed or while the neck is in an awkward position during sleep. Occasionally, a cervical disc that is probably already degenerated or weakened may rupture after trauma. This often occurs in association with traction of the arm or shoulder or after injury of the neck from flexion or extension. Rarely, a large extruded fragment may tear through the posterior longitudinal ligament medially with or without neck trauma and may present as a median or paramedian herniation compressing spinal cord or both spinal cord and nerve root. In this situation the patient may complain of weakness and sensory symptoms of lower limbs in addition to arm pain or quadriparesis may be present with varying sensory symptoms and no pain at all in the event of a median disc rupture compressing spinal cord alone. This is so unusual that it occurs in only about 2 percent of patients with herniated cervical disc.

Bilateral arm pain, however, does not occur from cervical disc rupture nor does cervical disc herniation occur at more than one level simultaneously. Cervical herniation should not be confused with cervical spondylosis, in which chronic degenerative disc disease results in ventral ridges and osteophytes at multiple levels, which can produce a more chronic form of myelopathy or myeloradiculopathy, especially in a person with a congenitally small cervical canal. However, even under these conditions, bilateral arm pain seldom occurs.

The radicular nature of arm pain in the patient with cervical disc herniation is readily demonstrated on examination. It is usually intensified, as are paresthesias, by extension of the head and especially extension with the chin turned toward the opposite side. Relief is often achieved by flexion. This finding, however, is less true of C5 and C8 nerve root compression, the two segments usually with less flexion and extension movement. At times flexion or lateral flexion of the head aggravates root pain. The so-called compression of the head to reproduce arm pain is not so reliable because the disc fragment causing root compression has already extruded from the disc space.

The other prominent findings on examination are those resulting from compression of the motor nerve root. Here again a pattern of abnormality is usually, although not invaribly, consistent. The patient with compression of the C5 nerve root exhibits primarily weakness of deltoid, supraspinatus, and infraspinatus musculature, which is demonstrated easily by comparison with the opposite side. At times the biceps muscle may be weak, but usually no loss of biceps reflex occurs. Compression of C6 nerve root results largely in weakness of biceps, brachioradialis, finger extensors, and sometimes wrist extensors. This is associated with decrease of the biceps and radial periosteal reflexes. Loss of C7 motor nerve root function is evidenced by weakness of triceps and the finger extensors, with decrease or absence of the triceps reflex. Weakness of finger extensors is common to C6, C7, and C8 nerve roots, indicative of the multiple innervation of this function, whereas selective weakness of finger flexion is seldom evident, probably because of a rich admixture of fibers in the brachial plexus. The clear differentiating feature of C8 motor nerve root involvement is the association of weak interossei. C8 root is similar to C5 root in its relation to biceps reflex, and only rarely does impairment of its function affect the triceps reflex. Despite the patient's sensory symptoms and even complaints of numbness in the fingers, objective impairment of sensation is not commonly found on testing for pain, temperature, or light touch.

DIFFERENTIAL DIAGNOSIS

Although this constellation of symptoms and signs usually discloses the diagnosis of herniated cervical disc within a few minutes, a problem in differential diagnosis may at times arise. Shoulder pain caused by arthritis, tendinitis, or, most commonly, adhesive capsulitis has often been mistaken for nerve root compression. Limitation of shoulder abduction and elevation of the arm is occasionally misinterpreted as deltoid weakness. However, the clear relation of pain to shoulder rather than cervical motions and the restriction of the shoulder itself, even on passive movement, easily localize the problem.

Compression of the C6 nerve root, in particular, sometimes produces radiating pain across the pectoral region and into the arm, and so this has been confused with angina when it occurs on the left side. Neoplastic processes, such as Pancoast's tumor, are usually associated with more diffuse signs, including Horner's syndrome, and more constant pain unrelated to neck movement. Intraspinal neurofibroma or meningioma, however, may require myelography to establish the correct diagnosis.

Probably the most common confusion has been in young or early middle-aged women with long neck, sloping shoulders, and small costoclavicular space referred to as the thoracic inlet. The neck pain in these patients is diffuse. Arm pain, although preponderant on one side, is often bilateral, and the paresthesias may affect both hands and may seem to be related to elevation of the arms and forearms. Usually little or no neurological deficit exists in these patients, and to assign the symptoms to a single cervical nerve root is almost impossible.

The common neck pain after injury from vehicular deceleration and rear-end collision is almost always caused by muscular and ligamentous sprain. Radiation is bilateral, diffuse to shoulders and scapulas, to the occipital region, and even as far as the frontal and retro-orbital regions. It is similar to the neck and head pain from muscle contraction or tension. Although arm pain and paresthesias may be present, neither conforms to a specific root pattern, and the neurological examination shows no objective abnormality.

DIAGNOSTIC PROCEDURES AND TREATMENT METHODS

Most patients with herniated cervical disc, probably 70 percent of those seen as outpatients, recover spontaneously and require no specific therapy or operation. The pain of nerve root compression is most intense during the first 4 to 5 days and usually has lessened to some degree by the time the patient is seen and referred for neurosurgical evaluation. Those patients who do get better usually are free of pain completely by 6 weeks. Mild residual weakness or sensory symptoms likewise clear in time.

Radicular pain is caused by swelling of nerve root from compression, and so conservative measures require that the neck be kept at rest as much as possible to avoid further trauma to nerve root and to allow spontaneous regression of swelling. Because extension by closing the

facets usually further reduces the aperture of the nerve root foramen, patients are best advised to sleep with several pillows, maintaining flexion as much as possible, and to use a soft cervical collar positioned so that the head is in slight flexion rather than extension. In those few patients who exhibit no relationship of their pain to neck motion and no relief with change in neck position, such measures obviously are useless, and more reliance is placed on use of analgesics.

Despite its widespread use, cervical traction has little, if any, value. If it can be applied with the head in flexion, it may be helpful temporarily, but for many patients hanging in doorways at home has aggravated rather than alleviated the problem. Also, hospitalization of the patient for traction alone when simpler measures serve equally well is unjustifiable.

Once recovery begins the patient can anticipate full relief and return of function with surprisingly little danger of recurrence at the same level. The nerve root swelling subsides, and extruded disc material contracts; some of it is resorbed and some forms fibrocalcific tissue, eventually becoming osteophytic. But if the quantity of herniated material has not been great, the nerve root finds more space and is relieved. The cervical myelography that showed such a herniated disc has been repeated as long as 16 years after the acute event in patients who had spontaneous recovery and has indicated a small residual asymptomatic defect.

The patient who is obviously improving does not require radiography or myelography of the cervical spine. These studies, although they might demonstrate some abnormality, would not influence selection of conservative treatment in any way. The major questions are when to abandon conservative treatment and what are the indications for operation. The decision to operate cannot be arbitrary or based on specific time limits. A patient with massive disc herniation, extreme pain, and severe deficit may require operation within 7 to 10 days; in another patient with lingering minor root pain and no neurological deficit, nonsurgical measures may be continued for several months. Median or paramedian disc rupture with symptoms and signs of spinal cord compression demands early or possibly urgent surgical intervention.

After 4 to 6 weeks of persistent nerve root compression without relief, it usually becomes evident that operation is required. This period of time does not preclude restoration of neurological function after surgical excision of the disc.

Radiography of the cervical spine is performed before myelography. It may show degenerative narrowing of one or more disc spaces, but does not give any indication of the level or degree of nerve root compression, nor does oblique radiography of the cervical spine traditionally interpreted by radiologists as demonstrating presumed encroachment on neural foramina have any value or any reliability in assessing nerve root involvement or compression. Cervical myelography remains the definitive procedure to confirm the diagnosis of disc herniation and also to establish for the surgeon its size and location. Although iophendylate (Pantopaque) myelography appears to provide better contrast, metrizamide (Amipaque) injected at C1–C2 is usually adequate to outline the lesion and eliminates the possibility of spinal headache.

Myelography must be performed on every patient before operation, not only because neurological signs may be misleading, but also because normal results on cervical myelography rule out herniated disc as a cause of the patient's problem, and other possible causes must then be investigated. Unlike the lowermost lumbar region, the cervical canal is too narrow for a herniated disc to escape detection by myelography.

Computed tomography does not achieve the accuracy of myelography in localizing a lateral fragment of extruded disc. It has little, if any, value when used without metrizamide but can be extremely helpful in those patients in whom the spinal cord is under compression to determine whether the compressive lesion is a soft midline disc or a hard ventral ridge or osteophyte. This information often assists the surgeon in determining the type of operative procedure to employ.

Electromyography has no value in the diagnosis of herniated cervical disc and adds only additional expense. Discography has been shown repeatedly to have no demonstrable benefit. Nevertheless, it is still being used by some, and those procedures referred to as discometry and analgesic discography have been believed to show abnormalities that were symptomatic in the absence of actual cervical disc herniation. Scientific evidence does not support such speculation. Surgical discectomy after these procedures has frequently been performed on patients with psychogenic neck pain or on those who have persistent pain after vehicular or industrial accidents.

OPERATIVE TREATMENT

Although many surgeons prefer anterior cervical discectomy by the Smith-Robinson or Cloward technique, many advocates of anterior operations employ no fusion bone at all, allowing the disc space to collapse and eventually to fuse after operation. Complications of anterior approaches to cervical disc lesions include resorption of fusion bone and possible damage to esophagus, recurrent laryngeal nerve, or vertebral artery. Many surgeons, however, continue to use a posterior approach, especially for laterally ruptured disc, combining hemilaminectomy with foraminotomy at the appropriate level. This type of operation allows a wide exposure and release of the nerve root, so that the extruded fragment of disc can be excised and the early osteophyte formation or even the hard spur can be cureted beneath the root to provide full decompression. The disc space itself is never invaded, and fusion therefore is not necessary. The operation is performed by most surgeons with the patient in the sitting position, which raises the issue of possible air embolism, but this risk, for the most part, has been overstated.

Regardless of technique or approach, the operation should be limited to excision of the symptomatic cervical disc. Myelography often discloses asymptomatic defects, and extending the surgery to two levels or bilaterally for radiologic reasons alone, regardless of the approach, increases the risk of damage to nerve root or spinal cord. It may be difficult to decide whether compression exist at the C6 or C7 root level because of confusing neurological findings and myelographic defects at both segments. Under this circumstance, operation at two levels may be justified. As stated previously, this limited type of operation for herniated disc should not be confused with the extensive and more hazardous operations necessary in patients with spondylotic myelopathy and myeloradiculopathy.

When operation becomes necessary for herniated cervical disc with nerve root compression, it results in prompt and gratifying relief of the intensive nerve root pain. Some residual neck discomfort may be expected in a small number of patients, but the risk of increased neurological deficit or operative nerve root damage is minimal. Unlike lumbar disc herniation, cervical disc herniation rarely recurs at the same level. Persistence or recurrence of radicular pain is more likely to be caused by a retained fragment than by a recurrent fragment.

SPONDYLOTIC MYELOPATHY

SANFORD J. LARSON, M.D., Ph.D.

Patients with functionally significant spondylotic myelopathy require surgical treatment. While general agreement exists concerning the need for operation, there is considerable difference of opinion regarding the approach, whether anterior or posterior, and in either case the extent of the procedure. With the posterior approach, the major question is whether laminectomy is sufficient or if the dentate liagments should also be divided. With the anterior approach, some surgeons favor resection of the spondylotic ridges only, while others consider resection of the midportion of the vertebral bodies and discs to be necessary.

The selection of the surgical procedures should depend on the pathologic anatomy. In these patients, the vertebral bodies become thicker, encroaching on the spinal canal, most prominently at the interspace where the spondylotic ridges develop. In patients with a congenitally narrow canal, the cord becomes constricted. More commonly, the developing osteophyte and thickened vertebral body displace the spinal cord posteriorly. Although in some patients the subarachnoid space remains patent posteriorly, the spinal cord is nevertheless flattened because it is fixed to the dura laterally by the dentate ligaments. The posterior displacement and the increased transverse diameter of the spinal cord increase the axial tension in the axons of the long tracts. The tension is proportional to the distance from the source of the deformity, which in patients with spondylosis is located on the anterior surface of the cord. Consequently, the tension is greater in the dorsal columns, which are displaced posteriorly, and in the corticospinal tracts, which are displaced laterally, than in the more central and anterior portions of the cord. These anatomic changes are consistent with the clinical findings of spastic quadriparesis and decreased proprioception with minimal disturbance of micturition and perception of pain.

The major problem, therefore, is deformity of the spinal cord with increased axial tension in the long tracts, and the goal of treatment is restoration of a normal configuration to the spinal cord and a reduction in axial tension. This requires restoration of normal relationships between the spinal cord and the spinal canal. To achieve this goal, it is necessary to define the nature and extent of the deformity. Until magnetic resonance imaging (MRI) becomes widely available, myelography will continue to be necessary. Of the contrast media available, Pantopaque is the least efficient because the cord is only outlined in the anteroposterior projection, and so in many instances the effect of the bony changes on the spinal cord must be inferred. Furthermore, Pantopaque lateral to the cord can obscure central defects. Because the procedure is done with the patient prone, the demonstration of spondylotic ridges may not necessarily mean that the spinal cord is deformed. Gas myelography with polytomography provide excellent demonstration of the spinal cord and of the contours of the spinal canal. If gas is present posterior to the cord, any posterior displacement of the cord could be related to gravitational force rather than tethering. To distinguish which of these is responsible for the deformity, at the conclusion of the procedure the patient can be placed in the supine position. Continued contact between the spinal cord and the floor of the spinal canal indicates that the cord is indeed tethered. Metrizamide demonstrates the available subarachnoid space and therefore is superior to Pantopaque. However, like Pantopaque, metrizamide lateral to the cord obscures central defects, and consequently either polytomography or postmyelographic CT scanning is necessary to outline the spinal cord. It is very likely that magnetic resonance imaging combined with lateral polytomography or CT scanning including sagittal reconstructions will obviate the use of contrast media. Three-dimensional images of the spinal canal derived from CT scans should also provide valuable in selecting the appropriate surgical procedure and determining its extent.

The anterior approach has a major theoretic advantage over laminectomy because the spondylotic ridges and thickened vertebral body are removed, restoring a normal relationship between the spinal cord and the spinal canal. However, in most patients with spondylotic myelopathy, the cord is involved at two or more levels. Because the entire vertebral body is thickened and because gas myelography has demonstrated that in many patients the soft tissue between the vertebral body and dura is hypertrophic, removal of the midportion of the vertebral body as well as the spondylotic ridges ensures a more satisfactory reconstruction of the spinal canal. Consequently, a long graft usually is necessary for fusion of three or more veretebral bodies, requiring postoperative immobilization in a rigid and nonremovable orthosis. If the spinal cord is severely constricted, particularly in patients with congenitally narrow canals, the cord may be significantly injured in the process of vertebral body resection. Furthermore, with the anterior approach, the recurrent laryngeal nerve may be injured and the esophagus may be lacerated. The major indication for an anterior approach is kyphosis associated with spondylosis. In these patients, laminectomy is ineffective because the cord is not able to move posteriorly and therefore remains deformed by forced contact with the floor of the canal. Another indication for the anterior approach is in patients who do not achieve the anticipated degree of neurological recovery after laminectomy and who have radiographically demonstrable persistent deformity of the spinal cord secondary to continued contact with the floor of the canal.

For most patients with cervical spondylotic myelopathy, laminectomy is the best procedure. Those who have a congenitally small canal with relatively small spondylotic ridges may need only a laminectomy, but it is usually advisable to add division of the dentate ligaments to the procedure. This adds little to the duration of the operation and does not increase morbidity. The dura can be opened, in almost all instances, without a significant opening in the arachnoid. The dentate ligaments are cut at the point of attachment to the dura, and therefore very little cerebrospinal fluid is lost and blood is not admitted to the subarachnoid space. A tight dural closure is advisable, particularly if the arachnoid has been widely opened. Some patients in whom the arachnoid has been opened and the dura has been left open have developed a pseudomeningocele with severe headache and prolonged febrile course secondary to aseptic meningitis. Rarely, a fascial graft may be necessary to avoid compromise of the spinal cord which has moved posteriorly.

The laminectomy is technically simpler if done with the patient in the sitting position because blood drains from the wound instead of accumulating in its depths. Even a small amount of blood can obscure the relevant anatomic structures, making the procedure more tedious and time-consuming. However, if the arachnoid is opened with the patient in the sitting position, the cerebrospinal fluid drains from the cerebral subarachnoid space, cisterns, and ventricles. Because many of these patients are elderly with some degree of cerebral and cerebellar atrophy, the bridging veins between the cerebral hemispheres and the sagittal sinus, and the superior surface of the cerebellum and the tentorium are placed in traction. If, for example, this traction is sufficient to tear one of the bridging cerebellar veins, air embolism could follow. Furthermore, substantial loss of cerebrospinal fluid is not well tolerated by some patients, who appear to develop headaches and confusion as a consequence. Whether the patient is operated on while in the sitting or prone position, it is equally important for the head and neck to be in a neutral position. Increased pathologic tension in the spinal cord secondary to flexion of the cervical spine appears to be a more likely explanation for postoperative increase in neurological deficit than is injury to the cord produced during the actual removal of the laminae.

During the immediate postoperative period, it is usually advisable to keep the patient recumbent for 2 to 3 days, turning at intervals from side to back to side. Return to the erect position should be gradual, moving from progressive elevation of the back of the bed, to sitting at the edge of the bed, to sitting in a chair, and to walking over a period of several days. The patient should not be left unattended in a chair, since postural hypotension may develop with loss of consciousness. The head may then fall forward with acute flexion of the neck. The combination of hypotension and increased tension in the cord may produce significant increase in myelopathy.

A late complication of cervical laminectomy is the development of progressive kyphosis or swan neck deformity. If pain is the only symptom, anterior interbody fusion to prevent further deformity and to prevent movement at the affected area is sufficient. However, this is not enough in patients with an associated increase in myelopathy. To decrease the axial tension and spinal cord deformity responsible for the myelopathy, the spinal canal must be shortened. This can be done by applying skeletal traction to improve vertebral alignment and then proceeding with anterior interbody fusion. If the malalignment persists, an anterior approach is necessary for resection of the midsagittal portion of the vertebral bodies in the affected area, followed by interbody fusion.

The results of surgical treatment are reasonably good. Most patients achieve a significant improvement in neurological function, and in those who do not improve, the progression of neurological deficit is usually arrested. A small number of patients may continue to experience an increase in myelopathy, but significant deterioration in neurological function as a result of surgery is rare.

CERVICAL SPUR

CHARLES M. HENDERSON, B.S., M.D., F.A.C.S.

When I agreed to review this topic for the editor of this compendium, I did so with some trepidation. In this chapter, I refer generously to data compiled previously as an in-depth review of 846 unilateral cervical foraminotomies, and then a secondary review of an additional 309 operative procedures (for a total of 1155 posterior-lateral operations). These data are available in two previous publications on this topic. I wish to express one further disclaimer. The opinions expressed here are my own and do not attempt to present a standard of care or to impugn any competent surgeon (either neurosurgeon or orthopedist) who prefers a different approach for the treatment of the signs and symptoms secondary to this pathologic condition. This is not only "how I do it", but more specifically, how I think about it.

Pain in the neck, periscapular area, chest, shoulder, arm, and hand is no respecter of age, sex, socioeconomic background, or work ethic motivation. When one superimposes actual and demonstrable weakness in the involved extremity, one has a patient in need of help—but by which modality? In this short review, I shall attempt to go through the step-by-step analysis of this problem, and what the attending physician might, could, or should offer these patients in an effort to try to help them.

The physiologic theories concerning disc degeneration (with or without a history of injury) and associated osteoarthritic spur or ridge formation are well beyond the scope of this review. Suffice it to say, for any and all reasons, intervertebral discs do undergo degenerative changes. Either as a by-product of these biochemical and anatomic changes or in association with them, bony proliferation can and does occur. In the vast majority of the population, these changes produce neither subjective nor objective signs or symptoms. However, in a small percentage of patients, the gradual increase in size of the bony spurs or ridges can insidiously encroach on the available space for passage of the neural structures. It is these patients I shall discuss. No effort will be expended concerning treatment options for the painful and/or stiff neck alone. Nor will specific treatment options be discussed concerning patients who manifest signs and/or symptoms of actual spinal cord disease or compression. These comments will be specifically restricted to patients with a painful neck and upper extremity with or without demonstrable weakness.

As the degenerative changes develop in the cervical spine, there is frequently bony proliferation involving the medial facet joints and further extension of this bony growth to involve the intervertebral foramina. Neural tissue can adapt to significant compressive forces without signs or symptoms until "something happens". That "something" is frequently ill-defined, and in our series, less than 15 percent of the patients had a history of a specific injury or incident precipitating the final acute episode. The natural history is usually one of increasingly frequent episodes of neck pain, with radiation to the periscapular area, shoulder, anterior chest region, and extremity. The episodes tend to last longer and occur more frequently. Although the mean age is in the mid to late 40s (47 years for men and 45 years for women), the condition can be present in patients as young as the late teens to as old as the 70s, or even 80s. In our own review, patients with this condition actually requiring surgery represented less than 4 percent of the total patient population in an active three-man neurosurgical practice. We found this to be a bit more frequent in women than in men (59% to 41%), and approximately equal regarding lateralization (47% on the left side and 53% on the right side). The mean duration of symptoms, as related by the patient, was considerable (50 weeks) with a mean of 42 weeks for men and 55 weeks for women. The most frequent presenting symptom is pain and/or aggravating paresthesias (tingling, burning, numbness). In our own patient group, this was present in over 99 percent of the patients. Demonstrable weakness in the arm or hand was present less frequently (68%). Neck pain is common (80%), but as noted earlier, this symptom alone will not be discussed. Approximately 50 percent of the patients have periscapular pain (either along the top of the scapula or, as more frequently noted, along the medial border). Eighteen percent of the patients had significant anterior chest pain, and a small group presented with actual "cervical angina". Significant headache was noted in less than 10 percent of the patients, as opposed to the primary neck pain problems in which headache is considerably more frequent. This is particularly true of patients with a traumatic liability or compensation-related history.

For a variety of anatomic reasons, the most frequently involved intervertebral spaces are C5-C6 and C6-C7. In our own patients, 44 percent had a primary problem at C5-C6, and 42 percent at C6-C7. In another 12 percent, we felt that the two spaces were equally anatomically involved at the time of operation. Involvement with C4-C5 or C7-T1 was unusual.

As one would expect, in patients with spurs at C5-C6, the pain and/or paresthesia was most frequently in the C6 dermatomal pattern; and with osteophytes or spurs at C6-C7, the C7 root was primarily involved. There was no hard and fast correlation, however. There was a specific correlation between the primary operated space and the pain or paresthesia pattern only 74 percent of the time. The demonstrable motor deficit (be it deltoid, biceps, triceps, or grip) was compatible with the primary operative space more frequently (85%). It is significant to note, however, that the pain and/or paresthesia need not be specifically dermatomal, and we found this to be true in 46 percent of our patients. In the patients with truly dermatomal pain/paresthesia patterns, 25 percent were in the C6 dermatomal pattern, and a nearly equal number in the C7 outline. In the patients with demonstrable preoperative weakness (68%), it was noted that the triceps was more involved than the biceps (38% to 28%).

In summary, the history, with or without trauma, of increasing pain in the neck, lateral cervical area, scapula, anterior chest region, and upper extremity should alert one to the possibility of nerve root pressure in the cervical region. One should attempt to document just where the pain and/or paresthesia is located, and specifically test the major muscle groups in the involved extremity. Obviously, other conditions must be ruled out, ranging from Pancoast tumor of the pulmonary apex through all the conditions presenting under the umbrella of "shoulder outlet syndrome" (e.g., cervical rib, scalenus anticus syndrome). The peripheral nerve entrapment syndromes in the upper extremity must also be considered, including ulnar nerve involvement in or around the medial epicondyle, and median nerve involvement at the wrist. With these conditions, electrodiagnostic testing may be extremely helpful. Although not common, injuries to the brachial plexus itself are also a source of concern.

After obtaining a good history, and with a complete neurological examination, the next step in the work-up is to obtain plain radiographs of the cervical spine, usually including oblique views. We have found plain films to be most helpful in a negative nature. Good films tend to rule out anatomic malalignment, fractures, neoplastic processes involving the bony structures by erosion or deformity, and the like. But even good plain films do not often make the diagnosis of a significant cervical spur. In the total population, radiographic evidence suggesting disc space narrowing, anterior or posterior spur formation, or actual foraminal narrowing is extremely common, and usually these conditions are entirely asymptomatic. In patients with cervical root symptoms, we have found only an approximately 50 percent correlation between the radiographically involved space and the truly symptomatic space, as documented at the time of surgery. Nevertheless, for multiple reasons (some of which are purely medicolegal), one usually obtains plain films and attempts to correlate these with presenting symptoms. On occasion, radioactive bone scans can be helpful, and there is every indication that CT scanning of the cervical spine (both with and without

In almost all patients with an acute process involving the spinal axis (whether it is cervical, thoracic, or lumbar), "conservative management" is advised. Advising "conservative management" is frequently easier than defining the term. Assuming one can define the term, conservative management for how long? I know of no absolute rules to guide one in this regard. In over twenty years in the private practice of neurosurgery, I have found rest, muscle relaxants, anti-inflammatory agents, and analgesic to be helpful in the majority of patients. One can also rely heavily on those two other famous physicians: Mother Nature and Father Time. I do not feel that cervical immobilization apparatuses have been particularly helpful, other than in restricting neck motion. In many patients, this form of treatment can be as aggravating as the disease process itself. As with most others, I have found cervical traction (using seven pounds of weight: in 45 minutes and out 15 minutes, out to eat, out to sleep, out for bathroom privileges) to be helpful in many patients. I have not found the "over the door" traction set-up to be particularly helpful, however; nor have I noted great benefit from so-called "intermittent traction", as used by physiotherapists. I have noted that patients frequently feel much better while in traction, only to relapse shortly after discontinuing the traction. The jury is still very much out regarding how long one will be able to justify in-hospital use of traction and other conservative modalities. If the patient does not present with specific demonstrable weakness in the arm or hand, I believe that "conservative treatment" should be used until the patient either becomes relatively symptom-free or states that he or she wants something done about the problem. There is no way to gauge objectively the degree of discomfort the patient is having. What may be an irritant to patient A, may be incapacitating to patient B. However, if the patient presents with motor deficit or if demonstrable motor deficit develops during the trial of "conservative treatment", one should be more concerned. Significant motor deficit should be treated aggressively, and increasing motor deficit should be treated even more aggressively.

Patients who require actual nerve root decompression (by whatever means) should, in my opinion, have a preoperative myelogram performed. We have used Pantopaque solution exclusively for these myelograms, and can document no difficulty with this contrast medium, either anecdotal or radiographic, other than the usual 5 to 10 percent incidence of postmyelogram headache. We have no experience with water-soluble media in the cervical region for this condition. Ninety-eight percent of our patients had a myelogram performed preoperatively, and in the other 2 percent, a myelogram was not performed because of either an iodine sensitivity or some purely technical reason. We do not perform outpatient myelograms because of the possibility of a significant postmyelogram response (e.g., headache, nausea, vomiting). As alluded to pre-viously, we do not perform myelograms on patients with this condition who are not strongly considered as operative candidates, and we have almost no experience concerning myelograms on patients with primary neck pain problems. We have not used discography in evaluating these patients, and have found the results produced by discography by others to be of extremely limited localization benefit. We do use the myelogram in an attempt to confirm clinical localization; to note incidence of more than one space being involved (12%); and to rule out other intraspinal causes of the symptom complex.

In my experience, the cervical myelograms range in interpretation (by the operating surgeon, not the radiologist) from normal (3%) to bilateral foraminal disease with anterior bar formation (4%). The vast majority show foraminal defects (mild, 12%; serious or significant, 60%) or "true disc defects" (12%). I have noted that approximately 9 percent of the patients have bilateral foraminal defects, although the patient's symptoms were strictly unilateral. It should be noted that the myelographic defect is not an indication for operative intervention; nor is the absence of a "true disc defect" on a myelogram a contraindication for nerve root decompression. A patient may well have incapacitating pain, frequently with significant motor deficit, in association with a minimal myelographic defect. To understand this, one must understand that the basic nerve root compressive problem is in the foramen itself, and usually not intraspinally. By the same token, one can have an extremely large defect, as documented on myelogram, on a nonsymptomatic side; and significant defects may be present after surgery in patients who are absolutely symptom-free.

The debate as to the operative procedure of choice for unilateral cervical radiculopathy has been with us since the popularization of anterior cervical approaches (as described by Cloward, using a bone dowel technique, and by Smith and Robinson, using a disc space filling bone graft). In recent years, a further debate has developed, even among those proponents of an anterior approach, regarding "to fuse or not to fuse". Data have been presented that would indicate that "simple" cleaning out of the disc space, and presumably the posterior osteophytes, will produce results approximately equal to those obtained with fusion (by whatever means). It is not clear why the pendulum has swung so far away from a posterior approach for this problem, and that approach is certainly the one of our preference. This decompression (or foraminotomy) is one reserved for unilateral (or rarely bilateral) radiculopathy (both sensory and motor). It is not the procedure of choice for trauma, instability, bony destructive lesions, or myelopathy. Each of these conditions is best treated by a different operation—some anterior, some posterior. I believe that the signs and symptoms secondary to cervical spur or osteophyte formation, or to unilateral disc herniation (either soft or hard), can be best treated by this posterior operation.

The operation I prefer for simple cervical radiculopathy can be described in simple and straightforward terms. After evaluation of the myelogram, the clinical situation is reviewed again with the patient (and frequently with members of the patient's family, as well). The operation is described, as well as the statistically potential complications, including the possibility of paralysis, weakness, infection, difficulty with either bowel or bladder control, drainage or recurrence. The anesthetic risk is also explained, including the possibility of death, as well as the possibility of bleeding or hemorrhage. Alternative methods of treatment are also discussed, and after all this, I dictate a further formal consultation note for the chart record and indicate the patient's presumably Informed Consent for the procedure.

The patient is visited by the anesthesiologist preoperatively, and he in turn explains the anesthesia to be given for the proposed operation.

On the day of surgery, the patient has either TED stockings or Ace bandages applied to the lower extremeties (including the feet, and up to midthigh). This is done in the hope that it will help to prevent venous stasis when the patient is in the sitting position during the operative procedure. He or she is then brought to the operating room, and appropriate general endotracheal anesthesia is induced. Using a standard operating table, the patient is gently brought up to a semi-sitting position. The head is held in place by means of a soft stabilization apparatus, and pins have not been used. Care must be taken to ensure that the lower arm of the cervical head holder does not press against the anterior chest wall, and that the endotracheal tube has neither slid nor become kinked. I have not used central venous pressure (CVP) monitoring, and feel that the complications of routine CVP insertion exceed the potential benefits of their placement. My nonuse of CVP is justified, both by nationally quoted statistics concerning complications of CVP and by an intensive review of these complications in our own hospital. Many notable authors (both surgeons and anesthesiologists) believe that routine use of CVP in all procedures performed in the sitting position is mandatory. I agree that CVP is strongly indicated for many procedures done in this position (e.g., posterior fossa explorations, cervical intradural procedures, cervical arteriovenous malformations). Since the procedure I am describing is entirely extradural and primarily extraligamentous, the likelihood of trouble with the cervical veins is truly minimal. Nonetheless, meticulous attention is paid to any and all bleeding points, whether arterial or venous.

A midline incision is made in the posterior cervical region, and this is carried down to the spinous processes in the mid and lower cervical regions. Intraoperative x-ray localization is essential. Next, the paraspinous fascia is incised in a vertically linear manner, and the paraspinous muscles are gently separated from the lateral aspect of the spinous process and the laminar arches. There is a tendinous extension of these muscles attaching on the posterior and posterior-lateral aspect of the spinous process. This is cut using either scissors or a conventional knife. The cutting cautery is not used; I have found this to be neither helpful nor desirable. The muscles are held back by means of a standard hemilaminectomy retractor, and the laminae themselves are then directly visualized. Since we have already obtained x-ray localization, only the involved laminae need to be exposed and cleaned.

At this point, a small dental dissector (Goldman-Fox Knife No. 7, Paul Brandt Company, Freehold, New Jersey) is used to establish an operating plane by dissecting the ligamentum flavum from the lateral aspect of the inferior portion of the superior lamina, and the superior portion of the lamina below. Once this ligamentous attachment has been dissected free, a small amount of the inferior aspect of the superior lamina and superior aspect of the inferior lamina is removed, usually using a 5-mm, 40°-angle Kerrison punch. Following this small amount of bone removal, the dental dissector is again used to explore the lateral aspect of the interlaminal space in order to identify the intervertebral foramen. It should be noted that there is moderate variability in the anatomic configuration of the foramen, both in its actual location in the vertical plane and in the degree of angulation in the anterior-lateral dimension. When this orientation has been established, a small (3-mm) 40°-angle punch is used to remove the posterior lip of the foramen. I do not use a power instrument for this portion of the procedure, although I certainly recognize how helpful this tool might be to a surgeon who uses it routinely for this type of work. I prefer the small punch for two reasons: (1) I am more comfortable with it, and (2) I believe that this bone removal can be done more slowly and meticulously by this manual means. Obviously, this is a personal prejudice and must be viewed in that context. A potential point of criticism of the use of this small punch is that the pressure of the punch on the posterior aspect of the root might well cause it further injury or harm. Although this criticism is theoretically valid, I have not found it to be important.

As one removes the bony ridge comprising the posterolateral aspect of the foramen, several anatomic landmarks must be kept in mind. At the point where the nerve root actually enters the foramen, one notes a change in the texture and appearance of the ligamentum flavum. This does not represent the full extent of nerve root compression, however. Two to 4 mm further laterally, one usually sees a small actual "step-down" in the appearance of the posterior aspect of the root. When one sees this second anatomic change, one is probably as far lateral as one needs to go. Two further anatomic clues are: (1) the appearance of a small vein laterally in the foramen, usually indicated by the sudden appearance of a small amount of venous oozing (a tiny pledget of Gelfoam inserted into the lateral aspect of the decompression nearly always controls the ooze without further problems); (2) the sensation that posterior pressure on the back of the root is lacking, as manifested by use of this same dental dissector. I would note that the space is explored using this small dissector after each bit of bone is removed. After one ascertains adequate nerve root decompression (by use of the dissector as well as by direct visualization of the back of the root), one simply stops with that space. If there is any question about a second space being involved, either above or below, it is explored by the same technique. This second space exploration and/or decompression seldom takes more than 10 minutes. In our experience, 12 percent of our patients had two spaces equally involved anatomically.

The facet joint is not disturbed, other than occasionally in its most medial aspect. Since the facet is anatomically intact, no additional instability is caused.

The incision is closed by means of absorbable suture material to reapproximate the muscle and fascia. This same material is used to reapproximate the subcutaneous area, and the skin itself is closed by whatever mechanism the surgeon prefers. A simple compression dressing is used, and I do not use any type of postoperative immobilization apparatus (either soft or hard collar). The patient is ambulated on the night of the day of surgery and increasing activity is encouraged beginning on postoperative day one. I generally remove the sutures on postoperative day 5, and the patient is discharged from the hospital on that same day. At the time of discharge, the patient is given prescriptions for a mild analgesic and for a muscle relaxant. He or she is asked not to get involved with any kind of significant exertion for the first month postoperatively, and is asked not to drive a motor vehicle during this time span. The vehicular restriction is purely prophylactic. A person who does not have good range of motion of his or her neck should not be behind the wheel of a motor vehicle. A rather lengthy list of detailed postoperative instructions is mailed to the patient's home, and these are to reinforce the verbal instructions.

When the patient is seen in the office after the first month, the majority of the restrictions are removed, and the mean length of time to return to work or other "normal" activities is 9.4 weeks from the day of surgery (9.3 weeks for men and 9.5 weeks for women). Many highly motivated individuals return to work prior to that time, and some within the first week or two postoperatively. It is of interest to note that in the statistical review of this population, there was no difference between "private" patients and the smaller percentage of either workmen's compensation or liability patients (15% of this total patient group) in this regard.

Further strictly technical points concerning this procedure must be included with this description. The ligamentum flavum is not opened. There is no attempt made to explore anterior to the root, even in patients with suspected soft or hard disc protrusion and/or herniation. There is no attempt made to remove any spurring anterior to the root. This decompression is posterior-lateral, purely and simply, and one should not make a bigger operation out of this procedure than is deemed necessary to achieve adequate nerve root decompression.

Analysis of this large group of operations (1155) confirmed my initial impression that this procedure is simple, safe, and good. I obtained 96 percent relief of sensory symptoms and 98 percent benefit regarding preoperatively present motor deficit, and I noted a true recurrence rate of 3 percent (same problem at the same space on the same side). I had a zero mortality, and a surgical morbidity of 1.5 percent (1.2% superficial wound infection, and 0.3% incidence of wound or muscle separation requiring secondary closure). All patients were done in the sitting position, and with a zero incidence of demonstrable air embolus (either by ECG, Doppler change, or clinical signs or symptoms).

It is obvious that a competent surgeon can obtain excellent results from an anterior approach, but analysis of available data would indicate that even the most favorable figures would either barely approximate, or fall short of, these figures. In addition, the complications associated with the anterior approach (involving damage to the great vessels, larynx, esophagus, recurrent laryngeal nerve, disc space infection, non-union, or pseudarthrosis) is not an inconsiderable percentage.

In summary, I would hope to present a case for re-evaluation of the posterior approach for simple cervical radiculopathy (either motor or sensory), with its associated benefits and very restricted complication rate. No operation is a panacea for all patients, no matter how definitively the diagnosis is established. Nevertheless, this procedure is, without question, the most gratifying one to both patient and surgeon.

MULTIPLE SUBTOTAL SOMATECTOMY

MARIO BONI, M.D.

Multiple subtotal somatectomy (MSS) is used, when necessary, to decompress the cord anteriorly at several levels. The operation has several important features: (1) in the somatectomy, the central part of the vertebral bodies is removed for about 15 mm, until the posterior longitudinal ligament is completely exposed; (2) body removal is subtotal, the lateral walls of the vertebral bodies are not removed; and (3) it may be multiple, involving several vertebral bodies. Decompression is followed by stabilization through somatic reconstruction with tricortical autogenous bone graft from the iliac crest modeled and inserted in diastasis.

INDICATIONS

Multiple subtotal somatectomy is indicated in the treatment of stenosis of the cervical canal caused by anterior compression. It is absolutely necessary to be certain that the problem is myeloradiculopathy caused by anterior cervical canal stenosis. The anterior compression producing a cervical canal stenosis can have different causes. The technique has the following indications: (1) *degenerative arthrotic (spondylotic) myeloradiculopathy*, when anterior compression at the level of three or more intervertebral discs is present; (2) *traumatic compression*, either in cases of multilevel somatic lesions with fragments anteriorly in the canal, or trauma with serious kyphotic deformity; (3) *severe instability* resulting from laminectomy and when, because of persisting anterior compression, laminectomy has failed; (4) *inflammatory compression*; (5) *neoplastic bone destruction* when it is necessary to remove the tumor and reconstruct the destroyed vertebral bodies for stabilization.

CONTRAINDICATIONS

The somatectomy operation is contraindicated in the face of serious cardiorespiratory disease and when the myeloradicular compression is posterior. The operation is usually not required for single-level compression, but it is not contraindicated.

PREOPERATIVE PREPARATION OF THE PATIENT

After the diagnosis has been made and the MSS recommended, the patient is prepared for the surgical procedure by starting respiratory therapy, active mobilization of the limbs (which has to be continued in the postoperative period), and, moreover, using the cervical brace that will be worn after the operation. The preparation of the patient for anesthesia and for the surgery itself is the same as for any neck surgery.

The operation is performed in two stages: (1) the taking of the graft from the iliac wing, and (2) the operation on the cervical spine. The patient is first laid supine on the table, with a pillow under the gluteal region, in order to better expose the iliac crest. After skin closure and dressing, the patient is prepared for the cervical second stage. The position of the neck and head is very important because the pharynx, larynx, trachea, esophagus, thyroid, and inferior laryngeal nerve should not be under tension, but easily retractable. Therefore, when the operation is performed at higher levels, the neck should be slightly flexed and the head in slight extension; when the operation is performed on the lower levels, the neck should be extended and the head slightly flexed.

A special aluminum support is fixed to the head device. This support is shaped to suit the posterior profile of the neck, so that a steady rest is provided during surgery. The definitive head position is completed by two side supports fixing the temporal regions, as well as by a large band that passes under the chin and is fastened to the head device. Skeletal fixation can also be used. In order to reduce bleeding, the surgical bed is tilted up by about 30°; hypotensive anesthesia has been used for the operation in our protocol. The lower limbs are wrapped with elastic bandages so as to prevent venous stasis due to the position.

SURGICAL TECHNIQUE

Stage One: Taking the Autogenous Graft From the Iliac Crest

The excision is usually performed on the right or on the same side as the operation on the neck. The skin is incised 1 cm below and parallel to the iliac crest in the central portion. A full-thickness graft is removed with an osteotome or an electrical saw. The transplant is about 2 cm wide. It is important to assess its length, which depends on the number of intervertebral spaces involved: approximately 18 mm should be calculated for each space to be operated on; since the graft is inserted in diastasis by means of a suitable distractor, 1 cm should be added to the length.

Preparation of the transplant is started: the graft consists of a three-sided cortical foil of hard bone which surrounds the inner spongy bone; it is freed from the residual soft tissue and is shaped with the bone forceps and rasp until it is made straight; then it is wrapped in blood-soaked gauzes and put aside for later use.

Stage Two: The Operation on the Cervical Spine

The operation is performed from the right. The skin is incised parallel to the anterior margin of the sternocleidomastoid muscle. The anterior longitudinal ligament is reached by passing between the neurovascular trunk and the visceral formations.

The neurovascular trunk is pulled laterally, while the visceral formation is pulled upward and medially. A soft retractor is used. For low exposure (T1), it is sometimes necessary to ligate the inferior thyroid artery; for high exposures (C2-C3), a section of the thyro-lingual-facial venous trunk is performed. This approach allows exposure of the cervical spine from C3 to T1.

An intraoperative roentgenogram is required at this point to localize the intervertebral spaces to be operated on. The anterior longitudinal ligament is then incised with an electric scalpel, detaching and opening it laterally. The operation is started from the more distal intervertebral space. Removal of the discs is first performed and, if protruding anterior osteophytes are found, they are removed by means of an osteotome. Several methods can be used to drill the vertebral bodies. In arthrotic disease or in posttraumatic deformities it is easier to use Cloward's instruments. The drill goes down to the posterior wall of the vertebral bodies, which is removed by means of curets until decompression of the posterior longitudinal ligament is carried out.

When there are protrusions of the uncus extending into the intervertebral foramina with compression of the roots, partial posterior uncusectomy is required. This partial transdiscal uncusectomy is performed with curets angled by 45° and 90° to remove the posterior part of the uncal spur after removal of the posterior walls of the adjacent vertebral bodies.

This procedure is repeated at each level requiring decompression. There will be three or more holes involving adjacent vertebral bodies separated by the residual of the central vertebral bone. These bone bridges are then removed by the bone forceps and the exposure of the posterior longitudinal ligament is completed by using high-speed drills and curets. In this way a broad trench 15 mm wide has been prepared, and in its bed the posterior longitudinal ligament and the dura mater are exposed.

In acute traumatic disorders or in neoplastic diseases in which Cloward instruments cannot be used, decompression is obtained by employing drills, bone forceps, and curets. In such cases an important consideration in the technique consists of preserving the vertebral artery, isolating the lateral portion of the vertebral body through a bilateral sagittal cut with high speed drill.

Once the posterior longitudinal ligament has been completely freed and all the causes of compression have been removed, the transplant site is prepared. By means of curets or a drill a suitable groove is cut into the body at the upper end of the trench and into that at the lower end, so as to make a hollow to accept and keep the graft in a fixed position after insertion. At this point, with a special distractor, a diastasis is realized. The length of the trench is measured with the special compass-like instrument and the depth with the Cloward gauge. On the basis of these measurements, the preparation of the graft is completed: it has to be a few millimeters longer than the bone trench (the correct length depends on the diastasis that is likely to be obtained) and the depth of the transplant is computed so as to make it lie, once it has been positioned, a few millimeters off the posterior longitudinal ligament. The ends of the graft are then modeled to make it fit perfectly in the groove prepared in the vertebral bodies. The graft is inserted into the trench in diastasis by pressing hard or with a hammer, and the distractor is removed. In this way the graft is firmly seated. If the graft has been modeled properly and embedded, no secondary means of fixation are required. However, in cases with severe instability (traumatic or neoplastic lesions involving several levels or with extensive laminectomy), it is advisable to fasten the graft anteriorly with plates and screws. Once the arthrodesis has been accomplished in this way, it is important to review the whole surgical field for impeccable hemostasis. The two bellies of the omohyoid muscle, the platysma, and the skin are sutured as well. If hemostasis has been adequate, no suction drainage is necessary.

Radiologic verification of the position is always performed in the operating room.

POSTOPERATIVE CARE

An orthopaedic brace (SOMI-brace) that has been fitted before the operation is applied to the patient on the surgical bed. With severe instability, a halo is utilized by cast or jacket. Forty-eight hours after operation, the patient is allowed to sit on the bed; on the third day (depending on the condition of the wound from which the graft was obtained), the patient becomes ambulatory. The evolution of the fusion and position should be periodically checked roentgenographically. The orthopaedic brace has to be worn for 90 days until the fusion of the graft is shown by radiographs.

GREATER OCCIPITAL NEURALGIA

NIKOLAI BOGDUK, M.B., B.S., Ph.D.

The term "greater occipital neuralgia" implies a painful condition of the greater occipital nerve, but in practice, it tends to be ascribed indiscriminately to virtually any complaint of pain in the occipital region. Consequently, undue emphasis has been placed on disorders of the greater occipital nerve as the cause of occipital pain.

In the first instance, the greater occipital nerve is not the only nerve that innervates the occiput. Its territory overlaps that of the lesser and third occipital nerves, and it is enigmatic that for all the theories implicating the greater occipital nerve as the cause of occipital pain, similar ones involving the lesser and third occipital nerves have not been equally popularized.

More significantly, however, a much neglected concept is that the occipital region is an area to which deep pain may be referred from a large number of structures. Experimental and clinical studies have clearly demonstrated that occipital pain can be produced by noxious stimulation of the dura mater of the posterior cranial fossa, the vertebral arteries, the periosteum of the occipital condyles, any of the upper cervical synovial joints and muscles, and even the C2-C3 and C3-C4 intervertebral discs. The common feature of these structures is that they are all innervated by branches of the first three cervical spinal nerves. It is therefore possible to summarize the differential diagnosis of occipital pain, succinctly and comprehensively, as any painful disorder of the structures innervated by the upper three cervical nerves or of the nerves themselves. Consequently, any diagnostic approach to occipital pain should be based on this comprehensive differential diagnosis and not restricted by any preoccupation with the greater occipital nerve and its disorders.

A useful diagnostic algorithm, used for other forms of headache, involves taking a general medical history to establish the context of the complaint; then the pain is defined in terms of the length of illness, its onset, site, radiation, quality, frequency, duration, associated features, time and mode of onset, precipitating or aggravating factors, and relieving factors. Each of these parameters offers clues that may indicate or exclude a particular diagnosis.

GENERAL MEDICAL HISTORY

A past history of illness or concurrent symptoms may reveal systemic disease of which occipital pain may be a presenting feature or only a component complaint. In this regard, occipital pain may occur when upper cervical arthritis develops in a patient with rheumatoid arthritis, ankylosing spondylitis, or degenerative joint disease. A history of vascular disease may suggest vertebral aneurysm. Features of spinal cord irritation implicate craniocervical instability as a result of congenital, traumatic, or destructive vertebral disease. A dental history needs to be considered because occipital pain may be a component of temporomandibular joint dysfunction.

LENGTH OF ILLNESS

The length of illness serves in a general sense to distinguish benign from threatening complaints. A long-standing static complaint is unlikely to be due to progressive disease such as tumor or aneurysm. A complaint of short duration is not in itself pathognomonic, but obliges exclusion of serious disease such as tumor, hemorrhage, or craniocervical infection. Herpes zoster affecting the C2 ganglion may be prefaced by pain a few days before the eruption of vesicles.

ONSET

An acute onset of severe pain may indicate cerebral hemorrhage or infection, but a gradual onset is of little diagnostic significance. A history of trauma invites an appraisal of what might have been injured. In this con-

text, occipital pain is frequently associated with hyper-extension or acceleration injuries to the neck, but it should be noted that anatomically, the greater occipital nerve is protected from direct damage in such injuries. Occipital pain following "whiplash" more strongly implicates damage to upper cervical musculoskeletal structures.

SITE

For present purposes, it is assumed that the principal complaint of pain is localized to the occipital region. In some cases, however, the pain may encompass other areas of the head or neck. Some patients complain of frontal headache, but interrogation can reveal that, in fact, the pain actually starts in the occipital region before radiating and focusing in the forehead (to be discussed).

RADIATION

Occipital pain may be localized, or it can be a component of a more widespread referral. Common patterns include occipital pain spreading around the temples to the forehead and eyes, or passing directly through the head to the frontal region. Conversely, frontal pain may spread backward to include the occiput.

The pattern of referral is in no way pathognomonic of either the source or the cause of pain. All that can be determined at this stage of the assessment is whether the pattern of complaint is suggestive of pain referred to the head, or whether the occiput is only incidentally involved in a more generalized headache such as migraine.

QUALITY

The quality of the pain is one of the keys to distinguishing between neuralgias and other causes of pain. Neuralgic pain tends to be felt superficially, at least in addition to any deep pain, and is of a shooting or lancinating quality. In contrast, referred pain from musculoskeletal or other deep structures is aching in quality and is perceived only deeply.

Throbbing pain has traditionally been regarded as indicative of vascular headache, but this characteristic is not reliable for it can occur simply by awareness of pulsation superimposed on other causes of pain.

FREQUENCY

Musculoskeletal pain tends to be constant, although in the early stages of an arthritic disorder, the patient may be subject to intermittent episodes of constant pain. This constancy, coupled with its deep, aching quality distinguishes referred musculoskeletal pain from neuralgic pain.

Neuralgia is episodic or paroxysmal. In this context,

it is noteworthy that true greater occipital neuralgia, consisting of paroxysmal attacks of lancinating pain, associated with cutaneous trigger areas, as in trigeminal neuralgia, is a rare condition. Other so-called greater occipital neuralgias, if they exist, are more strictly entrapment or irritative peripheral neuropathies. These may or may not be paroxysmal in nature, but they can be distinguished on the basis of their associated features (qv).

Headaches with a distinct periodicity, such as 2 to 5 days of pain occurring one to four times a month, are highly suggestive of migraine, but appropriate associated features must be present before this diagnosis can be ascribed with confidence.

An accelerating frequency of episodes of pain should alert the physician to serious conditions such as tumor, aneurysm, or hemorrhage.

DURATION

The duration of pain is meaningless in patients with constant pain, but attacks measured in seconds or minutes are suggestive of a neurogenic origin, and regular attacks measured in days are suggestive of migraine.

ASSOCIATED FEATURES

Associated features are probably the most reliable characteristics that permit the differentiation of the various causes of occipital pain.

Musculoskeletal causes of pain should not be associated with neurological signs, unless the spinal cord or spinal nerves are secondarily involved. The former is self-evident, and indicates craniocervical instability. With respect to the latter, it should be noted that the first and second cervical spinal nerves do not emerge through intervertebral foramina and so are not susceptible to compression as are other spinal nerves. Therefore, one must postulate unique lesions before ascribing neurological signs and symptoms to "compression" of the C1 or C2 nerve roots. Moreover, it should be remembered that the C2 spinal nerve is distributed to the neck and face, through its ventral ramus, as well as to the occiput, through its dorsal ramus. Therefore, signs should be present in both dorsal and ventral distributions before compression of the C2 roots is diagnosed.

The C2 ventral ramus also conveys proprioceptive sensation from the tongue, and this feature underlies the basis of neck-tongue syndrome, a condition characterized clinically by the sudden onset of occipital pain and ipsilateral numbness of the tongue following rotation of the head. In this condition, the pain is caused by subluxation of a lateral atlantoaxial joint, and the apparent "numbness" is caused by compression of the proprioceptive afferents in the C2 ventral ramus when this nerve is impacted against the subluxated articular process.

Other features suggestive of a musculoskeletal origin of occipital pain are restriction of active and passive movements of the upper cervical joints, especially if such movements aggravate the pain. Areas of tenderness in the upper cervical region are complementary in this regard, particularly if sustained pressure over a tender area evokes referral of pain to the head. The interpretation of tender areas, however, is fraught with ambiguity, for they can occur in a wide variety of headaches, including migraine, and may simply represent normal areas of tenderness. They may represent so-called myofascial trigger points, which however, may be either primary or secondary irritative foci. Tenderness overlying the articular pillars, particularly at the C2-C3 level, may indicate an underlying zygapophysial arthropathy.

With respect to entrapment neuropathies, except in true neuralgias (e.g., trigeminal neuralgia), there are no known mechanisms by which peripheral nerves can be irritated to produce only pain. Large-diameter afferents cannot escape mechanical irritation or ischemia, and so paresthesias and numbness are hallmarks of entrapment neuropathy be it painful or painless. It is therefore unjustifiable to diagnose entrapment of the greater occipital or other nerve in the absence of such cutaneous neurological features. Occipital pain, in the absence of other neurological symptoms, invites a search for a musculoskeletal or non-neurogenic cause.

Nausea, vomiting, and photophobia are associated features strongly suggestive of migraine, especially when coupled with periodic pain. Intermittent neurological signs may occur in vertebrobasilar or classic migraine.

Vague complaints such as blurred vision and dizziness are not pathognomonic despite the temptation to consider dizziness as a symptom of vertebrobasilar insufficiency. Other features of vertebrobasilar insufficiency should be established before this diagnosis is made because dizziness itself can be caused by disturbances to cervical proprioceptive mechanisms resulting from cervical trauma or arthritis, which in no way imply vascular insufficiency.

TIME OF ONSET

In other forms of headache the time of onset can be characteristic, as in the matutinal headaches of hypertension, but this parameter has not been shown to be of relevance in occipital headache. The only phenomenon perhaps worthy of mention is that headache occurring toward the end of the day would be consistent with tension headache or an arthritic condition aggravated by head movements during the day.

MODE OF ONSET

If not already constant, musculoskeletal pain tends to build up in intensity as the affected part is used during the day.

An explosive onset of pain should be alarming and warns of possible sinister conditions such as aneurysm, hemorrhage, or acute subluxation of the spine.

PRECIPITATING OR AGGRAVATING FEATURES

The precipitation or aggravation of pain by neck movements is strongly suggestive of a musculoskeletal cause. In this regard, the patient may volunteer that certain activities, such as reading with head bent forward or reversing the car, aggravate the pain. Otherwise, examination may reveal aggravation of the pain by passive neck movements.

When no aggravating factors can be identified, a musculoskeletal cause is unlikely, and an intracranial or idiopathic etiology should be considered.

RELIEVING FACTORS

Relieving factors are infrequently of diagnostic value, for usually the patient identifies none. However, if certain postures ease the pain, or if formal immobilization of the neck in a collar eases the pain, a cervical cause is implied.

PHYSICAL EXAMINATION

The physical examination relevant to the diagnosis of occipital pain has been described. Simply to summarize, a neurological examination should address signs of intracranial pathology, spinal cord injury, and sensory changes in the territory of both the ventral and dorsal rami of the cervical spinal nerves; the neck should be examined for mobility and tenderness, and ideally this should include an assessment of intersegmental motion, not just movement of the entire cervical spine.

INVESTIGATIONS

The purpose of formal investigations is twofold: to screen for occult or unsuspected disease, and to confirm or differentiate suspected disease.

Conventional investigations such as skull radiographs, nuclear scans, and computerized axial tomography may be used to assess possible intracranial disorders. Angiography may be indicated for vascular disease.

Plain radiographs of the cervical spine, which should include transoral views of the atlantoaxial joints and odontoid process, may reveal congenital abnormalities, bone tumors, and old or recent fractures. Computerized tomography may further resolve such changes and is particularly useful in identifying rotatory subluxations of the atlas. Conventional tomography may reveal arthritic changes not apparent in plain radiographs. Myelography may be required to resolve abnormalities of the upper cord and posterior cranial fossa.

In the absence of overt morphologic changes, diagnostic blocks provide the most valuable means of determining the source of pain, particularly in musculoskeletal disorders.

The traditional procedure in this regard is a superficial block of the greater occipital nerve, in which the nerve is injected at, or near, the site at which it crosses the superior nuchal line. Theoretically, relief of pain following such a block indicates that the source of pain lies at or distal to the block, but distal to the superior nuchal line; the greater occipital nerve is only cutaneous, and there are no known occult cutaneous causes of occipital pain. Consequently, a positive block implies a source of pain at the site of blockade.

Such deductions have been the cornerstone of diagnosis of entrapment and irritative neuropathies of the greater occipital nerve. However, certain pitfalls need to be recognized. First, diagnostic blocks become ambiguous if large volumes of anesthetic (e.g., more than 2 ml) are used, for the anesthetic possibly affects more than just the target tissue. Any relief obtained could be due to the anesthetization of suboccipital trigger points rather than the greater occipital nerve. Second, it has been established that anesthetization of the cutaneous nerves to an area of referred pain can appear to relieve the referred pain. Thus, a positive greater occipital nerve block may represent an illusory block of referred pain, rather than "greater occipital neuralgia". Any diagnosis of neuralgia or neuropathy, therefore, should not rest on the result of blocks alone. It should be made on the basis of clinical features consistent with, if not pathognomonic of, a neurogenic origin of pain.

Recent innovations have been the development of blocks of the deeper branches of the upper cervical nerves, particularly their dorsal rami, and of the upper cervical synovial joints themselves. Using fluoroscopic control, the C2 spinal nerve can be blocked where it lies dorsal to the lateral atlantoaxial joint. The third occipital nerve can be blocked as it crosses and supplies the C2-C3 zygapophysial joint, and other cervical dorsal rami can be blocked as they cross the articular pillars. Periarticular or intra-articular injections can be used to anesthetize individual cervical joints, and the upper cervical intervertebral discs can be tested by provocation and analgesic discography.

By a judicious application and interpretation of these several techniques, a detailed search can be made for most musculoskeletal causes of occipital pain. Nerve blocks can be used to delimit the source of pain to the territory of a particular nerve, and joint blocks can be used, if required, to further refine the diagnosis. In our own units, we have been struck by the frequency with which the C2-C3 zygapophysial joint proves to be the source of occipital pain.

A technique complementary to nerve blocks is the use of a stimulator. If a nerve block is being performed, the nerve can be stimulated electrically prior to anesthetization. Reproduction of the patient's pain by electrical stimulation complements the observation of relief of pain following blockade.

For diagnostic, research, or medicolegal purposes, diagnostic blocks and electrical stimulation can be controlled. There can be no doubt about the diagnosis if stimulation and anesthetization is positive for one particular nerve or joint, but not for adjacent structures, or if the patient responds appropriately to a random series of single-blind injections of local anesthetic and placebo.

TREATMENT

Whereas it is axiomatic that the proper treatment of occipital pain depends on an accurate diagnosis having been made, much of the literature on this subject is marred by ambiguity, neglect, or presumption of the diagnosis. This has led to the popularization of various and contrasting forms of treatment, often accompanied by partisan declarations of efficacy, but rarely has a particular form of treatment been elaborated with a defendable rationale, clear indications, and proven efficacy.

For some conditions, such as vertebral aneurysm, posterior fossa tumors, and craniocervical instability, the treatment is conventional and does not warrant discussion. For migraine, an extensive pharmacologic armamentarium is available in standard neurological practice. However, it is the treatment of apparent neuropathies and musculoskeletal disorders that remains controversial or undetermined.

The traditional neurosurgical therapy for so-called occipital neuralgia has been occipital neurectomy. The controversial aspects of this procedure are several, but the fundamental issue is its rationale. It is pernicious to perform neurectomy simply for referred pain. Not only does this invite unnecessary complications, but it also invites failure, for the source of pain is not treated. Neurectomy should not be entertained unless a neurogenic cause has been established and not confused with referred pain.

Even if entrapment or irritative neuropathy is the diagnosis, it is questionable whether neurectomy is indicated. Decompression would be a more logical procedure for entrapment neuropathy, but such tailored procedures have not been evaluated for occipital neuralgia. Instead, there seems to have been a preoccupation with destructive neurosurgery, paradoxically when no consistent neurogenic disease affecting the greater occipital nerve has ever been demonstrated.

Greater occipital neurectomy, in all its forms, risks serious complications. Simple neurectomy invites formation of a regenerative neuroma, and this condition becomes an additional differential diagnosis of recurrent pain after occipital neurectomy. More seriously, transection of a cutaneous nerve predisposes to the development of anesthesia dolorosa, and the risk of this debilitating complaint alone should temper any consideration of neurectomy.

The complications of, and lack of rationale for, greater occipital neurectomy should relegate neurectomy to the status of a rarely used procedure.

As an alternative to surgery, some authorities advocate the injection of local anesthetic and steroids into the greater occipital nerve. Although this is logical if an inflammatory neuropathy is presupposed, there are no established means of identifying cases of inflammatory occipital neuralgia. Occasionally, it may be rewarding to inject steroids as a trial of therapy, but no data justify the universal application of this form of therapy or guarantee the longevity of its efficacy.

Another major field of therapeutic approaches relates to various assaults on the suboccipital region. The earlier literature advocates the injection into the suboccipital muscles of local anesthetic and steroids, or sclerosants. More recently, this has been supplanted by radiofrequency occipital denaturation, a procedure in which large areas of the suboccipital region are coagulated with a radiofrequency electrode. Despite enthusiastic reports of the efficacy of all these varieties of treatment, their liability is that they have not been evaluated by independent investigators and their rationale is ambiguous. These treatments presuppose some form of disease in the soft tissues of the suboccipital region, sometimes interpreted as traumatic degeneration, but no disease has ever been formally demonstrated. In the absence of an attractive rationale, it is difficult to advocate or endorse such destructive therapy.

That arthritis of the upper cervical spine can cause occipital pain has been recognized since the turn of the century. Efficient treatment of this phenomenon, however, has been hampered by both the lack of means for precise diagnosis and an fundamental lack of knowledge of the mechanisms and causes of arthritic pain.

Collars, physiotherapy, acupuncture, and transcutaneous nerve stimulation may be palliative, but these techniques do not address the cause of pain. Analgesics and nonsteroidal anti-inflammatory drugs conspicuously appear poorly effective for chronic spinal pain. Manipulative therapy or cervical mobilization is arguably rational for arthritic conditions, but no trials have established the efficacy of manual therapy for head pain of proven cervical origin. Moreover, injudicious manipulation, particularly of the atlantoaxial joints, carries with it the risk of vertebral artery thrombosis.

The development, in recent times, of selective nerve and joint blocks, coupled with the use of high-resolution tomography, has improved diagnostic capabilities for arthritic conditions of the upper cervical spine. Blocks, correlated with radiologic changes, can pinpoint individual joints responsible for occipital pain, but we are still left with the problem of how to deal adequately with joint pain. Those trying to cope with this problem have employed a variety of approaches, each of still undetermined value, but each attempt carries with it at least a hope that a reliable treatment may be perfected.

If blockade of a particular dorsal ramus successfully relieves pain temporarily, percutaneous radiofrequency coagulation of that nerve or its branches may be entertained. Some advocates of this therapy report good success rates at 1-year follow-up. In our experience, patients with occipital pain due to arthopathy in the C2-C3 zygapophysial joint can expect 4 to 6 months of complete pain relief if the third occipital nerve is coagulated at its origin. Regeneration of the nerve seems to be the factor that limits the efficacy of this procedure, but in the event of regeneration, the procedure is repeatable. Current research efforts are being directed toward a means of impeding or delaying regeneration. To this end, I have tried open neurectomy, but have met with painful neuroma formation, and so I have abandoned this approach until a reliable means of preventing neuroma formation is established.

Another recent innovation for pain of zygapophysial joint origin is the use of intra-articular steroids. Some early reports claim relief of pain for up to 9 months in patients whose pain can be relieved by diagnostic joint blocks.

HERNIATED THORACIC DISC

THOMAS DUCKER, M.D.

Intervertebral thoracic disc herniation resulting in a neurological deficit is not nearly so common as those in the cervical and lumbar area. The thoracic spine is less mobile because of the rib cage. In most clinical reviews, it is the reason for less than one percent (1%) of all the disc operations. It tends to occur in those aged 35 to 55 years, in both sexes, and is rarely seen in children or senior citizens. When an elderly patient presents with a clinical picture of thoracic disc herniation, it is commonly associated with thoracic spondylosis, thoracic spinal stenosis, and compression from a degenerative disc and osteophyte formation rather than a true disc herniation. The only population that tends to have a high incidence of this disorder is that of achondroplastic dwarfs.

CLINICAL PRESENTATION

In most patients, thoracic disc herniation has an insidious onset. The disorder starts spontaneously without trauma. The mid and lower thoracic spine is more commonly involved; the upper spine from T1 to T5–6 is rarely afflicted with this problem. The initial symptoms are usually pain on bending or lifting and other complaints that are difficult to localize. Numbness is a common complaint. Soon thereafter, the patient describes unsteadiness and stiffness of gait. Although the triad of mechanical low thoracic back pain, numbness in the lower extremities, and subsequent unsteady gait in a patient who is free of malignant disease is the most common presentation, it certainly is not the only presentation. Some patients simply present with a gait disturbance without numbness or pain.

The diagnosis is easily missed and other medical problems are considered. When there has been some radicular component to the pain, the patients have been studied for pancreatitis, ulcer disease, and other intra-abdominal or retroperitoneal disorders. A spinal epidu-

ral tumor is more common than a disc herniation. The older patient is more likely to have spondylosis with spur and degenerative disc disorders associated with a spinal stenosis. The fact that nearly one-half of these cases are misdiagnosed and ineffectively treated by astute clinicians attests to the difficulty in recognizing this disorder.

On physical examination, the most sensitive index to thoracic compression is hyperreflexia in the lower extremity compared to the upper extremity. The gait disturbance or motor deficit can best be detected by having the patient either run in place or hop on one foot. On testing for motor strength, it is often difficult to define the problem, and a sensory examination may not be convincing for organic disease. For all of the aforementioned reasons, it is important to listen to the patient's complaint in order to suspect the disorder. The problem can be further compounded by the fact that in older patients who have spondylitic spur formation, the neurological deficit may be asymmetrical and indicative of a Brown-Séquard syndrome.

Plain roentgenograms are helpful. In the younger patient, the disc space may be calcified, with actual shifting of the calcium toward the canal. In the older patient, the osteophytic spurs can be appreciated. Computerized tomography is helpful if the exact disc space involved is known. The newer magnetic resonance imaging technique appears to be an even better tool. Once the space is identified, the CT scan can confirm the disorder. Often these noninvasive radiologic techniques provide the clinical diagnosis.

Myelography remains an important diagnostic tool. Differentiating between medical and surgical disorders may be difficult, and Pantopaque myelography is still the most accurate method. If a water-soluble contrast material is used, follow-up computerized tomography is usually needed. Even with good myelography, computerized tomography, and other diagnostic tools, the diagnosis is not easily made. The block can be suggestive of an epidural tumor.

TREATMENT

The goal of treatment is to stop the compression and short-circuiting of the neural elements. The standard decompressive laminectomy is no longer the procedure of choice once the proper diagnosis is made. Other procedures have had a higher success rate in achieving good results. Our standard decompressive laminectomy cures or improves 40 to 60 percent of the patients, whereas more posterolateral, lateral, and anterolateral approaches have a higher degree of success, in the range of 85 to 90 percent. No particular procedure has a 100 percent success rate. The choice of procedure depends on the surgeon's experience and clinical training.

The speed with which one recommends operative decompression is directly proportional to how fast the disorder is advancing. For a long standing disorder with minimal symptoms, there is sufficient time to carefully plan an operative approach and to allow the patient to consider informed consent. A few patients deteriorate rapidly, demanding urgent diagnostic studies. In some of those cases, the myelographic procedure itself may cause further deterioration. It is in these hurried circumstances that difficulties arise in diagnosis, treatment, and a full comprehension of the disorder.

Although a laminectomy is not the preferred procedure, it has been safely carried out in many patients. The posterior approach for laminectomy must be carefully accomplished without introducing any instrumentation beneath the lamina. Such techniques as using the rongeurs parallel to the cord and/or high-speed air-drilled decompressive laminectomy need to be considered if one has not ascertained whether the diagnosis is thoracic disc disease or epidural tumor. If one has already accomplished the laminectomy only to discover that the major problem is a herniated thoracic disc, the procedure should be converted to a paravertebral posterior approach by one of two techniques:

1. A lateral incision is made, extending in a T-shaped fashion from the previous laminectomy incision to permit a more direct posterior approach parallel to the previous exposure. By means of a high-speed drill, the lateral wall of the spinal canal is drilled away. Through this more lateral opening, the disc fragments can be removed.
2. By means of a transpedicle approach through the facets and the pedicle, the lateral aspect of the canal and the lateral portions of the vertebral body itself are exposed. The interspace can be entered through this approach and the disc material removed.

If the proper preoperative diagnosis is made, one should choose an operation that does not entail a laminectomy. There are basically three choices: (1) a paramedian lateral approach, basically referred to as the transpedicle exposure, (2) a posterior lateral costotransversectomy type of operation, and (3) a lateral exposure to the disc space through a thoracotomy.

The transpedicle exposure, which has been partially described above, can be used in conjunction with a laminectomy. However, when the correct diagnosis is made preoperatively, the preferred procedure is hemilaminectomy and facetectomy, through a midline incision posteriorly with the paravertebral muscles reflected and exposed only on one side. By removing the facet and the pedicle, one can create a cavity to expose the lateral aspect of the canal and the disc itself. The interspace can be entered and the disc material removed from this more posterior or paramedian approach. The decompression is accomplished without any dura sac and/or cord manipulation.

The posterior lateral costotransversectomy is a well-accepted procedure for the treatment of thoracic disc protrusions. The patient is placed in a lateral prone position, usually with the right side up, unless the preoperative studies show the disc herniation to be confined to one side. The incision is paramedian and curvilinear. Because it is curved at its apex away from the spine, a flap can be reflected toward the spine over the rib area leading to the disc space. It is usually the rib below in the numbering that leads to the proper space. For example, the tenth rib leads to the 9–10 interspace, but in many cases, to get good exposure, it is necessary to remove the more proximal end of the rib above and below. When the rib is being removed, the tissues are reflected toward the pleural cavity. The posterior aspects of the facet and transverse process are rongeured away. The head of the rib is removed to expose the intercostal nerves, which can be traced back to the dura sac at the foramen. Once that is accomplished, the tissues can be reflected off the vertebral body so as to expose the disc space itself. The lateral aspect of the spinal canal can be drilled away to expose the dura and root sleeve. At the disc space, the disc can be identified and carefully curetted away from the dura sac and canal. In the majority of cases, the pleura is not violated and there is no significant pneumothorax and, consequently, no need for a chest tube postoperatively. In some cases, evacuation of the air with a small chest tube for 24 hours postoperatively is needed. Even though the incision may appear lengthy, its paramedian position is not so painful as anticipated. Patients make a good recovery without having undergone either a laminectomy or a thoracotomy. The only limitation in the procedure is a less clear definition of the anatomy via the posterolateral approach, causing difficulty in dissecting the tissues away from the vertebral bodies.

The third option is a lateral exposure through a transthoracic transpleural approach. A standard right posterior and lateral thoracotomy is used. Since the major blood supply to the cord in that area often enters on the left side, most surgeons prefer to use a right-sided thoracotomy. When one is concerned about discs higher in the thoracic spine, it is best to be away from the heart. Once the chest cavity is entered, the vertebral bodies are readily identified, along with the various intercostal nerves and their vascular support. The head of the rib is identified as it approaches the disc space. A marker is placed in the disc space, and an intraoperative roentgenogram is taken before the head of the rib is removed to confirm one's positioning. Then the intercostal nerves are dissected away, adjacent ligaments are freed, and part of the sympathetic chain is cut away or retracted before the head of the rib at the disc space is removed. Next, part of the bone of the vertebral body itself, just anterior to the foramen, is drilled away. This exposes the neural foramen and intercostal nerve, along with the disc space itself. The disc now can be safely removed from this lateral exposure, always curetting anteriorly and away from the dura sac. Once the canal is successfully decompressed, fusion with a bone plug usually is not needed, but if there is an adjacent piece of rib that will readily fit into the joint space, this can be impacted to prevent any further collapse. The rib graft used as a bone plug may or may not be incorporated into solid bone in due time. The thoracotomy is closed in the standard fashion. Chest tubes are required when this exposure is used.

CONCLUSION

Thoracic discs are not common and proper diagnosis is often difficult. If one is so unfortunate to be in the predicament of already having performed a laminectomy only to find a thoracic disc, then the operative exposure has to be converted by taking down part of the facet and pedicle in order to achieve a more lateral exposure to safely remove the disc. While there is earlier literature to recommend a transdural removal of the disc,

this has not been very successful in the hands of experienced clinical operators. If the proper diagnosis can be made preoperatively,, then one has to choose between a paramedian lateral exposure, a posterolateral approach through the costotransversectomy, or a lateral exposure through a thoracotomy and transplural exposure. Each of these other more lateral exposures are more successful than the laminectomy. Each of these procedures has its advantages and disadvantages. My own personal experience working with my colleagues has dictated that the posterolateral costotransversectomy approach has been the most common. Working with ones thoracic surgeon, especially in a community hospital, the transthoracic, transpleural operation certainly has its advantages in achieving a clean exposure to a thoracic disc with a high degree of safety and no significant complications. As is the case with all thoracic cord compression problems, the chances of operative deterioration are in significant numbers, approximately five percent. This is because the small size of the spinal cord with attentuated blood supply, which could be further comprised in any of the above listed exposures.

LOW BACK PAIN WITH OR WITHOUT SCIATICA

BERNARD E. FINNESON, M.D.

Back pain is an ancient symptom. Specialists in anthropology speculate that when man's prehistoric ancestors assumed the upright position, varicose veins, hemorrhoids, and low back dysfunction were created. The problem appears to be increasing in frequency, or at least, increasing numbers of patients are being seen in physician's offices and emergency clinics with this complaint. Reasons for the increase are conjectural. Our "automated" life style may be a factor. Most individuals usually ride rather than walk, take elevators rather than walk up and down stairs, and use mechanical lifting devices to avoid physical stress. When the coddled muscles, tendons, and ligaments are called on to perform an occasional vigorous activity that will cause stress to the low back, it is possible that these structures are not quite up to the task. Possibly today's patient is less willing to put up with the pain and wants corrective measures instituted with dispatch. Litigation and disability are other imponderable factors.

ASSESSMENT OF THE PATIENT WITH LOW BACK PAIN

The most important tool in assessing the patient with low back pain is a careful history. Pain, the most subjective of symptoms, can be appreciated by the physician only by listening carefully to the patient's description of his symptoms.

The physical examination, although not to be slighted, is not so important as the history. The examination provides the physician with information regarding lumbar muscle spasms, lumbar mobility, reflex, and sensory or motor changes in the lower extremities.

A variety of x-ray studies are available to supplement our clinical impressions. These include roentgenograms of the lumbosacral spine, computerized tomographic scanning of the lumbar spine, and bone scans using radioactive isotope. X-ray invasive procedures, such as myelograms and lumbar venograms, are usually reserved for patients who are being considered for surgery.

MANAGEMENT

Approximately 85 percent of all low back ills improve with so-called self-care methods and without requiring professional medical intervention. These measures are as follows:

...ve low back discomfort ...nctively attempt to avoid. The method and extent of ...e severity and nature of the ...a limited activity program ...g, prolonged forward bend- ...d prolonged auto trips) to the ...est.

...by a variety of methods is the ...m of therapy. Heat relaxes ...ove local muscle nutrition by ...d may be analgesic. It is fre- ...ng the muscle spasm of low ...wers or tub baths, heating ...-fashioned hot water bottle ...'do-it-yourself' patient with ba...

...f massage has its roots in anti... ...ul in modern day conserva- tive ... ...ck dysfunction. Paraspinal muscl... ...d by gently performed deep knead... ...ne beneficial effects include increase... blood flow, muscle relaxation, and improved muscle tone. A spouse or friend may administer this method of treatment.

Mild Analgesic Medication. Mild analgesic medication, such as aspirin or some of the other analgesics that can be purchased without a prescription, is quite effective in relieving low back pain and is usually found in the medicine cabinets of most low back pain sufferers.

Occupation Changes and Modifications in Activities of Daily Living. A patient can often relate the onset of low back symptoms to specific activities performed either at work or in daily living. Modification of such activities may alleviate or improve symptoms, obviating more intensive management. Many patients change occupation and alter home activities without physician guidance. Frequently, it is the patient and not the physician who takes the lead in this regard. A physician must continue to remember that it is often the patient's activities that precipitated the low back dysfunction that requires treatment. Such activities should be modified. If a patient has had a longstanding low back dysfunction and is performing work that involves stress on the low back, treatment of the presenting symptoms without attempting to modify the stress-producing work is unrealistic. When the patient is eventually freed of pain following treatment, it is short-sighted to permit a return to the same conditions that originally produced the pain.

LUMBOSACRAL STRAIN

Acute Lumbosacral Strain

This condition is caused by stress or injury to the low back. The precipitating episodes vary and may include lifting excessive loads or lifting when the body is in a mechanically disadvantageous position. Direct trauma to the low back or aborted falls in which the lumbar muscles, tendons, and ligaments are stretched by the sudden torsion movements of the body to avoid falling may cause this syndrome. The precipitating trauma usually causes immediate low back discomfort. Often the initial pain is not especially severe and is appreciated mainly as a stiffness in the low back area. The patient may continue to remain active in the hope that this mobility will "work away the muscle spasm". The reverse may occur, and the pain worsens so that the patient may eventually become completely incapacitated as a result of increased activity.

Examination reveals severe bilateral or unilateral spasm of the lumbar paraspinal muscles. Both flexion and extension of the lumbar spine increases the discomfort and lumbar mobility is limited. Reflex, motor, and sensory examination of the lower extremities are usually normal. X-ray films of the lumbosacral spine are usualy normal, but may reveal some straightening of the normal lumbar curvature. When the muscle spasm is unilateral, a lumbar list or mild scoliosis may be noted.

Management. Rest, heat, gentle massage, and analgesic medication are the basic methods of treating this problem. Occasionally the pain is so severe that oral analgesic medication may not be strong enough to reduce the acute muscle spasm, and injectable narcotics are required.

Chronic Lumbosacral Strain

This syndrome is characterized by chronic recurrent episodes of low back dysfunction. These episodes may be related to mechanical stress on the lumbar area, and at other times similar symptoms may occur quite spontaneously without obvious cause. The symptoms vary considerably in both intensity and frequency. A prolonged interval of rather mild discomfort may be disrupted by a severe exacerbation of pain of varying duration. At times, the mild persisting pain remains largely in the background and is ignored by the patient who considers this a "normal state". However, the patient may remain mindful of the potentially latent nature of the pain and may live quite defensively in an effort to avoid precipitating a severe and incapacitating flare-up of back pain. The term chronic in this syndrome relates to a history of recurrences rather than the duration of each specific attack. The pain often covers a wide area, is not usually of great severity, and is commonly described as somewhat annoying or even mild. In many cases, the posture, body habitus, and general carriage of the individual with chronic lumbosacral strain is less than satisfactory. The patient may be overweight, and the truncal musculature may be generally atonic and somewhat flabby. Whether these associated findings are a significant cause of the syndrome or merely an effect of longstanding back dysfunction and defensive living is conjectural.

Examination reveals relatively mild paraspinal muscle spasm in the lumbar area. The lumbar spine is rarely fixed and severe paraspinal muscle spasm is not a common finding. Lumbar motility may be fairly good. A significant increase in the lumbar lordosis is often noted. Lower extremity reflexes, motor power, and sensation are normal, as is straight-leg raising. X-ray films of the spine may reveal a slight increase in the normal lumbar lordosis.

Management. In dealing with any chronic low back problem, a thorough work-up is essential to rule out visceral or pelvic disease. Appropriate laboratory studies, x-ray films of the spine, and possibly a bone scan may be advisable.

Corrective low back exercises designed to increase the strength of the trunk musculature must be regularly performed. If the patient is overweight, a gradual weight reduction program is initiated. A moderate decrease in heel height is advisable for women who are accustomed to wearing extremely high-heeled shoes. Instruction regarding low back hygiene, including explanation of the body mechanics involved in standing, walking, sitting, lifting, and other activities of daily living is helpful. Because it is difficult to alter postural habits that have become established over many years, the patient should be informed that it usually requires at least 6 months before improvement is appreciated. Sometimes it is necessary to utilize a lumbosacral corset designed to assist in truncal support. As lumbar muscle tone and strength improve, the need for this support is reduced.

HYPERTROPHIC OSTEOARTHRITIC DEGENERATIVE CHANGES

Hypertrophic degenerative changes involving weight-bearing joints including the lumbar spine is a natural aspect of the aging process. The presence of this condition is demonstrated by spine films, but degenerative changes are not necessarily symptom-producing. Lumbar spine films of the patient population of any nursing home probably would exhibit considerable hypertrophic osteoarthritic degenerative changes, but most of these patients have no complaints related to their low back. Occasionally, when an elderly individual complains of low back pain and hypertrophic osteoarthritic degenerative changes can be seen on lumbar spine films, the physician assumes that the osteoarthritis is the cause of the symptoms and is in danger of overlooking another more serious condition which may be responsible for the low back pain.

STENOTIC LUMBAR SPINAL CANAL SYNDROME

Some individuals who are born with relatively small spinal canals and subsequently develop hypertrophic degenerative spurring, which further decreases the capaciousness of an already small canal, may eventually develop a stenotic lumbar spinal canal syndrome. This occurs when the reduced size of the spinal canal causes stricture to the neural elements within. Patients suffering from this condition are unable to lie in either a flat supine or prone position and are comfortable only when lying on one or the other side with hips and knees in flexion. Individuals with a stenotic lumbar spinal canal syndrome may walk about in a rather conspicuously stooped forward position and cannot comfortably assume a completely erect posture. The pain described by the patient may be limited to the low back, but often is associated with lower extremity pain, either unilateral or bilateral.

Management of this problem may require intermittent wearing of a nonreinforced lumbosacral support and an exercise program utilizing the so-called Williams' lumbar flexion maneuvers, which are designed to flatten or reduce the lumbar lordosis. Occasionally, when the patient cannot sleep in a flat bed, it is necessary to rent a hospital bed, which can be positioned with the knees in flexion and the head of the bed elevated, to maintain the lumbar spine in the position of lumbar flexion. In rare situations, when the problem does not respond to an adequate conservative management program, myelography is necessary, and in some cases, a decompressive laminectomy may be required.

LUMBAR DISC HERNIATION

Most people with a herniated lumbar disc syndrome give a history of having varying degrees of low back pain initially with subsequent development of sciatic pain in association with the low back pain. As the sciatic pain increases in severity, the low back component of pain eases so that by the time the patient consults the physician, there is relatively little or no back pain and the predominant symptom involves the gluteal region or buttock and extends down the course of the sciatic nerve. Usually weight-bearing, whether in walking, standing, or sitting, aggravates the pain, and bed rest eases the pain.

Examination reveals some paraspinal muscle spasm of the lumbar region with significant limitation of lumbar motility both in flexion and extension. Straight-leg raising of the involved extremity is usually painful, indicating nerve root irritation. The two most common sites for lumbar disc herniation are the two lowest interspaces, the L4–L5 and L5–S1 disc spaces. A disc herniation at the L4–L5 interspace is associated with numbness over the dorsum of the foot extending to the great toe, with demonstrable weakness of the great toe extensor. A disc herniation at the L5–S1 interspace is associated with numbness along the lateral aspect of the involved foot with a diminished or absent Achilles reflex.

Conservative management of this problem requires an adequate interval of rest, which can be carried out in the patient's home. The patient should either lie in bed, lie on the sofa, or lie on the floor with a pillow. Walking, standing, and sitting must be avoided as much as possible. Analgesic medication is helpful, and if the pain is severe, narcotics may be required. During the interval of conservative management, a CT scan can be obtained on an outpatient basis. The area scanned is best deter-

mined by the clinical picture, and the most frequently scanned levels are the L3–L4, L4–L5, and L5–S1 interspaces. An adequate interval of conservative management would include at least 3 weeks of rest at home. If the patient's symptoms do not improve after this interval of time, it may be necessary to obtain additional information in the form of a metrizamide myelogram. If the clinical picture and the x-ray studies indicate nerve root pressure from a herniated disc, aggressive management may be in order. This would involve consideration of either intradiscal chymopapain or lumbar disc surgery.

NEOPLASMS OF THE SPINE

Almost 70 percent of all spinal tumors are metastatic; the remaining 30 percent are divided between primary spinal tumors and direct tumor invasion from adjacent structures. Low back pain as the first symptom caused by the occult or unsuspected malignant tumor is always a concern to the physician. A patient who is middle-aged or elderly, who has never previously experienced low back dysfunction and complains of severe low back pain, requires careful assessment with the occult neoplasm in mind. In addition to lumbar spine films, a bone scan is advisable to rule out such a problem. If the bone scan is abnormal and this finding cannot be clearly explained by lumbar spine films, a careful medical evaluation to rule out neoplasm is in order.

PSYCHOLOGICAL FACTORS

Because pain is such a subjective phenomenon, evaluation of this symptom is sometimes difficult. Differentiation of organic from psychic factors is often a problem since both factors usually contribute to the final expression of pain, and the proportion of contribution by somatic and psychic spheres changes constantly. It is in this area of evaluation that the "art of the physician" is most severely challenged and is almost impossible to subject to quantitative evaluation and criticism. Questions as to the consistency of pain, its interferences with performance of duties, and how it affects vital functions such as sleep must be answered and evaluated clearly by the physician.

Prolongation of symptoms in the face of secondary gain is a fact acknowledged by all physicians. The issues involved are complex and often vary. Compensatory or work-related injuries produce symptoms that are clearly quite different in comparison to similar injuries where there is no secondary gain. This is a complicated problem and one that should be recognized clearly by the physician involved in the care of such patients.

The physician should also bear in mind that from the patient's point of view, there is no such thing as a "psychogenic backache". Patients are completely satisfied that the back pain that brings them to your office is caused by "that accident", and they assume that the physician will support them in this belief. The management of such patients is a complex process. A few specialized programs are making progress, but overall this remains an unsolved clinical problem.

HERNIATED LUMBAR DISC

RUSSEL W. HARDY, Jr., M.D.

The symptoms of lumbar disc herniation were known in ancient times, but it was not until surprisingly recently that the origin of these symptoms was recognized. Even in the late nineteenth century, sciatica and back pain were attributed to spurious disease of the sciatic nerve or lumbosacral joint.

Interestingly, surgeons who first operated on lumbar disc protrusions recognized that these lesions caused sciatica, but falsely assumed that the herniated discs were neoplastic in origin. The traumatic and degenerative etiology of disc herniation was first postulated early in this century, and in a classic paper published in 1934,

Mixter and Barr described the surgical treatment of herniated lumbar discs.

A review of the pathology of disc protrusion is useful in understanding the medical and surgical management of this condition. The intervertebral disc consists of two parts; (1) the cartilaginous nucleus pulposus and (2) the annulus fibrosis, composed of connective tissue. The annulus surrounds the centrally placed nucleus, which acts as a cushion between adjacent vertebral bodies. In young individuals, the nucleus has a relatively high water content, but with aging it loses water as nuclear degeneration takes place. Disruptions of the annulus occur in response to a single traumatic event or to the "wear and tear" of aging. The result is that fragments of the nucleus protrude through the annulus, thus causing the herniated disc. The herniations usually occur laterally, but may also occur in the midline of the spinal canal.

When a disc herniation occurs, a number of symptoms may appear, and a number of outcomes are possible. First, it is very likely that backache, either acute or chronic, is an early manifestation of disc herniation. (However, it is important to realize that backache per se may also arise from sites in the spine other than a ruptured disc, and backache by itself is rarely an indication for operation on the lumbar spine.)

When the herniated disc protrudes laterally into the spinal canal, it may stretch and compress the nerve root crossing the disc space and give rise to radiating leg pain, and perhaps to neurological symptoms such as paresthesias, motor deficit, and reflex change. Central disc herniations are much less common than bilateral protrusions; when these occur, they may cause symptoms of cauda equina compression such as bilateral pain, sphincter disturbance, saddle sensory loss, and diffuse lower extremity weakness. Fortunately, neurological catastrophes from central lumbar disc herniations are distinctly rare.

Following herniation, the disc fragment may gradually lose water content and thus decrease in size. It is unlikely that large disc protrusions actually "go back into place", but subtle changes in the relationship of fragment to root may occur. In any case, various mechanisms lead to spontaneous reduction in root compression in many individuals. If this occurs, the patient's symptoms resolve over a period of several days to many months. Thus, if left untreated, it is probable that a large number of patients with herniated discs will recover. Nonoperative therapy (to be described) is designed to facilitate the reparative processes following disc protrusion. If such reparative processes do not occur, or are insufficient, active intervention is usually required to treat neural compression.

As noted, the presenting symptom of a herniated disc is pain, beginning usually in the back but rapidly evolving into sciatia. Pain from root compression is usually sharp and fairly well localized. It is often increased by motion of the spine or by standing, sitting, coughing, or straining. Frequently, but not always, back and leg pain are decreased by recumbency.

In addition to pain, the patient may experience other symptoms of root compression such as paraesthesias, loss of sensation, and weakness. Sphincter disturbances may occur from cauda equina compression from midline disc, but bladder disturbances may also occasionally accompany a lateral disc.

Physical examination may reveal a variety of findings. Inspection of the back may show flattening of the normal lordosis, with scoliosis toward or away from the affected side, depending on the relationship of the herniated disc to compressed root. Motion of the spine may be restricted and usually is painful. The most important sign of a ruptured disc, pain on straight-leg raising, is caused by further stretch of an already compromised root when the extended leg is flexed at the hip. This test is positive in the vast majority of patients with acute disc protrusions. In some instances, patients may have a crossed straight-leg raising test, usually a sign of very large protrusion situated under or medial to a root. Finally, patients with upper lumbar herniations may have pain on straight-leg extension rather than flexion.

Neurological changes are both of diagnostic and localizing value. Paresthesias and sensory loss may follow a specific root distribution: numbness on the lateral foot suggesting an S1 root lesion; paresthesias or pain in the great toe are quite specific for L5 compression. Motor deficit is more specific than sensory disturbance: weakness of plantar flexion occurs with an S1 lesion, loss of dorsiflexion of the foot or toe with an L5 lesion, and quadriceps weakness with an upper lumbar root compression. Reflex changes are also specific, with an absent ankle jerk signifying an S1 lesion and a reduced knee jerk indicating an L3 or L4 root lesion.

As noted earlier, the symptoms of a herniated disc may range from very mild to severe; the severity of symptoms dictates the extent of work-up and the type of management. Patients tend to fall into one of three groups: acute, relapsing, or chronic. Patients with acute symptoms have pain of relatively sudden onset and may have associated neurological deficit. Patients with relapsing symptoms have pain-free intervals interspersed with acute attacks which then resolve. Individuals with chronic symptoms have more or less continuous back pain and sciatica, but are able to function to some degree in spite of their symptoms.

The management of these three groups of patients differs and will now be considered separately.

Patients may develop acute pain in response to trauma, or the symptoms may appear spontaneously. Usually a brief interval of back pain is followed by sciatica. Rarely, in older individuals, there is leg pain with little associated back pain. The evaluation of these patients consists of a physical examination and lumbar spine films (done mostly to exclude tumor, infection, or other causes of back pain). Treatment consists initially of complete bed rest, either flat or in a semi-Fowler's position. Mild narcotics (codeine or Percodan), supplemented by muscle relaxants (Valium or Robaxin), usually suffice to keep the patient comfortable. High-dose steroids have also been advocated in acute situations and may merit a trial for a limited period. Medications and bed rest may be supplemented by local heat; conversely, an ice pack may serve to alleviate muscle spasm. Exercises are specifically not employed except in the recovery phase, when the patient may be started on a "pelvic tilt" exercise designed to improve abdominal tone.

Generally, bed rest is continued for at least a week before surgical therapy is considered. Usually a patient who is going to recover with bed rest shows distinct signs of improvement within 7 to 10 days, and if this occurs, nonoperative treatment should be continued until recovery is complete or until it is obvious that the patient has reached a plateau.

If the patient has not shown signs of recovery within one week, as evidenced by a decrease in pain and neurological symptoms, surgical intervention may be necessary. The first step consists of additional diagnostic tests, a CT scan of the spine, and probably a myelogram. A CT may be the sole diagnostic test if the herniation is clear-cut and is compatible with the clinical picture. In most instances a myelogram is also required to confirm the diagnosis and to help plan surgical management. A myelogram is absolutely mandatory if there is a doubt about the diagnosis. This myelogram should include the conus medullaris (up to a lower thoracic vertebral level) as well as the cauda equina.

Once the diagnosis has been confirmed, a decision is required regarding the type of surgical therapy to be undertaken. It should be emphasized again that persistent signs of root compression (leg pain and neurological signs and symptoms) are the indication for surgery. Back pain alone is seldom an indication for disc surgery, except in rare cases of upper lumbar or very large central extruded discs which may be accompanied by little or no leg pain. At present, two options are available. The first is lumbar hemilaminotomy and excision of the disc. This time-honored operation should be highly effective (90%) in relieving symptoms when a clear-cut herniated disc is present. In expert hands it normally has a low morbidity and very low mortality rate. Recent enthusiasts have advocated the use of the microscope in disc incision, but this is not mandatory, and "microdiscectomy" differs little from the conventional operation. Indeed, some would argue that an adequate disc exploration requires a generous exposure of the disc, nerve root, and dural sac in order to be certain of a complete disc removal.

An alternative to operation, chemonucleolysis with chymopapain, has recently become available. This material was first used clinically in the 1960s by Lyman Smith. It was later taken off the market because of questions concerning efficacy and complications. Controlled studies have recently demonstrated that chymopapain injected into herniated discs relieves symptoms approximately 70 to 80 percent of the time. Relief of pain may be immediate or occur in the several weeks following injection. The major risks are anaphylaxis, which has been fatal in a few patients, and transverse myelitis and subarachnoid hemorrhage, perhaps related to the inadvertent subarachnoid injection of the material.

Recent experience suggests that chemonucelolysis may be a reasonable alternative to surgery. It has the possible advantages of avoiding an incision and anesthetic, and possibly a shorter hospitalization. However, chemonucleolysis is possibly less effective than laminectomy, and there is concern about potentially serious complications. Chemonucleolysis is not a trivial procedure. Its indications are the same as for operation: it should not be used indiscriminately to treat back pain in the absence a demonstrated disc protrusion. In addition, certain patients—those with complete blocks, those with evidence of cauda equina compression, or those with sequestered disc fragments—are not candidates for chemonucleolysis.

The preceding paragraphs outline treatment for patients with acute sciatica with no or modest neurological deficits. In patients with evidence of cauda equina compression (as evidenced by sphincter involvement or bilateral pain or motor deficit), the situation is much different. In such individuals urgent operation is required to avoid a permanent severe deficit. The same statement applies to individuals with severe footdrop, in which case early operation may be indicated.

2) Patients with relapsing sciatica present a somewhat different management problem. Such individuals may have only a limited number of acute attacks and recover from each with appropriate bed rest. If recovery is complete, and the episodes are infrequent, surgical intervention may never be required. When recovery is prolonged or incomplete, or when the frequency of attacks constitutes a disability, operative intervention may be indicated.

Patients with relapsing symptoms should be placed on a program of back exercises during asymptomatic periods and given common sense instructions in avoiding symptoms. These include care in lifting heavy objects, use of a firm sleeping surface, and avoidance of prolonged sitting or bending.

3) If an individual presents with chronic backache and sciatica, a careful history is in order, particularly in the elderly. Patients with chronic sciatica may be harboring a spinal or retroperitoneal tumor (e.g., metastatic prostatic carcinoma), and the initial work-up should include an abdominal and rectal examination. Individuals with lumbar canal stenosis or a lateral recess syndrome complain of pseudoclaudication, that is, leg pain increased with walking or standing, but relieved by sitting. This must be distinguished from ischemic claudication secondary to peripheral vascular disease, which produces leg pain aggravated by walking, but relieved by standing.

Assuming other causes of sciatica have been excluded, patients with chronic symptoms may be treated conservatively and expectantly. Patients with chronic symptoms should be managed somewhat differently than those with relapsing sciatica. Many of these patients have mechanical back pain rather than a herniated disc, and can be managed with a program of postural exercises. If done properly and consistently, these exercises relieve symptoms in a large percentage of cases. One of the best forms of exercise for patients with problem backs is swimming (crawl stroke), which relieves symptoms by improving abdominal tone and thus improving posture.

Occasional patients with chronic backache and sciatica are helped by a well-fitted lumbar corset or brace. Of greater importance is a firm sleeping surface, particularly if the individual wakes in the morning with backache. For patients who must sit or drive for prolonged periods, a portable back support (inexpensive and commercialy available) reduces backache. Again, common sense advice, such as telling the female patient to avoid high-heeled shoes, is important and often overlooked.

In a limited number of patients with chronic sciatica, or in patients with mild acute episodes, a caudal epidural block, containing local anesthetic and corticosteroids, is effective in relieving symptoms. The epidural block presumably relieves symptoms from the mechanical effects of the block plus the anti-inflammatory effect of the steroids. Generally, the patient obtains relief from the first block or not at all, but in some individuals, two or three blocks may be needed. If no relief occurs after three blocks, spaced a week apart, the treatment should be abandoned. If caudal blocks are employed, they should be given by an individual skilled in this anesthetic technique.

If chronic sciatica persists and is unrelieved by nonoperative therapy, surgical intervention may be required, depending on the amount of pain and the tolerance of the individual. (If the history has suggested lumbar canal stenosis or a lateral recess syndrome, early operative treatment is necessary since osseous nerve root compression is not ordinarily relieved by nonoperative measures.) Patients who may require surgery should have a CT and myelogram as part of their evaluation. Again, it is important that the meylogram be extensive enough to exclude upper lumbar or lower thoracic lesions, which can also produce sciatica; every busy neurosurgical service has seen patients who had incomplete myelography and underwent a disc excision, when the real cause of sciatica was a spinal cord tumor not detected on the original study.

Patients with chronic sciatica may be candidates for either surgery or chymopapain, if the problem is a herniated disc. However, many of these individuals have at least a component of spondylitic compression instead of, or in addition to, a ruptured disc, and in such patients surgery is the treatment of choice.

One category of patients not previously discussed consists of symptomatic patients with a history of a prior laminectomy. If those patients did well after their first disc excision, and then developed new sciatica, they may have a recurrent disc at the original or a different level. Such patients should be handled no differently than other patients with sciatica, treated first conservatively and then investigated for a surgical lesion if they do not respond.

A much more difficult group are those with "failed back" syndromes. Many of these patients never responded to surgery, and a careful history may show that the original operation was inappropriate. Patients with chronic back pain and sciatica should be investigated for a treatable lesion, such as a recurrent disc or previously undiagnosed tumor. If this is not found, further surgery is unlikely to help. A rare patient obtains relief from a rhizotomy or dorsal column stimulator, but generally such operations fail. Some patients may benefit from a comprehensive pain management program, including detoxification, transcutaneous stimulation, biofeedback therapy, and investigation into psychosocial components of pain. Such programs are more likely to benefit the "failed back" patient than multiple spinal operations; unless a very clear reason for further surgery is present, the physician can do the patient a service by helping him to cope with his chronic pain rather than advising further surgery for doubtful indications.

CONGENITAL AND ACQUIRED SPONDYLOLISTHESIS

JOSEPH A. EPSTEIN, M.D., F.A.C.S.

Spondylolisthesis, essentially displacement of the lumbosacral vertebra, has three essential anatomical patterns. The first, dysplastic spondylolisthesis, consists of a congenital deficiency of the superior sacral or inferior fifth lumbar facets or both and is responsible for gradual slipping of the vertebra forward. In the second spondylolytic type, the defect occurs in the pars interarticularis, permitting forward displacement of the fifth lumbar vertebra; however, the lamina and inferior facets remain behind so that the spinal canal itself is not significantly narrowed. The defect in the neural arch can occur as a fatigue fracture, as an elongation of the pars which may eventually separate, or as an acute fracture occurring through the isthmus.

The third, degenerative spondylolisthesis, primarily occurs in the fifth and sixth decades of life and in women far more frequently than in men. The displacement occurs primarily at the L4–L5 level and is limited in forward subluxation at approximately 1 cm. It is associated with marked overgrowth (arthrosis) and locking of the posterior articular facets, which tend to stabilize the lesion at this degree of listhesis.

Spondylolysis and spondylolisthesis occur in 5 percent of the general population. The incidence increases until the age of 20 years and is then static. A more frequent occurrence is noted in individuals performing arduous weight-lifting and in football players. There is a high rate of occurrence among family members, and it is unusually common in some Eskimo tribes.

INSTABILITY WITHOUT NEURAL COMPRESSION

The first two types occur primarily in children and in adolescents and may present with back pain, usually manageable by bracing and physical therapy. When the degree progresses to approximately one-half of the vertebral body and continues forward with stress, spinal fusion is usually indicated. It is rare in these younger individuals to have evidence of nerve root entrapment such as that caused by a herniated disc or by stenotic changes in the area of the pars or by fibrosis in the area of pseudoarthrosis.

WHEN NEURAL COMPRESSION IS PRESENT

When neural entrapment occurs with radiculopathy, usually in more mature individuals, a more aggressive approach is required with decompression of the nerve root in the specific zone where stenotic or fibrotic changes occur. Myelography is mandatory in all patients who exhibit evidence of radiculopathy. This may indicate the degree of stenosis associated with these various anomalies and may exclude the presence of neoplasm, which can well occur in the area of the cauda equina and produce similar symptoms. Laminectomy is indicated by the presence of a complete block in the myelogram and signs of cauda equina involvement. With instability, a bilateral-lateral column or transverse process fusion is the procedure of choice. If Harrington rod distraction is to be employed, there is risk of trauma to the cauda equina, but with adequate laminectomy and decompression this complication is less likely to occur.

One must be aware of the fact that multiple anomalies may coexist involving the lumbar and sacral segments, such as an elongated pars or a malformed series of facets, which may make satisfactory reduction and decompression more difficult.

Of those dysplastic patients in whom the neural arch of L5 remains intact, the arch moves forward with the vertebral body and approximates the superior sacral margin with obliteration of the spinal canal. Cauda equina compression follows, often with bowel and bladder disturbances. This type requires laminar decompression in addition to the appropriate fusion. A variety of procedures have been recommended to stabilize this area or to lift the subluxed vertebra into a more normal position. Harrington rods and various plates both anteriorly and posteriorly combined with bone fusion are all recommended; no single procedure is completely satisfactory.

NEURAL COMPRESSION WITHOUT INSTABILITY

Of greater concern to the neurosurgeons are older patients in the fourth and fifth decades who develop signs of neural compression when the degree of olisthesis has been relatively stabilized. In this group, bony decompression is extremely helpful because of narrowing of the spinal canal, either centrally or laterally in the area of pseudoarthrosis where neural entrapment occurs. Curiously, after the age of 30, the degree of olisthesis is said to be relatively fixed; this may not be so, and if there is considerable back pain, spinal fusion should be done as a supplementary procedure. Again, the type of fusion is preferably posterolateral, over the

transverse processes, and at times must be combined with anterior fusion. The combined fusion, both posterior and anterior, provides the greatest degree of stabilization. An adequate support is extremely important in the postoperative management of patients who require fusion.

When a pure monoradicular pattern of entrapment is present and a myelogram shows evidence of a lateral lesion, the decompression may be confined to one side. Should the myelogram indicate the presence of a herniated disc, simple removal of the disc with laminotomy and neural decompression will suffice without disturbing the opposite side or changing the anatomy in any significant way. This is an infrequent occurrence. More often the symptoms are bilateral or more severe on one side than on the other and the more appropriate Gill procedure is required. In the presence of a complete block of the spinal canal with marked stenosis, the greater degree of decompression is indicated. Laminectomy or a modified Gill procedure is never indicated in children and young adults without including fusion. Removal of the articular facets may result in further subluxation if arthrodesis is not done.

THE DEGENERATIVE PROCESS

Degenerative spondylolisthesis with an intact neural arch is becoming increasingly recognized as a cause of low back pain with radiculopathy and the syndrome of intermittent neurogenic claudication. Although spondylolisthesis may be asymptomatic for many years, with increasing age the symptoms are being recognized more readily now as a common problem amenable to decompressive surgery. Degenerative disc changes precede the development of the prominent apophyseal arthrosis so characteristic of this disorder. Initial degeneration of the disc is followed by unique stress on the posterior facets, which become severely arthrotic with ultimate subluxation of the entire vertebra forward to the limits imposed by the locked facets. This results in a segmental form of stenosis with back, buttock, and lower extremity pain as evidence of radiculopathy, or cauda equina ischemia and symptoms of intermittent neurogenic claudication. With the latter, patients develop diffuse and increasing low back and extremity pain on ambulation or while simply standing erect, followed by limping with numbness and weakness. The symptoms are relieved with remarkable rapidity by sitting down or by recumbency, differing in this regard from symptoms caused by vascular occlusive disease. Degenerative spondylolisthesis may occur in conditions other than degenerative disc disease, such as osteogenesis imperfecta, agenesis of the articular facets, following trauma, and at levels above a spinal fusion. It has also been observed in tuberculosis, cancer, and Charcot's disease. There are very few associated neurological abnormalities and rarely restriction of straight-leg raising. The claudication symptoms can exist for many years. The distance for which walking is tolerated slowly decreases, and eventually ambulation may be limited to only a few steps. Even then neurological abnormalities are unusual. It is rare to find an associated herniated disc. The onset is insidious, and progression is frequently associated with a rather characteristic postural change in which the patient walks in an increasingly flexed position, often called the "Groucho Marx" gait. The patient usually stops walking and tries to sit down as weakness occurs and the warning pain and dysesthesias become apparent.

In the presence of rapid progression, conservative measures are rarely helpful. The use of flexion exercises, a flexion type of back support, and anti-inflammatory drugs may provide some measure of relief.

Obesity, hyperlordosis, osteoporosis, and other factors may increase the severity of the neuropathic changes. In patients with chronic, nonspecific back and leg pain, the development of intermittent neurogenic claudication is often the precipitating factor in the need for surgical decompression.

Simple x-ray studies and tomograms in the AP and lateral views provide eloquent evidence of the olisthesis, which is usually limited to about 1 cm with evidence of severe arthrosis of the posterior articular facets and narrowing of the foramina. This is further confirmed by CT scanning. The most important study, however, remains the myelogram, which confirms the segmental stenosis at the level of olisthesis, often revealing a complete block. It is possible to further evaluate the entire lumbar and cervical canals if necessary.

Surgical decompression provides adequate relief in at least 80 percent of these patients if performed before irreversible changes occur in the roots of the cauda equina. Obviously, urgency is indicated when bowel and bladder incontinence and evidence of distinct neurological defect occur. Peripheral vascular disease may be an associated abnormality, especially in older individuals, and must be studied appropriately. The presence of a peripheral neuropathy, so commonly encountered in diabetics and alcoholics, may contribute to the disability and cannot be relieved by surgery. Nonetheless, these patients should not be denied a decompressive procedure if the myelographic findings and the history remain suggestive of spinal stenosis. Electromyographic and nerve conduction studies are especially helpful to differentiate these diseases.

The interspaces above L4–L5 may also be involved, but the common changes occur at L4–L5, rarely at L5–S1, the latter being the most common site of the congenital type of spondylolisthesis previously described in adolescents and young adults. The operative procedure relates to the degree of stenosis and arthrosis, and the levels involvement. The nerve root most frequently involved is the L5 root as it passes over the step-like deformity in the floor of the canal, with the superior articular facet cradling the nerve roots in the lateral recess. The associated inferior articular facet of L4 causes greater encroachment on the canal in the more central portions and may also compress the L4 roots laterally. Therefore, to be effective, laminectomy must include both the L4 and L5 levels; the lower half of L3 may also be excised if there is evidence of involve-

ment of the suprajacent nerve roots. Each nerve root must be decompressed and followed out on through the foramen since the deformities of the superior articular facet are extensive and may extend medial to the pedicle, inferiorly and laterally.

The nerve root is the essential guide, and both the L4 and L5 roots must both be carefully observed in order to make certain that appropriate release of these structures has been accomplished. Generous free fat grafts or pedicle grafts should be applied over the defects created by the laminectomy and by the medial facetectomy and foraminotomy.

It is rarely necessary to sacrifice an entire facet during this procedure, and by using an undercutting technique with appropriate thin-tipped angulated Kerrison punches and upbiting curets, the major supporting structures may be preserved. Since these joints are also severely arthrotic, a great deal of stability can be retained in this pattern, and it would be most unusual to have evidence of further subluxation if enough joint surface can be maintained. Since the findings are usually more severe on one side than on the other, the procedure needs to be less extensive on the less symptomatic or asymptomatic side. It is unusual to find evidence of a herniated disc, and because of this, the annulus should be preserved along with the posterior longitudinal ligament, providing further stabilization.

Patients are given steroids for 4 to 7 days; the initial dose of 10 mg of dexamethazone is given at the time anesthesia is induced or the day previously if symptoms are severe. The dose of dexamethazone is gradually reduced, beginning with 4 mg orally every 6 hours. It is discontinued in 4 to 7 days. Nonsteroidal anti-inflammatory drugs may be used for longer intervals if needed. Physical therapy and adequate psychosocial support are mandatory in older individuals who require a great deal of reassurance. The use of a physiatrist may be extremely helpful in the postoperative management.

In patients in whom the disc has been obliterated because of the advanced spondylosis, the spine is quite stable and more generous decompression may be performed; facets may be sacrificed if necessary to provide a proper neural decompression. When the disc is intact although degenerated, specific preservation of this structure remains important in maintaining stability. Secondary intertransverse fusion may be a needed adjunct in individual cases.

Adhesions between the capsular ligaments, yellow ligaments, and arthrotic facets may be difficult to separate, and care must be taken to avoid lacerating the dura, which would result in escape of spinal fluid and its associated complications. Injuring an incarcerated nerve root, which may be fixed in an extremely tight subarticular position can be avoided with proper instrumentation. The small, angulated, sharply filed-down Kerrison punches and upbiting curets are indispensable.

Our patients have undergone surgery in the crouch position, and transfusion has not been required. The advantage of an almost bloodless field is extremely important in protecting the dura and nerve root during the dissection and decompression. The use of steroids hastens ambulation so that patients can be up within the first 24 hours, and they rarely require catheterization.

Patients are discharged within 5 to 7 days after surgery, at which time they can take care of their simple needs. Within 2 to 3 months, they are capable of performing without specific restrictions. The problem patient is the individual with extreme obesity, hyperlordosis, a long history of back pain, a dense neurological deficit, an associated peripheral neuropathy, or a history of diabetes or alocholism.

THE UNSTABLE LOW BACK

DAVID L. FILTZER, M.D.

The dictionary defines "unstable" as "not stable; not firmly fixed, firm, or steady; liable to fall, change, or cease."

In years past, many loosely applied terms such as "sciatica", "sacroiliac disease", and "lumbago" were frequently used to indicate diagnoses, whereas, in retrospect, they were merely a description of symptom complexes. As we became more scientifically sophisticated, and aided by startling medical advances, we were able to establish more accurate diagnoses based on newly perceived pathologic entities. We now realize that low back pain is not simply "lumbago", but may result from numerous different pathologic conditions, that "sciatica" is not lower extremity pain per se, but may be caused by a variety of pathologic entities including lumbar radiculopathy, sacroiliac joint disease, lumbosacral plexus neuritis, and others. Lumbar radiculopathy itself has many origins, such as disc protrusions and extrusions, arachnoiditis, epidural scar, and spinal stenosis, to mention only a few.

Similarly, the term "unstable low back" is often a misnomer when applied to nontraumatic situations. Our discussion here will deal solely with the nontraumatic aspects of lumbar spine disease which may result in instability.

In 45 years of clinical orthopaedic experience, I have witnessed the gradual evolution of more exact diagnoses of so-called instability of the low back. Retrospectively, I have come to realize that what we frequently formerly termed "instability" was not instability at all. It is now my firm conviction that compressive factors involving the cauda equina and nerve roots are the cause of most nontraumatic disabilities involving the lumbar spine, and that currently there is only a limited role for stabilization of the lumbar spine by spinal fusion.

At one time, not long ago, the major indication for spinal fusion in lumbar discogenic disease and/or spondylosis was that the patient had had two or more unsuccessful explorations with disectomy and/or foraminotomy. We now refer to these unfortunate individuals as having the "failed back" syndrome. Formerly, when nothing startling was discovered on exploration of the back, we tugged on a spinous process with a Kocher clamp, saw what we considered to be abnormal motion at that particular segment, decided the trouble was from "instability", and proceeded to carry out a spinal fusion. We were not clinically sophisticated enough at that time to realize that the fundamental problem was foraminal constriction, lateral recess stenosis, or lumbar spinal stenosis; nor did we stop to consider that there would be some increased mobility at the explored segment because we had removed the liagmentum flavum, and had stripped the capsule from the facets, frequently had excised the interspinous liagment as well, and/or had carried out a laminectomy or a wide laminotomy. Therefore, not knowing what else to do, we all too often fused, compounding the basic problem because of additional bleeding, the formation of more epidural scar, and/or arachnoiditis. The attempted fusion commonly ended up with a pseudarthrosis as well, further complicating matters. I point all this out retrospectively, for at that time we had no concept whatsoever of these pathologic entities that are so obvious to us today.

That many of these arthrodesed spines made reasonably satisfactory recoveries was no cause for self-congratulation. These recoveries can be explained on the basis of two possibilities: either (1) the patient did not need the fusion to begin with and he would have improved without the fusion, or (2) according to a currently realized more basic concept, neural tissue compromised in a constricted bony canal can usually accommodate itself to that constricted canal in the face of rigid immobilization. (This concept explains why symptoms from compressed nerve roots sometimes improves as a result of relatively inefficient simple bed rest or the use of a back support).

Today, the name of the game is *decompression*, and stabilization is seldom indicated if adequate decompression is carried out, unless the decompression is so radical as to cause instability. Of course, there are other special conditions (e.g., spondylolisthesis) in which there is true instability and in which, in most instances, decompression should be combined with stabilization.

I would emphasize that errors in diagnosis and the subsequent performance of an inappropriate or inadequate surgical procedure cannot be rectified by a superimposed spinal fusion. The excision of a degenerated intervertebral disc rather than of a protruded or an extruded one, the failure to recognize a root constricted in a tight lateral recess or in a narrowed intervertebral foramen, the inability to perceive spinal stenosis, epidural scarring, and arachnoiditis—none of these can be corrected by resorting to a spinal fusion.

In my years of practice, I have seen the pendulum swing back and forth several times between discectomy without fusion and discectomy always combined with fusion. I can vividly remember operating, as a young house officer, with Dr. Walter Dandy, the Neurosurgeon-In-Chief, and Dr. George E. Bennett, the Orthopaedic Surgeon-In-Chief at the Johns Hopkins hospital. What Dandy then called a "concealed disc", we now realize is a ventral bar or a foraminal spur. At that time, and even many years later, spinal fusion was carried out routinely following discectomy because we did not recognize any of the indications of which we are now aware.

I have attempted to emphasize the importance of total, thorough, and complete decompression, even if it results in instability of the spine. In spinal stenosis, laminectomies should be wide and complete, and the compressed roots traced into the foramina and decompressed there even if it means partial or complete facetectomy and unroofing of the foramina. Such a radical procedure is not often necessary, but if one is to err, one should do so by decompressing so as not to run the risk of leaving compressed neural tissue behind. If wide decompression causes instability, so be it; a fusion should then be carried out.

There are times when partial facetectomy and unroofing of the foramen would not result in instability and therefore a fusion would not be necessary. In general, the older the patient, the more ligamentous hypertrophy and fibrosis are present, and often these elements alone ensure stability, rendering arthrodesis unnecessary. However, if one must err in such instances, opt for stabilization rather than run the risk of another operation to stabilize such a back.

My own experience has been that a unilateral major facetectomy results in instability, and such a segment should be fused. One cannot rely on the intact facets on the other side because the torsional effect of a major unilteral facetectomy frequently gives rise to residual pain, from compression of the nerve root in the contralateral intervertebral foramen.

PREOPERATIVE EVALUATION OF INSTABILITY

One is often able to demonstrate instability preoperatively and make a tentative determination regarding the necessity for a spinal fusion. I cannot overemphasize the importance of obtaining a full set of preoperative plain films of the lumbar spine, including dynamic stress views and oblique views. I reject the contention now held by so many of my colleagues that a CT scan is all that is needed to ensure a definitive diagnosis. A CT scan gives no indication of possible abnormal mobility at one or more segments, cannot document a pseudarthrosis, and does not always demonstrate a pars defect, either because the slices are too far apart or because the obliquity of the cut is not gauged so as to permit visualization of the partes interarticulares. Although one can most often see a pars defect on the plain lateral and AP views, this is not always so, particularly when there is a scoliosis and/or an acute lumbosacral angle. In such cases, the

pars is often obscured by other superimposed bony structures. Therefore, I urge that an integral part of any work-up should include a full set of plain x-ray films.

Such roentgenographically demonstrated preoperative instability does not necessarily indicate the need for an arthrodesis. This decision should be made at the operating table and must depend on the abnormality found, the ability to correct this abnormality, the degree of abnormal motion discovered, and the age and medical condition of the patient. In short, we must rely on our experience and clinical judgment at the operating table. In many instances, in elderly patients of questionable risk, we may opt to carry out only that decompressive procedure which is absolutely essential, and elect not to perform an arthrodesis even though we may believe that it is indicated. In such instances, one may depend on postoperative bracing for stability. The continued use of a rigid back support or body cast postoperatively depends on the patient's postoperative symptoms and his ability to function without such a back support.

Spondylolisthesis is a major cause of low back instability and almost always involves the fifth lumbar vertebra, which slips forward on the sacrum. It may be either congenital or acquired and should not be confused with spondylolysis.

In spondylolysis there is a unilateral defect in the pars interarticularis or bilateral defects in the partes interarticulares *without displacement or forward slipping*.

On the other hand, spondylolisthesis is associated with a forward displacement of the body, including all of the anterior elements of the vertebra, secondary to bilateral defects in the partes interarticulares of that vertebra. The degree of slip is indicated by grades: grade I implies a forward slip of 25 percent or less of the involved body on the segment below; grade II indicates a slip of 25 to 50 percent; grade III means that there is a slip of 50 to 75 percent; and grade IV constitutes a slip of over 75 percent. The treatment of a major spondylolisthetic slip is a subject unto itself. In general, reduction is carried out by bringing the sacrum into line with the body of L5, rather than by attempting to line up the body of L5 onto the sacrum. A variety of manipulative measures, including the use of traction, casting, and placement of distraction and/or compression rods, have been utilized, combined with a spinal fusion. More recently, for a complete slip, some authors have described a vertebrectomy using a combined anterior and posterior approach, followed by fusing L4 to the sacrum, with combined interbody and posterolateral arthrodeses.

Controversy exists whether these defects in the partes interarticulares are congenital or acquired. The consensus is that most of these are acquired and result from a series of stress fractures, usually in childhood, when these fractures occur through the cartilaginous partes interarticulares. However, they may also be acquired in the teens or in early adult life in the same manner. A study of football players made several years ago indicated that interior linemen were more prone to this condition, the theory being that the partes interarticulares are subject to multiple stresses during violent contact in their play. Stress fractures then occur and frequently heal with sclerosis, lenghthening, and thinning of the partes interarticulares. The same process is repeated over and over again until eventually non-unions of these stress fractures occur, in some instances with resultant defects. It is also believed that a small number of spondylolistheses are congenital in origin, such defects having been described in the neonatal state.

Bilateral spondylolysis has the potential of slipping and becoming an actual spondylolisthesis. Spondylolysis is most often asymptomatic, although in physically active individuals it may give risk to low back pain, but rarely is there an associated radicular component.

The diagnosis of a spondylolisthesis can be suspected in the clinical examination when one palpates a deep hollow where the spinous process of L5 is usually felt. The slip, however minor, is visualized on the plain lateral x-ray film and the defects are generally apparent on the AP and lateral films, although they are much more likely to be observed in the oblique views. The CT scan may show the defects in the partes interarticulares, and one may also visualize the so-called double margin sign. This appears when the outline of two vertebral bodies is seen on the same slice of the CT scan; one body forward to and superimposed on the other.

Spondylolysis, on the other hand, may be easily missed. If proper cuts are made, the defect(s) may be apparent on the CT scan, but they may not be visualized on the plain AP and lateral views, and careful study of the oblique views may be necessary for demonstration.

Patients with spondylolysis usually never come to operation. However, if the back pain becomes incapacitating and fails to respond to conservative measures, one can consider two surgical options: (1) spinal fusion, or (2) a newly described procedure which appears to have considerable merit. In this latter operation one passes braided wires from the transverse processes to the spinous process of that single involved vertebra, thereby compressing the defects in the partes interarticulares. At the same time, small inlay bone grafts are inserted across the defects. This procedure has the advantage of avoiding arthrodesis of one or more segments, thereby not limiting spinal motion and not placing excesive stress and strain on the pivotal joints above and below.

One should not jump to the conclusion that every diagnosed case of spondylolisthesis requires operation or even active conservative treatment. Many of these patients, even at times those with a grade II slip may have only intermittent episodes of back and leg pain. Such attacks may be controlled by a few days of inactivity or bed rest, analgesics, and local counterirritants such as liniments, local heat, or ice. Recent thinking has suggested that the local application of ice is more effective than heat. We frequently use a well-fitting, molded body jacket as a therapeutic trial. If such external immobilization relieves symptoms it is reasonable to assume similar relief by internal immobilization with a spinal fusion.

Such individuals once identified, should be checked periodically for possible further slippage. In particular, children with this condition must be observed frequently, especially during periods of active growth, for a possible increase in the slip.

In those spondylolisthetics who have more frequent and more incapacitating symptoms, an initial conservative regimen is indicated. However, they must also be watched carefully for possible progression. If obese, they ought to be placed on a rigid reducing diet so as to mechanically reduce the stress and strain on their vulnerable backs. Back and abdominal strengthening exercises are to be utilized in order that these strengthened muscles may act as external splints for their backs. While building up these muscles a flexion type back brace may be employed, particularly in patients with a radicular component. These patients are usually more comfortable sleeping supine in the flexed position, either with hips and knees flexed over pillows or on their sides in the fetal position. I would emphasize that most of these patients can be managed successfully by conservative means.

When do we elect to operate on a patient with a spondylolisthesis? This depends on the severity of symptoms, his need to be physically active, the frequency of recurrent attacks, whether he has developed a neurological deficit, and whether the degree of slipping has increased.

In spondylolisthesis, the cause of radiculopathy is twofold; (1) nerve root drag by the forward slip of the body, and (2) compression of the nerve roots by the formation of hypertrophied ligamentous and fibrocartilaginous masses about the intraspinal portion of the defects.

There are several operative choices for the surgical management of spondylolisthesis. These include the Gill procedure (removal of the posterior "floating" element) alone, the Gill procedure combined with lateral transverse process fusion, interbody fusion through the posterior, retroperitoneal, or transperitoneal approaches, or bilateral foraminotomies at L4–L5 without excision of the posterior "floating" element, combined with a standard posterior fusion from L4 to L5 to the sacrum. The intervertebral disc at L4–L5 is usually degenerated but should not be excised unless there is a demonstrated protrusion or extrusion. Excision of the intervertebral disc at L4–L5 may make for further instability and increased slipping, even if an arthrodesis is carried out. The intervertebral disc at L5–S1 is rarely involved.

Fusion should be carried out in situ in a grade I slip and in most cases of grade II spondylolisthesis without the necessity of reduction.

My own perference is to combine the Gill procedure with bilateral lateral fusions from the transvere processes of L5 to the alae of the sacrum.

Degenerative spondylolisthesis is a condition not associated with defects in the partes interarticulares. It results from degenerative changes in the facets and almost always involves slipping forward of the body of L4 on L5. The normal obliquity of the facets, which precludes forward slipping, is changed to a transverse alignment due to wear and tear over the years, with resultant degenerative disease in the facets, so that the body together with its posterior elements slips forward. This occurs mainly in the sixth and seventh decades of life, when degenerative changes are most prevalent. It is manifested by low back and radicular pain due to nerve root drag as well as degenerative changes in and about the facets and intervertebral foramina, causing root compression.

A diagnosis of degenerative spondylolisthesis is made by observing the slip on the plain lateral x-ray film, by seeing the changes in the facet joints on the plain oblique x-ray films and on the CT scan, and by the typical hourglass contracture on the myelogram. The double margin sign may also be observed on the CT scan.

My preference for treatment of degenerative spondylolisthesis is to perform a laminectomy of L4 and bilateral foraminotomies at L4–L5, combined with bilateral transverse process fusions from L4 to L5.

In degenerative disease of the lumbar spine, retrolisthesis is not uncommon and may be a contributing cause of spinal stenosis. This can generally be treated by laminectomy alone, and an arthrodesis is rarely, if ever, indicated.

TYPES OF FUSION

The *Albee spinal fusion* was designed to perform an arthrodesis in the tuberculous spine. Accordingly, an attempt was made to obtain fusion without entering the infected areas in the intervertebral discs and vertebral bodies. It is an extra-articular fusion and consists of making a midline incision in the lumbodorsal fascia, splitting the middle of the spinous processes of two or more vertebrae down to the laminae with a sharp osteotome, wedging the two halves of the split spinous processes apart without fracturing them, and inserting a single cortical tibial graft in the open spinous processes of the vertebrae to be fused, securing the graft in place by suturing the lumbodorsal fascia over it. Today, there is no longer any indication for the use of this type of arthrodesis since, with debridement of infected and diseased bone and the use of antibiotics, we are no longer afraid to attack infected bone and discs directly.

The Albee fusion was succeeded by the *Hibbs fusion*. In this type of arthrodesis, the spinous processes are amputated, the laminae cleaned carefully of all soft tissue and then decorticated. Local chips from the decortication and the amputated spinous processes are used as grafts. Usually, we do not attempt to fuse the facets in this type of arthrodesis. Care should be taken that the small bone chips used as grafts do not fall through the interlaminar defect made for exploration of the intervertebral disc. Today, we may sometimes utilize this type of fusion, but mostly when the patient's condition does not permit prolonging the operative procedure. However, it is not the ideal way to ensure union.

The modified Hibbs fusion is an excellent procedure and, in my opinion, need not always be abandoned for the lateral fusion described by McElroy. There are times when the modified Hibbs fusion can be utilized to advantage, and the complication of a postfusion stenosis occurs, in my opinion, less often than generally publicized.

The modified Hibbs arthrodesis is performed in the same manner as the original Hibbs fusion, except that instead of utilizing local bone as graft material, one obtains corticocancellous strip grafts harvested from a posterior iliac crest. Personally, I prefer to spare the spinous processes and decorticate them together with the laminae, despite the fact that this makes the procedure somewhat longer and technically more difficult. However, it provides a far greater surface area of raw, bleeding cancellous bone into which the grafts can incorporate. I find that the fusion rate is enhanced when I use matchstick-size grafts of cancellous bone alone, avoiding the cortical grafts. I lay my grafts in a lattice-like fashion across the denuded laminae and spinous processes. The facets are denuded of cartilage and small chips of cancellous bone inserted therein.

The *H-graft* has been utilized to bridge a laminer defect. A piece of corticocancellous iliac bone is shaped like an "H" and placed so that each notched end surrounds a spinous process of the intact posterior elements above and below the vertebra with the laminar defect. This procedure is to be avoided; more often than not it results in pseudarthrosis. It is too much to expect that such a single large piece of bone can be revascularized and incorporated into the posterior elements of the host vertebrae.

The Albee arthrodesis, both types of Hibbs fusions, and the H-graft fusion involve only the posterior elements of the vertebrae, and all are referred to as posterior fusions.

McElroy described a *lateral fusion*, which bridges the travserve processes and extends to the alae of the sacrum if the sacrum is to be included in the arthrodesis. This was originally used as a salvage procedure when the posterior elements had been excised, as with a Gill procedure, a laminectomy, and/or a factectomy, and when there was insufficient bone stock posteriorly to accept the grafts. More recently, however, it has been utilized as a primary procedure even when the posterior elements remain intact. This can be carried out with a midline incision or by bilateral paravertebral muscle-splitting incisions; if the latter incisions are utilized, it is surprisingly easy to approach the facets and laminae so as to carry out interlaminar explorations; in this way, supporting ligamentous structures compromised by the midline approach can be spared and stability maintained. The transverse processes, as well as the lateral aspects of the facets and the posterolateral surfaces, of the vertebral bodies are cleaned of all soft tissue and decorticated. Decortication of the transverse processes alone does not prepare an adequate bed for acceptance of the grafts. These structures can be best decorticated by means of a large sharp curet. However, care must be taken to avoid fracturing the transverse processes, which can happen easily. If fracture does occur, fusion may be jeopardized. I like to insert a single rectangular piece of the outer table of the ilium, with only a minimal amount of cancellous bone therone, anterior to the transverse processes and wedged into a slot in the sacrum made by a sharp osteotome. This prevents the cancellous strips of graft from falling anteriorly out of position, and is a particularly valuable technical adjunct when performing this operation in a grade I or II spondylolisthesis, where the forward displacement of the body with its transverse processes makes for a deep hole in which the grafts can be displaced or lost. A profuse amount of cancellous bone should be used as graft material so as to completely fill this defect. Care must be taken to pile up the grafts along the lateral sides of the posterior aspects of the bodies and facets. The facets should be denuded of cartilage and small grafts inserted therein. This type of operation is termed a transverse process fusion, or a lateral fusion, or a posterolateral fusion, since it includes the lateral elements of the posterior portions of the vertebrae.

The ideal arthrodesis is a combination of the standard modified Hibbs fusion and the posterolateral fusion. It should be remembered that the posterior portion of such a fusion cannot be performed when the Gill procedure has been done or when a laminectomy has been carried out.

At times control of gross instability, such as follows bilateral total facetectomies, may require the use of internal fixation devices such as rods. Only in demonstrable gross instability need this adjunctive procedure be considered. Because of the higher pseudarthrosis rate of a lumbosacral fusion, some individuals have reinforced this kind of fusion with various types of plates. Personally, I rarely see an indication for their use.

It should be realized that metallic fixation alone, be it wire, rods, or plates, can never be depended on to permanently stabilize the spine. Such fixation is adjunctive only and fixes the spine only long enough for the fusion to take hold. Used alone, such fixation will invariably fail; it either bends, breaks, or cuts out of the bone with time.

Attention is called to the fact that the more levels fused, the greater the incidence of pseudarthrosis at one or more levels.

I am still conservative in my approach to postoperative care. Most orthopaedists allow their patients to get out of bed a day or so after operation and avoid bracing, but I strongly believe that this contributes to the pseudarthrosis rate. I insist on 6 weeks of bed rest with the patient flat in bed for the first 2 weeks, without a back brace. During this time the patient may turn from side to side, but may not sit. Thereafter, a rigid back brace is worn 24 hours a day for 3 months postoperatively. Six weeks postoperatively I allow my patients to get out of bed while wearing a brace. After wearing the brace 24 hours a day for 3 months, they are permitted to sleep without it, but must wear it when ambulating. I do allow them to remove it to take a shower, but at such times they are to avoid any bending whatsoever. Usually, it takes a full year for the fusion to solidify, and I have my patients wear the back brace until solidity is demonstrated on the dynamic x-ray films. Following the repair of a pseudarthrosis, I commonly apply a body jacket to include one thigh, with the hip in slight flexion. This ensures complete immobilization which simply cannot be obtained in a body cast or in a back brace alone. One theory holds that postoperative immobilization may militate against fusion and that a solid arthrodesis occurs more readily without immobilization and by encouraging activity. I disagree. My experience has been otherwise, and my fusion rates have proved this to my satisfaction.

One should clearly understand why it is necessary to fuse two interspaces in a posterior fusion and only one interspace in an interbody fusion or in a lateral transverse process fusion. When one does a posterior fusion, one is bridging an unstable segment that is not intact, so that the weight-bearing thrust must be carried from the intact segment above to the intact segment below. Therefore, if there is instability or disease at L5, for example, one must carry the posterior fusion from L4 to L5 to the sacrum. However, in the interbody fusion or in the transverse process fusion, one is using the anterior elements of the vertebrae. Accordingly, one need only stabilize the involved segment to the intact segment below. Consequently, in a spondylolisthesis of L5, one merely needs to stabilize L5 to the sacrum either by an interbody graft or by a lateral fusion from the transverse processes of L5 to the alae of the sacrum.

I have been disappointed with my results following interbody fusions in the lumbar area. These can be done via a retroperitoneal approach or via a transperitoneal approach, or by the posterior technique of inserting grafts between the bodies on either side of the thecal sac, the goal being incorporation of a large chunk of corticocancellous bone into the host bone between the vertebral bodies. However, in interbody grafts that may appear to be absorbing initially, arthrodesis may become solid on the x-ray films after 12 to 18 months. The use of an anterior interbody fusion in male children and young male adults is to be cautiously considered because of the possibility of interfering with sexual function by damaging the sympathetic/parasympathetic chain. This is more theoretic than real, since a recent worldwide survey of anterior interbody fusions has shown a very small percentage of impotence following such procedures. Bohlman and McAfee have developed a promising solution to the problem. They carry out a discectomy through a transperitoneal approach, insert a fibular peg graft across the two vertebral bodies to be fused, and place interbody iliac grafts in the intervertebral space on either side of the transfixing fibular peg graft. They have utilized this technique for grade I and grade II spondylolisthesis, and often they are able to reduce the spondylolisthetic slip either partially or completely by simple thumb pressure on the slipped vertebral body. This operation carries the potential of materially increasing the fusion rate in anterior interbody lumbar arthrodeses when performed for reasons other than spondylolisthesis as well as for spondylolisthesis itself. Dr. McAfee has graciously allowed me to describe this work even though it is as yet unpublished.

Instability resulting from neoplastic invasion of the lumbar vertebrae may jeopardize the cauda equina and nerve roots causing a neurological deficit. Such potential or actual instability may be attacked by stabilization with rods, plates, wire, and resin cement products such as methyl methacrylate. The exact technique depends on how much bone is involved and the location of the involvement. In general, these devices are anchored into the intact vertebrae above and below the involved one. Rarely, is this type of stabilization to be combined with spinal fusion. I have found it valuable, when stabilizing posteriorly, to utilize wire, wire mesh, and/or Kirschner wires to act as a framework into which the resin cement is impregnated.

Only rarely does an infectious process result in spinal instability. In such instances, thorough debridement, the insertion of bone grafts, and the use of external immobilization rather than the insertion of metallic or other foreign materials is the method of choice, coupled with the use of appropriate antibiotics.

Spina bifida occulta, sacralization of the fifth lumbar vertebra, and other congenital anomalies are rarely, in themselves, the cause of instability or an indication for spinal fusion. There are some exceptions, such as hemivertebra or a major anomaly that may result in listhesis, deformity, or torsional effect.

It must appear incongruous and even ambiguous that an orthopaedist, whose entire professional training involved arthrodesing spines, now decries the use of spinal fusion except in special circumstances. But the advancement of our knowledge and our current sophisticated techniques, with the ability to diagnose conditions undreamed of in the past, has led me to the unalterable conclusion that decompression is preferable to stabilization by arthrodesis, unless there is a definite indication for such a fusion.

THE FAILED BACK SYNDROME

RICHARD B. NORTH, M.D.

The "failed back syndrome" is a euphemism for the "failed back surgery syndrome" of persistent or recurrent low back pain, with or without sciatica, following one or more lumbar operations. A surgical failure may indeed reflect technical error, but it relates more often to the choice of operation, and in particular to the decision to operate at all. Inappropriate patient selection is recognized as the most common reason for a poor result from lumbar surgery.

The failed back presents as a fait accompli, in which the sequelae of surgery are superimposed on whatever remains of the underlying problem, compounding the difficulties of diagnosis. A surgical history obliges the physician, in a sense, to rule out a persistent surgical problem, but like most patients with low back pain, most with failed backs do not require surgical intervention.

Clinical evaluation of the failed back requires complete background information as to the patient's original presentation, the details of previous examinations and diagnostic studies (including actual films), and operative notes. This indispensable information should be obtained on referral, before the patient's initial visit. At issue are not only technical details of which the patient may be unaware, but also a broad perspective of prior interactions with the health care system, which cannot be obtained reliably from the patient alone. In this context, the initial interview is better directed and more revealing.

Examination of the patient begins in a sense with eliciting the history. Interactions with family or friends who may accompany the patient should be observed carefully. Pain behavior, postural abnormalities, impairment of range of motion, and elements of neurological deficit all may be evident before the formal physical examination begins.

Psychosocial factors such as job satisfaction, issues of secondary gain and compensation, and underlying personality disorders or family problems play a role in many patients. Unless a straightforward, treatable organic problem is evident, psychiatric evaluation and participation in management should begin early and routinely.

A complete history includes a description of the location, quality, and temporal variation of pain, aggravating and relieving factors, and associated subjective manifestations of neurological deficit. The proportion of axial, nonradiating low back pain, as opposed to referred or radicular pain, is important to determine; the latter has some localizing value, but may be misleading. Some symptom complexes suggest specific pathologic entities: For example, pseudoclaudication in lumbar stenosis, burning dysethetic pain in arachnoiditis, nocturnal pain in intraspinal tumor or vascular malformation, and morning pain and stiffness in ankylosing spondylitis.

A thorough general medical history and physical examination are important, but sometimes overlooked, parts of the evaluation of any patient with low back pain, which may reflect extraspinal disease such as abdominal aortic aneurysm, gynecologic disease, prostatic tumor, or renal or rectosigmoid disease. Stigmata of arthritic or autoimmune disease also should be noted.

Electrophysiologic testing (electromyography, nerve conduction studies, H reflexes, and somatosensory evoked potentials) and thermography, although no substitute for a careful neurological examination, have a role in certain clinical settings, although their sensitivity is limited. Neurological deficit which is equivocal clinically may be shown objectively; primary neuromuscular disease or peripheral entrapment may be demonstrated. In the failed back patient, paraspinous EMG may be expected to show nonspecific postsurgical changes.

Management of the failed back follows certain general principles in all cases, regardless of anatomic diagnosis and attendant prospects for surgical intervention. First, intercurrent psychiatric and social issues must be addressed, as previously noted; hospitalization (ideally in a multidisciplinary pain treatment program) may be necessary. Abuse of medications, particularly narcotics and benzodiazepines, must be curbed; withdrawal may require hospitalization for support, observation, and ancillary pain therapy. All patients deserve careful instruction in body mechanics and an appropriate exercise program; this must be deferred, of course, when an active surgical problem exists.

In some patients the failed back surgery syndrome is best managed by further surgery. In the absence of psychiatric contraindications, a clinical syndrome accompanied by, and reasonably consistent with, any of the following common anatomic lesions is an indication for repeat surgery:

1. Decompression
   a. An extradural mass consistent with retained, recurrent, or new disc herniation, which may be accompanied by epidural fibrosis
      b. Lateral recess and/or foraminal stenosis
      c. Lumbar spinal canal stenosis
2. Fusion
   a. Pseudarthrosis of prior fusion
   b. Segmental instability (e.g., iatrogenic spondylolisthesis). A trial of rigid external immobilization will help to resolve equivocal candidacy for fusion
3. Neurolysis. Microsurgical lysis of arachnoid adhesions is a formidable procedure with significant morbidity, perhaps best reserved for patients with clearly progressive neurological deficit endangering bladder and bowel function.
4. Ablative procedures. Monoradicular pain attributable to irreversible injury and not amenable to decompression, but reproducibly responsive to single root blocks, is an indication for dorsal root ganglionectomy. Rhizotomy, by comparison, is ineffective.

When indications for surgery are absent or equivocal, or are overshadowed by medical or psychiatric contraindications, less invasive methods may be useful. Lumbar facet blocks and radiofrequency denervations may be adequate treatment for mechanical low back pain (whose patterns of referral may mimic radicular pain). Recurrence of symptoms after this procedure is common, but it is sufficiently benign to be repeated safely. Similar considerations apply to epidural injections of steroids, local anesthetics, and/or narcotics, whose efficacy is a matter of controversy.

Transcutaneous electrical nerve stimulation (TENS) is helpful in many patients in all phases of the failed back syndrome, from perioperative to chronic. Selection criteria predictive of a favorable response are poorly defined, but this is of little importance for so benign a form of treatment, which may simply be applied empirically.

Implanted spinal stimulators may be considered for inoperable organic problems such as arachnoiditis, or in patients whose medical condition precludes major surgery to correct an anatomic problem. Selection criteria include psychiatric screening and a trial of stimulation with percutaneous electrodes. A patient who has not obtained adequate relief from TENS, but tolerates wearing the device, may still respond to an implanted stimulator.

In summary, the diagnosis and management of the failed back syndrome, although occasionally straightforward, often requires sophisticated diagnostic testing and multidisciplinary input. Many patients are best served by a comprehensive pain treatment program.

Certain aspects of the routine muscoloskeletal and neurological examination, the basics of which are well known, merit discussion. The straight leg-raising test in the supine position is usually inadequately recorded, in terms of production of true sciatic pain and of any protective position assumed by the patient. A "positive" straight leg-raising test is most consistent with root entrapment when accentuated by foot dorsiflexion, popliteal compression, and neck flexion, and when it is reproduced by knee extension when the patient is seated (Michelle's flip sign). Exacerbation of pain by axial compression, trunk rotation, and other mechanisms without apparent physiologic basis are among the "Waddell signs", which are predictive of a poor outcome from any intervention. "Nonphysiologic" sensory loss and "give-away" weakness also are noteworthy.

Diagnostic study of the failed back requires, as a minimum, plain x-ray films of the lumbosacral spine, including A-P, oblique, and lateral flexion-extension views. The latter may be compromised by poor effort or paravertebral spasm or splinting. When symptoms are postural, the examination should be designed to include appropriate dynamic conditions, such as standing versus supine views. If plain film examination is unremarkable, conservative or minimally invasive treatments such as lumbar facet blocks may, in appropriate patients, be undertaken before further study to rule out a surgical lesion. The residual patient population (i.e., patients who are not "appropriate" or who fail to respond to conservative treatment) will deserve such study, if not on the basis of clear symptoms and signs, then simply because postsurgical anatomy requires definition.

Although plain CT examination of the spine increasingly is replacing myelographic study, postoperative scarring in the failed back patient confuses its interpretation, even with intravenous dye enhancement to demonstrate vascular scar tissue. Intrathecal water-soluble contrast (e.g., metrizamide) helps to resolve this. Film screen examination (conventional myelography) before CT may be a more sensitive method for detecting certain extramedullary vascular malformations and for visualizing arachnoid and root sheath adhesions. CT, on the other hand, better demonstrates lumbar canal and lateral recess stenosis, and is uniquely able to show lateral disc herniations and other lesions lateral to the extent of root sheath opacification with dye.

In the failed back patient who has undergone fusion, conventional polytomography may still be useful when CT is equivocal. Radionuclide bone scanning is helpful in demonstrating pseudarthrosis, spondylolysis, and other metabolically active bony lesions, including disc space infections.

Alternative imaging methods generally are less useful. Magnetic resonance imaging improves upon CT in some ways, such as direct sagittal formatting, but poorly defines bone and, in the current state of the art, individual nerve roots. Epidural venography is compromised by postsurgical changes. Discographic imaging, and reproduction of symptoms by disc injection, are controversial and of equivocal value.

As a simple screen for discitis and inflammatory or autoimmune disease, every patient with failed back syndrome deserves an erythrocyte sedimentation rate, if not more extensive rheumatologic screening.

LUMBAR ADHESIVE ARACHNOIDITIS

HAROLD A. WILKINSON, M.D., Ph.D.

Lumbar adhesive arachnoiditis (LAA) is a painful, disabling, yet controversial disease. It is controversial for three principal reasons. First, even though the physical and myelographic changes of LAA are well recognized, not all neurosurgeons agree that it is a major, primary cause of pain and disability. Second, its pathologic spectrum is extremely wide, varying from simple nerve root blunting to multisegmental obliteration of the subarachnoid space, so that its clinical picture varies accordingly. This adds considerably to the uncertainty regarding its incidence and its clinical significance and must be kept in mind in reviewing the medical literature. Third, the etiology of LAA remains unclear. Both spontaneous and familial cases have been reported, but claims continue to appear in the medical literature that LAA is caused principally by myelography or by surgical trauma. The charge against myelography as a major causative factor in LAA is difficult to sustain, since LAA rarely occurs at the site of spinal puncture done at the time of myelography or in the caudal sac where Pantopaque (iophendylate) droplets gravitate, and LAA is extremely rare in patients who have undergone myelography for cervical disease. The possibility that LAA is the result of lumbar disc rupture per se has been less frequently considered.

Pathologically, LAA consists of fibrous and, rarely, osseous scarring in the subarachnoid space with thickening of the arachnoid membrane. Even though the term "arachnoiditis" implies an inflammatory process, leukocytic infiltrates are not found. In its simplest form, sometimes referred to as type 1 arachnoiditis, the process is limited to one or two adjacent nerve root sleeves. Myelographically, this causes a defect that can mimic the defect caused by lumbar disc rupture. The type of arachnoiditis more commonly seen in severely symptomatic patients, so called type 2 or type 2A, consists of circumferential or complete transverse obliteration of the subarachnoid space limited to one or two spinal levels. This usually occurs at the site of previous disc rupture or spinal surgery. The caudal end of the thecal sac commonly remains open and may contain movable droplets of Pantopaque (iophendylate). The more uncommon but most extensive form, sometimes called type 2B or type 3, consists of circumferential or transverse obliteration of the subarachnoid space which extends over multiple segmental levels. This type may be more common in the spontaneous or congenital version of the disease. Myelographically the circumferential forms appear as a ragged narrowing of the subarachnoid space with nerve roots plastered laterally against the walls of the spinal canal. The transverse form is characterized by complete obstruction of the subarachnoid space with a characteristic ragged upper margin. CT scans are usually incapable of diagnosing this condition, though scans done with contrast enhancement of the spinal fluid (CT myelography) are able to demonstrate complete obstruction or narrowing of the lumbar subarachnoid space.

Clinically, pain is the most constant feature of LAA. The pain usually involves a combination of back pain and radiating sciatica, the sciatica being bilateral in more than half of all patients. The sciatic pain is commonly characterized as burning, aching, or tingling. Both lumbago and sciatica are aggravated by activity, but are usually only incompletely relieved by bed rest. Coughing or sneezing, which distends the thecal sac, can be extremely painful. Neurological deficits are common. Single nerve root motor and sensory loss is common in type 1 LAA, but also may be encountered in type 2 or 3. Complete cauda equina syndromes with bilateral motor and sensory loss and loss of control of bowel, bladder, and sexual functions may be encountered in severe cases of type 2 or 3 LAA.

LAA usually becomes symptomatic within a few weeks or months after back surgery. However, symptoms may begin spontaneously, without surgery, myelography, or other spinal instrumentation. In these cases, LAA may be diagnosed as disc rupture, but of course the patient remains unrelieved following discectomy. Once symptoms develop, the patient may worsen progressively, but symptoms usually stabilize after 1 or 2 years. Exacerbation may follow minor injury or even an episode of violent coughing. After a year or 2, at least half of all patients begin a period of gradual recovery. Over the next 5 to 10 years, some patients gradually and spontaneously improve sufficiently to return to near-normal activity.

LAA can also be a clinical problem when it is asymptomatic. Extensive arachnoiditis, largely obliterating the subarachnoid space to myelographic examination, can seriously hamper detection of underlying recurrent disc ruptures. Furthermore, a patient's symptoms may be attributed to LAA and alternative treatable diagnoses may be overlooked—diagnoses such as lateral recess bony stenosis, painful facet joints, pseudomeningocele, fusion pseudarthrosis, or inflammatory discitis.

The diagnosis of LAA involves both detection of the physical presence of the disease and a determination of the symptomatic significance of its presence.

The physical changes of "primary" arachnoiditis should be suspected in the patient with a clinical picture suggesting lumbar disc disease but a myelogram showing unusually large, irregular, or bilateral defects. This is especially true if the CT scan shows little or no convincing evidence of disc herniation. Unfortunately, some patients with primary or early secondary arachnoiditis do, in fact, have a significant disc herniation as well. If such patients are studied only by CT scan and myelography is not done, the diagnosis of associated LAA is likely to be missed. Thus patients should be considered for myelography even in the presence of a significant disc bulge on CT scan if their clinical picture is atypical for lumbar disc disease, especially if symptoms are bilateral or if multiple nerve roots seem to be involved. The physical changes of LAA can be detected almost exclusively by myelography, preferably with water-soluble agents to prevent loculation of oily Pantopaque (iophendylate) and possible aggravation of the arachnoiditis. Pantopaque droplets are occasionally found trapped in LAA, and the diagnosis of LAA is occasionally made by demonstrating extensive loculation of Pantopaque within the lumbar spinal canal on plain radiographs.

The symptomatic nature of LAA is often difficult to confirm and often depends on exclusion of alternative diagnoses. In patients with the "failed back syndrome", LAA must be differentiated from all of the alternative diagnostic possibilities mentioned earlier. This may necessitate (1) CT scan with or without intravenous contrast to help differentiate epidural scar from ruptured disc material, (2) facet nerve or joint injection to rule out facet syndromes, (3) contrast or anesthesia discography to rule out discogenic pain or rupture of an unoperated disc, (4) epidural nerve blocks to localize the level of nerve root involvement, and (5) flexion-extension and tomographic back radiographs, isotope bone scans, and/or a trial of external steel bracing to rule out symptomatic fusion pseudarthrosis.

The therapy of LAA can employ either nonspecific or specific modalities. The nonspecific modalities are symptom-directed. Specific therapy is aimed at surgical correction of the structural abnormality of LAA.

Nonspecific therapy may be either noninvasive or needle-invasive. Sciatic pain can be treated with antineu-ralgia therapy. Dilantin, Tegretol, or thiamine, for example, effects a gradual reduction of pain, often requiring as long as 2 weeks to achieve good effectiveness. Nonsteroidal anti-inflammatory drugs (NSAIDs) are particularly useful for lumbago, but may bring some relief of sciatic pain as well. The multiplicity of these drugs which are currently available attests to the considerable variability in patient response which they elicit. All can cause significant side effects, most notably gastrointestinal distress, but the severity of side effects and the quality of good effects vary greatly from patient to patient. Blood levels rise rapidly as body enzymes become saturated, and so a steady intake at dosages adequate to produce either beneficial results or intolerable side effects is important, and failure to obtain benefit without side effects from one drug does not predict a lack of better response to some other NSAID. Bed rest is advisable only for acute flare-ups of this chronic disease, but limiting back motion through use of a canvas corset or steel brace can limit some of its symptoms. Intrathecal corticosteroids (I prefer Depo-Medrol, 80 mg/ml) seem to work better than epidural steroids and can bring dramatic relief to at least half the patients. This relief may last from a few weeks to many months. Although I am unaware of any proven instances of patient injury (other than sepsis) through the use of intrathecal Depo-Medrol, there are at least theoretic dangers, and injections more than three or four times annually probably should be avoided.

Specific therapy of LAA entails microsurgical lysis of adhesions, freeing individual nerve roots. This can be undertaken as a major operative intervention in patients with extensive transverse or circumferential LAA or as part of the exploration of a single nerve root defect demonstrated on myelography.

In my series of laminectomies and extensive microsurgical lysis of LAA, 80 percent of patients obtained short-term improvement of pain and neurological deficits, but by the end of one year only 50 percent of the total group remained improved. One technical problem associated with surgical lysis is that of preventing reformation of the arachnoiditis. This has been attempted through intrathecal or systemic administration of corticosteroids, but there is no firm proof that this is effective. Intraoperative use of enzymes to remove the thickened arachnoid and scar is probably contraindicated because of the resulting potential for chemical injury and accelerated scar formation. Decompressive grafting of the overlying dura also is rarely necessary and seems to add significantly to postoperative complications (notably spinal fluid leakage) without adding appreciably to the beneficial results. Patients should be cautioned that perhaps 10 percent might experience increased difficulty following surgery. This can vary from increased pain (sometimes caused by decompression of injured nerve roots, restoring them to painful partial function) to increased neurologic deficit, such as weakness, impotence, or incontinence.

Microsurgical lysis of adhesions in the nerve root pouch around a single nerve root has received little systematic study. There is no question that some cases of

LAA begin as single nerve root defects in patients in whom no disc rupture is discovered during extradural exploration. It has been suggested that intradural exploration and microsurgical lysis of adhesions be considered in patients with large myelographic defects who are found on extradural exploration to have no disc rupture, and perhaps if extensive extradural adhesions are encountered with or without disc rupture. This suggestion presumes that type 1 LAA is likely to be confirmed in these patients, but the risks and benefits of such surgical intervention have not yet been quantitated.

NONOPERATIVE TREATMENT OF THE FAILED BACK SYNDROME PRESENTING WITH CHRONIC PAIN

HUBERT L. ROSOMOFF, M.D., D. Med. Sc.

It must be stated that the failed back syndrome which eventually becomes chronic pain represents not a failure of the patient and his back, but rather a failure for the practioners of medicine and surgery. Invariably, the patient has been misdiagnosed and improperly treated, and the results are long-term disability, drug dependency, lack of productivity, behavioral disturbance, and for some, social and economic catastrophe.

The saga starts with the history. All too often the events leading to injury have not been recorded properly, and thus a series of erroneous conclusions ensue. It is now recognized that back pain and its allied disorders rank first among health problems in the frequency of occurrence. Eight of 10 people have, or have had, significant back pain. It is the leading cause of disability and lost work days in the working years. Cost—based on lost earnings, worker compensation or disability payments, and expenses for medical care—exceeds that of any single health disorder. The frequency and impact are expected to increase over the next decade, as longevity and average age of the work force increase.

Traditionally, the symptom complex of back pain with extension into the leg, or sciatica, is conceived as being due to a herniated disc, i.e., pinching or compression of one or more spinal nerve roots. By one estimate, more than 450,000 operations are performed annually for this presumed condition. Physiologic studies, however, demonstrate that, except for transient pain when first impacted, sustained nerve root compression, or "pinching", does not produce further pain. There may be numbness or loss of function, as when one's leg "falls asleep", but it is not a painful event. Therefore, other causes must be considered as agents giving rise to pain, and these causes are sought in the overlying soft tissues. It is a fact that, anatomically, the spine is surrounded by a large mass of muscle, fascia, and integument designed for protection. Embedded deep within these structures are the spinal canal, the intervertebral discs, and the contiguous nerve structures. The soft tissues bear the brunt of forces applied to the spine, and therefore soft tissue injury is an obligatory component of any spinal trauma.

Once the history has been obtained, the usual physical examination centers about the neurological system; 75 to 97 percent of these patients are found to have no neurological deficit at this time. Although the examination includes movement of the back and a sciatic stretch test, such as the Lasègue maneuver, this portion of the examination is done all too quickly and without full appreciation of the potential pathology to be identified. When done thoroughly, however, examination reveals multiple areas of tenderness, trigger points, and restricted range of motion in the back, hips, and legs, which result in mecahnical dysfunction, continuing strain, muscle fatigue, and pain. Superimposed on this initial set of events is the personal background that the patient brings to the injury. The profile of the "low back loser" includes a self-defeating personality with a poor work history, poor social interrelationships, a low sense of self-esteem, and a focus on painful bodily cues. This is a patient that often has poor skills, never likes his job, blames the employer for his injury, and eventually becomes angry with the insurance company that does not appear to tend to his needs. He is depressed, and there is a nonadaptive personality style. He is passive-aggressive and, very quickly, a "retirement syndrome" evolves in which there is the perception of the system "owing him" something or everything. The patient is angry at himself, his family, his employer, his physician who has failed him, his lawyer who has not provided him with a generous settlement, the insurance company who has made "his life difficult", and a social and legal system which he does not understand. He is fearful, particularly of reinjury and further loss of function. He is further concerned that he will be unable to perform his job for which he will be terminated with a loss of benefits. He is a target for failure. To this is added the problem of other dependencies, such as narcotics, barbiturates, muscle relaxants, and "street drugs", supplemented by alcohol abuse, withdrawal, retirement from life, and addiction to back braces, support equipment, television, and video games. The family circle commonly aids and abets this disability by subjugating their own needs while assuming the patient's responsibilities. They, too, are frightened, angry and protective. His physicians have failed to relieve him of his pain and mental burdens, having passed him through a series of unrewarding studies and treatments, including bed rest, traction, ineffective physical therapy, drugs, roentgenograms, myelograms, tests for nervous system dysfunction, and unsuccessful surgery. This iatrogenic failure is transmitted to the patient when the patient is asked to seek psychiatric help and is told that he, the patient, is the reason for failure, and it is implied that "it is all in his head". Meanwhile, the employer may be compounding the issue by an unsympathetic pose, a threat to fire the worker, and a refusal to modify the job to accommodate the injured. To boot, a poorly informed lawyer may advise his client inappropriately, and an uncaring insurance adjustor also comes to blame the patient for the lack of success in treatment. The patient now has chronic pain, is impaired physically, is weak and inactive, is drug and alcohol dependent, is hostile, untrusting, frightened, feels helpless and hopeless, is dependent, has sexual problems, and is anxious, depressed, and angry. Marital problems result; there is no job and no motivation; and he becomes disability-oriented. Where does one start to treat such a patient?

To begin, the treating physician must recognize the nature of the injury so as to prescribe proper diagnostic testing and treatment to follow. Most important to this analysis is the recognition that pain is derived most commonly from soft tissue disease, utilizing the nervous system only as a communicator to the brain for the signal of disturbance in the periphery. Once understood, the soft tissue or myofascial syndromes are easily recognized; treatment can be swift and efficient. In the low back, the common gluteal myofascial syndromes produce trigger points over the hip at the trochanteric bursa, creating sciatic referred pain. The other ends of this muscular arrangement are at the sacroiliac area and the ischial tuberosity. These syndromes feature painful weight-bearing, and sitting, standing, and walking become torture. Injured muscles such as the quadratus lumborum go into sustained contracture as a result of the trauma, resulting in a pelvic tilt or antalgic scoliosis. The paraspinal muscles of the back participate both posteriorly and anteriorly, and mechanical malalignment occurs when iliopsoas contracture induces sustained anterior flexion. These abnormalities then are worsened by the injudicious choices of bed rest, muscle relaxants, and excesive analgesia, which augment the mechanical dysfunction by disuse and deconditioning. The appropriate treatment consists of mobilization with intense and aggressive activation and a physical therapy program that stretches and releases the contracted muscles and their accompanying restricted joint motion. Physical modalities such as ice, not drugs, to desensitize and reduce the inflammation in the affected areas are available and easy to use. Ice, as a therapeutic modality, has long been overlooked as a primary mode of treatment for reaction to injury and inflammation. Heat is best used to soften tightened structures in preparation for physical therapy. Supplementary use of prostaglandin inhibitors to reduce inflammation and to inhibit the chemical interactions which lead to pain is important. Aspirin remains the keystone drug, and it is inexpensive.

Traditional diagnostic tests have failed to result in a successful therapeutic approach; plain roentgenograms, computerized tomography, and myelography, which are the studies commonly utilized, have either failed to show significant disease or have demonstrated some abnormality that has been acted upon without benefit. It is important to note that 50 percent of the population, at all ages, have CT scans which, technically, may be interpreted as showing an abnormality—one for which there are not symptoms; and 30 percent to 60 percent of myelograms have been demonstrated to be abnormal in individuals who have no back complaints. It therefore follows that clnical acumen continues to the major diagnostic tool. Other diagnostic testings—electromyography, thermography, discography, and venography—should be mentioned. Their reliability with respect to producing a diagnosis leading to successful therapeutic outcome is low, and their utilization has proved to be unrewarding. The failed back patient obviously has not responded to surgical intervention by laminectomy, fusion, electrical implantation for pain, facet rhizotomy, or assorted other techniques. The most current method, chemonucleolysis, has also proved unrewarding, and an increasing number of serious complications contraindicate its use.

The sedentary life style of modern living and a lack of physical fitness have been demonstrated to be the prime causal agents leading to low back injury. When the behavioral consequences are added to the physical, we have the ingredients for failure.

When the failed back patient has become disabled with chronic pain, treatment requires a multidisciplinary approach. No one physician has the expertise or resources to affect this complex, catastrophic condition. The components include aggressive intense physical medicine, understanding and dedicated behavioral medicine, and vocational rehabilitation with a therapeutic goal of a return to economic and social productivity on completion of treatment. Physical therapy begins with reduction of trigger points by the use of physical modalities; judicious injection with saline, steroid, or anesthetic agent; muscle stretching and strengthening to restore range of motion and endurance; gait training; and realignment of posture. Instruction on how to prevent reinjury, recognition of limitations of functional capacities as applied to job requirements, and maintenance of a continuing home conditioning program are essential. In a chronically established failed back, such a program requires at least 4 weeks of intensive management with an initial inpatient program, progressing to an outpatient program only when the first painful stretching and early conditioning period have been mastered. Occupational and recreational therapy, as a component of physical medicine, are likewise important. These disciplines deal with establishment of sitting, standing, walking, and driving tolerances; pacing with respect to daily and work activities; energy-saving techniques, and an indoctrination in the use of proper body mechanics. These are absolutely essential, for it is the inappropriate use of the body that precipitates injury that is avoidable. A complete therapeutic program should include job simulation as the patient improves with therapy. The patient is taught to properly perform his job assignments and is thus assured that he is capable of carrying them out. Furthermore, the patient and the treating physican are thus able to certify the work tolerances that can be accomplished. In fact, there are established techniques and criteria for measuring strength and the ability to move weight, as required by the job. These are to be found under the heading of "ergonomics" and "industrial engineering". One myth to be dispelled is that a sedentary job is better than one that is active. In fact, all investigation has shown that the sedentary jobs (e.g., clerical) produce major strain and force application to the back, whereas action type jobs with intermittent walking, standing, and sitting provide the best composition for injured back placement. Access to a good vocational counseling service is invaluable in developing good simulation and choice of occupation. Placement prior to completion of the therapeutic program with a goal of a return to work without "down time" between the completion of treatment and the return to full activity and/or work is a keystone to success. Most individuals can be returned to full activity, including hard labor, although some job modification may be necessary during an interim transitional period. Transferable skills, which require less exertion, may be a substitute choice.

The role of behavioral medicine is integral to a successful outcome. Almost without exception, all individuals who reach the status of the failed back syndrome have behavioral consequences, most commonly anxiety, depression, or both. Drug dependency or addiction is addressed immediately. Rapid withdrawal can be achieved when detoxification is integrated with the intense activation of an aggressive physical medicine program. Few or no withdrawal symptoms are noted. Coping mechanisms for the pain, disability, and affront to the ego must be treated. Attitudes toward work and disability must be altered in favor of wellness. Marital difficulty must be resolved, and so counseling becomes a major effort, and the impact of this injury to the individual and family unit must be managed. Formal psychotherapy is of little value, except for the occasional individual who has a background history of a major disorder which requires treatment in its own right. There is probably no such entity as psychogenic pain. There is invariably a physical basis upon which the personality structure and environmental circumstances leading to behavioral maladjustments are appended; these must be recognized and corrected. Another important tool that behavioral medicine employs is the use of relaxation and biofeedback techniques. The goal here is to reduce muscle tension in already injured, sensitized tissue and to develop the ability to relax such muscles when they are being maximally employed for movement and weight displacement. This may seem paradoxical, but all students of muscle physiology appreciate that fluid, efficient movement can only be achieved with a relaxed, steady, properly programmed sequence of muscle action. Otherwise the muscles become fatigued, crampy, and painful. Finally, when possible, the use of industrial engineers or ergonomists to adapt the patient to his work environment by selection, training, or modification of the work or its site can be invaluable. Prevention of reinjury is the key to both health and work satisfaction. Such an educational effort applies both to the employee and the employer, provided the latter will listen.

It is possible, even in the most severely disabled failed back, to return such individuals to full functional capacity and to work with a properly designed and directed multidisciplinary therapeutic program. This statement applies regardless of length of history, age or sex, number of therapeutic interventions, or all other parameters that have been investigated, exclusive of behavior. It does take a motivated, well-managed patient, who complies and makes the effort to rehabilitate, to achieve success. Seemingly, the one deterrant is the intractable behavioral disorder which does not yield to treatment or, more commonly, which the patient does not allow to be treated. Total patient effort is required to effect weight control, physical conditioning, the home maintenance program, and proper body mechanics, with pacing and energy-saving techniques, upon return to work. Education to prevent reinjury is essential. Drug intake and other dependent activities must remain interdicted. Behavioral modification, biofeedback, and relaxation skills must be maintained, along with stress management and coping techniques. Vocational counseling and job planning for immediate return to work on completion of treatment appears to be quite necessary for, as "down time" increases, the results of treatment progressively move toward failure. Maintenance of full activity and the healthy influence of a return to work and the attendant social/economic atmosphere become the assurance of a continuing, long-term successful result. Such a program, in combination with a dedicated staff and a motivated patient who accepts the responsibility and makes the total effort required for rehabilitation, can provide a return to full functional activity and a return to work in 86 percent of the population so managed. The failed back does not have to fail forever.

PAIN

SPINAL INJURY PAIN

ALLAN H. FRIEDMAN, M.D.
BLAINE NASHOLD, Jr., M.D., F.A.C.S.

Pain severe enough to disrupt a patient's normal daily activities frequently afflicts those who have suffered a significant spinal cord injury. The proportion of spinal cord injury patients who suffer intractable pain varies greatly among reported series. It is our opinion that dysesthesias of some form are common after a severe injury to the spinal cord. In up to 40 percent of cases, patients describe dysesthesias bothersome enough to disrupt their normal activities at least some of the time. Ten percent of patients rate the pain as severe. Painful syndromes are most likely to develop in patients with damage to the conus medullaris or cauda equina.

Although the etiology of pain following spinal cord injury is unknown, several hypotheses have been proposed to explain its origin. Even though each theory suggests a specific form of therapy, no single therapeutic maneuver has proved applicable to all patients with this kind of pain. Indeed, researchers who have examined a large number of patients with pain following spinal cord injury have noted that the patients' complaints are not identical, but tend to follow one of several different patterns. Instead of trying to separate patients by their pathophysiology, it is more useful clinically to separate patients according to recognized pain patterns.

Most patients suffer local pain at the site of the spinal injury. This pain is no different from the pain suffered by patients who sustain a spinal injury without concomitant spinal cord damage and is most likely secondary to fractured vertebrae, torn ligaments, or contused muscles. This pain generally abates spontaneously within 2 weeks of injury, although the occasional patient may continue to have some very low-grade persistent local discomfort. If the pain persists, the physician must be concerned about the possibility of an unstable spine with progressive deformity, a nonunion of a fracture with a painful pseudoarthrosis, or an infection with progressive bony destruction.

Patients may experience the acute onset of hyperesthesia and hyperpathia immediately following spinal trauma. In these cases, a concomitant, spontaneous burning pain occurs at the dermatomal level of the injury and extends caudally for a variable number of spinal segments. The burning pain is exacerbated when the painful area is touched. Although this type of pain may occur as a result of a complete spinal transection, it most often accompanies an incomplete spinal cord injury. Fortunately, this pain is self-limited and usually subsides spontaneously within 2 weeks.

Another group of patients suffer from chronic pain, which also begins at the level of the spinal cord injury and extends caudally for a variable number of dermatomes. The pain predominates in the border zone between normal and abnormal sensation and involves areas in which the sensation is impaired. It is sometimes referred to as "terminal zone pain". Although some authors postulate that this pain is secondary to nerve rootlet injury at the level of the spinal lesion, this pain is usually refractory to rhizolysis or rhizotomy. This pain may be symmetric, but frequently involves one leg more than the other. We have noted that a high percentage of patients who have a delayed onset of this type of pain have a spinal cord cyst. It is particularly important, when the pain has a burning quality, to distinguish unilateral localized pain from the diffuse or predominantly sacral pain, which will be described next. This pain usually has two components. The patients note a chronic, relatively dull, boring, aching, and sometimes burning pain. Superimposed on this baseline pain are waves of severe stabbing pain. These paroxysms of stabbing pain last from minutes to one-half hour. The paroxysms are generally aggravated by tactile stimulation of the area in which the pain is perceived and may also be provoked by prolonged activity or distention of the patient's viscera. Some patients emphatically note that the pain is decreased by rest or massage of the painful area. This pain syndrome is most common following high lumbar or low thoracic spinal injuries. It is usually chronic and persistent, worsening with time in a high percentage of patients.

Diffuse burning pain is all too frequently associated with paraplegia and occasionally with quadriplegia. This pain usually involves the entire corpus and limbs caudal to the level of the injury and may be particularly severe in the sacral dermatomes. Although the pain may vary in intensity at random intervals, the patient usually cannot recognize an exacerbating or quieting factor. In some patients the onset of the burning pain is delayed for many months; in more fortunate patients the pain begins soon after the injury and subsequently diminishes in time to a more tolerable level. This pain syndrome is most common following conus medullaris and cauda equina injuries.

Phantom sensations are common among patients with spinal cord injury. The phantom is most vivid immediately after the injury, and as time from the injury increases, the phantom sensation diminishes. Although the patient may feel that the phantom limb has assumed an awkward position, this phantom is seldom painful, unlike the phantom sensation which follows limb amputation.

Some authors describe visceral pain following spinal cord trauma. Whether this pain represents physiologic sensations indicative of distention or hyperactivity of the hollow intra-abdominal viscera or whether it represents referred pain resulting from the spinal cord injury itself is uncertain. In our experience, visceral pain usually indicates an independent intra-abdominal problem.

Therapy for each of the aforementioned pain syndromes is somewhat different. The acute pain associated with a spinal fracture can usually be quelled with a short course of narcotics. Because of the possibility of further neurological deficits resulting from vertebral canal impingement at the site of an unstable spinal column, assessment of the fracture and appropriate stabilizing procedures must be instituted prior to embarking on pain management. Narcotic analgesics at high doses may be necessary until approximately the fourth postinjury or postoperative day, when the patient's pain usually begins to abate. Transcutaneous nerve stimulation has been reported to ease local pain. Patients complaining of persistent local pain should be evaluated for instability, nonfusion, or infection.

Severe hyperesthesia occurring concomitantly with the spinal cord injury appears to be resistant to narcotic analgesia. Several pharmacologic manipulations have been employed in an attempt to treat this condition, but their efficacy is difficult to assess. Fortunately, this severe pain syndrome appears to be self-limited, disappearing spontaneously within 2 weeks of the injury.

Patients suffering with aching pain extending caudally from the level of injury, the so called "terminal zone pain", may be managed by a number of different approaches. Patients with low-grade pain that only occasionally interferes with daily activity can usually be managed with non-narcotic analgesics. Dr. Guttman, a leader in the treatment of spinal cord injured patients, has postulated that "end zone" pain is secondary to skeletal disease tht is avoidable by the proper care of patients in the immediate postinjury phase. This theory has not been corroborated by other physicians. Attention should be paid to the possibility of an underlying depressive or anxiety state, which can intensify relatively innocuous pain. Such conditions should be treated with appropriate pharmacologic and psychiatric therapy.

If the patient develops deterioration in his neurological status, investigation should be instituted for a possible traumatic syringomyelia. Posttraumatic syringomyelia occurs in approximately 2 percent of paraplegic patients. Most patients with traumatic syringomyelia note an intensification of pain and an enlargement of the painful area. In classic cases, the pain is exacerbated by coughing, sneezing, and straining.

In patients with disabling end zone pain which is refractory to medical management, dorsal root entry zone (DREZ) lesions should be employed. This microsurgical procedure, in which the dorsal root entry zone is coagulated, has been shown to be effective in relieving the pain of two-thirds of patients. Although rhizotomy, or intrathecal alcohol or phenol in glycerine injections, may afford some patients short-term pain relief, such local therapy seldom yields long-term relief from pain. Cordectomy has been shown to be successful in some patients with a distal conus medullaris lesion. In most clinics, such radical surgery is usually avoided. Cordotomy may help the patient with end zone pain, but the pain relief is often temporarily limited.

Persistent burning pain involving the entire body below the level of the injury remains a difficult problem to treat. This chronic pain syndrome requires thoughtful management aimed at avoiding drug dependence. The deleterious effects of insomnia, anxiety, and depression must be addressed in establishing a successful therapeutic regimen.

Although the use of narcotic analgesics is not to be condemned per se, patients with chronic diffuse burning pain usually only receive pain relief from large doses of narcotic analgesics and require escalating doses of medication to maintain this level of pain relief. The resultant addiction only compounds the patient's problem. Medications that enhance natural pain suppression pathways such as L-tryptophan, doxepin, and amitriptyline are helpful adjuvants which also help combat insomnia and depression. Doxepin and amitriptyline are generally effective in treating pain disorders at doses lower than those required to treat depression. Anxiety is best treated with a tranquilizing drug such as hydroxyzine (Vistaril) or fluphenazine (Prolixin).

Anticonvulsants have been employed in the treatment of spinal cord injury pain based on the theory that disinhibited neurons proximal to the site of the spinal cord injury act as hyperactive foci, initiating impulses that spread throughout the pain pathway. This situation is thought by some to be analogous to the epileptic focus which results from cerebral cortical trauma. Although this theory is far from proven, carbamazepine, clonazepam, and valproic acid have all been reported to be of limited benefit in treating this condition.

Diffuse burning pain has proved particularly resistant to surgical therapy. Rhizotomies, intrathecal alcohol, and intrathecal phenol are of no benefit in patients suffering with this condition. Some authors have theorized that painful sensations are propagated along sympathetic neurons, thus bypassing the spinal cord lesion. Although this line of reasoning was strengthened by early success in relieving the burning pain of paraplegia with sympathectomy, subsequent literature has demonstrated a lack of consistent results with this mode of therapy. Although anterior cordotomy has occasionally been reported to relieve end zone pain and localized unilateral burning pain, it is ineffective in quenching chronic diffuse burning pain or burning pain localized to the sacral dermatomes. Posterior cordotomy and midline myelotomy have also been employed without success.

Cordectomy has been proposed as a method of isolating the damaged area of the spinal cord and to disrupt any remaining occult spinal pathways which may carry painful signals from the area of injury. Surprisingly, this method of therapy has not been effective in relieving diffuse burning pain associated with paraplegia.

It has also been postulated that the burning pain results from a disinhibiting of the pain-producing signals. This theory assumes that certain ascending spinal pathways that normally inhibit pain signals are lost at the time of the injury. Such a situation could be remedied by augmenting the remaining pain-inhibiting pathways. This augmentation has been attempted by employing electrical stimulators. A review of the few cases reported in the literature seems to indicate that dorsal column stimulation is not effective in alleviating burning pain. Central nervous system stimulation is a theoretically appealing method of treating pain of deafferentation, but further evaluation is necessary before it can be recommended for the treatment of the diffuse burning pain of paraplegia. A review of the limited number of cases of burning postparaplegic pain treated by posterior thalamus, internal capsule, or periaqueductal grey stimulation indicates that central stimulation is less beneficial in treating this syndrome than in treating other forms of deafferentation pain.

DEFINING THE CHRONIC PAIN SYNDROME

BENJAMIN L. CRUE, Jr., M.D.

The recognition of the existence of chronic pain as a syndrome is a very recent development. It has been estimated that patients incapacitated by chronic pain are costing society in this country almost 100 billion dollars a year. Many patients with chronic pain are not being adequately diagnosed or adequately treated. This has been a failure of both the medical profession and the health care delivery system. From a socioeconomic standpoint, many patients suffering from chronic pain may be deprived of optimum care because of exclusions in the patient's insurance contract, whether it be private insurance, Medicare, Medicaid, or Workman's Compensation. Therefore, both the "evaluation" and the "management" of a patient with chronic pain must be viewed in this light.

The diagnosis and treatment of patients with chronic pain is of interest not only to neurosurgeons (who for years have received referrals of end-of-the-road patients with chronic pain), but also to some physicians in other specialties, such as anesthesiology, neurology, rheumatology, and psychiatry. There is almost no branch of medical practice that has not, at one time or another, been involved in the treatment of patients with chronic pain syndromes. This has given rise to a new (and as yet unofficial) multidisciplinary specialty known as "algology".

It also has produced the multi- and interdisciplinary pain team concept. Chronic pain therapy may be delivered in the setting of an outpatient pain clinic, an inpatient pain unit, or in a truly comprehensive chronic pain treatment center.

Pain itself defies definition, being a subjective complaint that accompanies many types of illness and almost all injury. Nevertheless, chronic pain can be considered an entity unto itself and various pain syndromes classified in a taxonomy. If this concept of chronic pain as a clinical entity is adopted, we do not have to talk about various types of pain syndromes that may or may not accompany various specific forms of underlying disease or injury. Chronic pain itself can be treated as a clinical problem. The adjective "chronic" merely means that it has gone on for a considerable length of time. Often a pejorative connotation is inferred when the therapist talks about an "unusual", "unreasonable", "unexplained", or "unacceptable" duration of pain, considering the particular etiology of the original pain. Chronic does not mean severe. The amplitude factor is not implied, and yet, if the pain were not significant subjectively to the patient, the patient would not be incapacitated by his suffering. The acceptable duration of pain before it can be labeled as chronic is generally 6 months. This is obviously arbitrary in any given case.

Acute pain is the subjective perception of hurt that immediately follows tissue inflammation or injury. This is not the place to discuss the recent advances in understanding of the peripherally acting mechanisms underlying the peripheral induction of this nociceptive input. The modern discoveries of the central endorphin and enkephalin mechanisms and the feedback loop from the higher central nervous system to the region of the dorsal horn for modulation of nociceptive input are not known to be important in chronic pain. It is understood that in acute pain with known nociceptive input the treatment is usually analgesic or narcotic (peripheral or central pharmacologic therapy), while the body is allowed to heal, and the nociceptive input presumably turns itself off, resulting in amelioration of the perceived pain. At times medicine can aid this process; for example, by removal of a kidney stone impacted in the ureter (a common source of severe acute pain from presumed nociceptive input over a *visceral* afferent system), or by the splinting of an injured extremity (and by immobilization, decreasing the nociceptive input over the *somatic* afferents), allowing the injured area to undergo a process of repair. However, this short-lived nociceptive input in the acute pain medical model is not the subject of this article. The question that remains is what relation this well accepted acute pain model has to the patients incapacitated many months or years from a so-called *chronic pain syndrome*.

At this point let me introduce a classification of pain:

Acute
Up to a few days' duration
Mild or severe
Cause known or unknown
Presumed nociceptive input
The "fix me" medical model
Subacute
A few days' to a few months' duration
Though no longer an emergency, in most ways treat like acute pain
Recurrent acute
Recurrent or continued nociceptive input from underlying chronic pathologic process, e.g., arthritis (rheumatoid or osteoarthritis)
Ongoing acute
Due to uncontrolled malignant neoplastic disease
Continued nociceptive input
Chronic benign
Non-neoplastic
Usually >6 months' duration
No known nociceptive peripheral input
Pain often made more severe by any type of subsequant sensory input
Basically a "central" pain
Seemingly adequate coping by the patient
Chronic intractable benign pain syndrome (CIBPS)
Chronic pain with poor patient coping (i.e., pain becomes the central focus of the patient's existence)

Two groupings (ongoing acute and recurrent acute pain) in this classification are of extreme interest to neurosurgeons in many instances, but should *not* be labeled chronic pain. Continued nociceptive input due to continuing disease from ongoing peripheral tissue destruction, as in uncontrolled neoplastic disease, in which the malignant tumor continues to invade in spite of therapeutic attempts, is often accompanied by continued pain. This is considered (incorrectly) by many to be a chronic pain syndrome. I believe that since there is continued nociceptive input, this pain of cancer should be considered as an ongoing acute pain process. When supportive techniques, antidepressants, anti-anxiety tranquilizers, and sociologic support mechanisms (e.g., family, health care team) have failed in pain amelioration, anesthesiologic or neurosurgical intervention (e.g., nerve block, rhizotomy, chordotomy) is indicated and usually gives reasonable results. By trading numbness for pain, what time the patient has left is improved. This may be an important part of the neurosurgeon's pain practice, but this is not done for "chronic" pain.

Even more confusing is the pain due to continued nociceptive input from underlying *chronic disease*, as is often found in arthritis. For example, in rheumatoid arthritis, where, in a younger person, there is recurrent flare-up of the redness, swelling and pain from the affected joints; or, in degenerative osteoarthritis in the spine in the region of a foramen for the entrance of a sensory nerve root, there may well be build-up of hypertrophic tissue that may somehow "irritate" the afferent fibers and initiate some type of recurrent nociceptive input, leading to continued or recurrent clinical pain. However, it is our contention that this is a chronic pathologic condition with recurrent acute pain in the nociceptive input model, and this should not be confused with a chronic pain syndrome.

I consider *chronic pain to be a syndrome only in the absence of demonstrated continued nociceptive input*. This then presumes some type of underlying central nervous system generator mechanism to continue the perception of pain. This viewpoint has been labeled as the *centralist concept of chronic pain*. All such chronic pain is considered real. However, there is no question that some central pains are more organic than others. The concept of real versus psychological pain has no meaning. The pain of causalgia and trigeminal neuralgia, and the post-stroke pain of the Dejerine-Roussy syndrome, may be of central nervous system origin, but these clearly organic problems are not the typical chronic pain syndrome. I would like to limit the present discussion to those patients with chronic pain with no known continued nociceptive input, in which cases there have been only functional or psychological environmental factors in the genesis of the pain, either predating the etiologic initiating injury, or reinforcing the ongoing disability.

It must also be pointed out that I am not talking here about the psychogenic or mental or imaginary pain that may accompany functional disorders as in a psychotic depression or schizophrenic break with reality. There is no question that pain can be part of such a functional disorder. This mental or psychogenic pain is best treated by addressing the psychiatric condition itself, and is usually not referred to as a "chronic pain syndrome". The chronic pain syndrome appears where there was originally disease or injury (and nociceptive input) in the acute pain model, where, for some reason, the pain does not turn itself off, but the suffering continues and becomes chronic. If this continues long after the peripheral etiologic nociceptive source has healed, it can be called a chronic pain syndrome.

I am concerned only with the patients in whom chronic pain has become incapacitating. These patients are no longer adapting and able to cope; they may have lost their very ability to survive; they may be so demoralized as to have no hope. The pain has become the central focus of their very existence, and indeed, the pain can be called "intractable". Although it was originally of nociceptive origin or "somatopsychic", I now consider it to be entirely a central phenomenon, and thus *all chronic pain is by definition "psychosomatic*. The treatment of such pain is not by nerve blocks or neurosurgical procedures to interrupt the supposed continued nociceptive input, which has long since ceased to exist. The treatment of these patients with chronic intractable benign pain syndromes thus becomes largely psychological or psychiatric. However, most patients and many physicians find this approach to therapy in chronic pain unacceptable as they do not understand it. The delivery of proper treatment under these circumstances becomes difficult indeed.

The diagnosis of a patient with a full-blown chronic intractable benign pain syndrome rests on the following criteria: The pain cannot be shown to be causally related to any active pathophysiologic or pathoanatomic process; has an antecedent history of generally ineffective medical and surgical intervention in the pain problem; and has come to be accompanied by disturbed psychosocial function, which includes the pain complaint and the epiphenomena that accompany it. The epiphenomena that accompany this syndrome can be listed to include at least the following:

1. Substance use disorders of varying severity, with their attendant CNS side effects.
2. Multiple surgical procedures or pharmacologic treatments, with their own morbid side effects separate from those related to above.
3. Escalated decrease in physical functioning related to accompanying pain and/or fear that this pain is a signal of increased bodily harm and damage.
4. Escalated hopelessness and helplessness as persistent or increased dysphoria does not give way in the face of mounting numbers of "newer" or different treatment interventions.
5. Emotional conflicts with medical care delivery personnel (doctors, nurses, therapists, technicians) that result in therapeutic goal interference.
6. Interpersonal emotional conflicts with significant others.
7. Escalated withdrawal and loss of gratification from psychosocial activity.
8. Decrease in feelings of self-esteem, self-worth, and self-confidence.
9. Lasting unpleasant mood and affect changes.
10. Decreased ability to obtain pleasure from the life process, reflected in the presence of profound demoralization and, at times, significant depression.

Once we recognize and diagnose a chronic intractable benign pain syndrome we must determine how the patient can be approached. It must first be understood that there is an unconscious dysphoric defense mechanism at work. *The patient has an unconscious need to continue to hurt.* This must *not* be interpreted to mean that the patient *wants* to hurt; the patient with chronic pain does have real pain and does not want to hurt. The need is an unconscious mechanism. Some unresolved, unconscious, emotional conflicts seem to be potentiating and keeping the central generator mechanism of chronic pain active.

In my experience the chief unresolved emotional conflict is *unresolved grief,* usually over loss. This may well be due to loss of a loved one by death, divorce, or desertion. It may well be loss of one's ability to do things, loss of one's youth, and so on. In these cases, all the ancillary considerations of narcissism and borderline personality play a role. Many symptoms of the chronic pain patient that accompany the subjective perception of pain are generally recognized unconscious mechanisms of defense, such as the conversion reaction seen in hysteria, a monoparesis, or the "stocking" or "glove" hypalgesia seen in chronic pain patients.

Probably the second most common unresolved emotional conflict underlying chronic pain is unexpressed or unresolved anger and rage. This is especially true in the younger male chronic pain patients, often injured on the job and covered with compensation, or injured in an automobile accident, where litigation is still involved. There are many other contributing factors of an emotional nature, including anxiety, depression, guilt, and shame. Total understanding of the particular patient and his particular chronic pain syndrome is often never fully obtainable. The question then becomes: How do you manage such a patient, incapacitated with chronic pain?

If this definition of chronic pain and some of the psychodynamic mechanisms of chronic pain are accepted, it becomes obvious that the treatment is not intervention, but psychotherapy. However, most patients with chronic pain are often absolutely opposed to psychiatric or even psychological referral.

A comprehensive pain center should have, in addition to an inpatient pain service, an outpatient pain clinic where these cases can be diagnosed and treated on an outpatient basis. Physical therapy, rehabilitation, reconditioning, psychological evaluation, and group psychotherapeutic programs are all important. Group psychotherapy is the treatment of choice in patients with chronic pain syndrome. These patients often learn more (and accept more) from their pain peers than from any member of the treating team. Unfortunately, there are currently only a few truly comprehensive pain centers in existence. Furthermore, in attempting to ascertain a correct referral for patients with chronic intractable benign pain, the attending physician or neurosurgeon is often faced with an inability to evelute for himself the appropriateness of the pain treatment clinic or center under consideration. Unfortunately, patients with chronic intractable pain often are refractory to even the best management currently available. Many even refuse referral to a chronic pain center. The individual physician, under these circumstances, must decide whether he wishes to persevere with supportive measures or to terminate the doctor-patient relationship. The individual patient derives no benefit from prolonged inappropriate treatment, such as the continued issuance of prescriptions for large doses of narcotics, analgesics, or anti-anxiety tranquilizers. However, if an individual physician is willing to take the time, and does have the inclination and patience,

he or she may well be able to, on an individual basis, make a profound difference and change for the better in the individual patient by being supportive, where such support is not inappropriate.

CHRONIC PAIN SYNDROME

DONLIN M. LONG, M.D., Ph. D.

Patients complaining of chronic pain can be categorized into three basic groups. There are those who have a recognized pain syndrome with an organic cause that is understood or presumed and for whom some definitive therapy is available. Examples of such patients are those with metastatic cancer, a pain syndrome such as trigeminal neuralgia, or chronic back pain and sciatica from a compressive neuropathy. Psychosocial factors in this group are relatively unimportant. There is a second small group in whom the complaint of pain is apparently related to a disturbance of thinking. Such patients have diagnosable affective disorders. Endogenous depression, conversion reaction, and somatization disorders are common. The third and largest category of patients are those who may or may not have a significant, ongoing, diagnosable cause for the pain complaint, but in whom psychosocial factors have assumed a dominant role in the disability. These factors are discussed in detail by Crue in his chapter, *Defining the Chronic Pain Syndrome*.

Many physicians approach the complaint of pain in a simplistic way, using only the medical model for disease. An organic cause of the pain is assumed, appropriate diagnostic procedures are done to define that organic cause, and then specific interventional therapies aimed at the presumed cause of the pain are employed. The psychiatric and psychosocial factors are generally ignored. Since this approach is truly applicable only to about one-third of all patients complaining of chronic pain, it is not suprising that the therapy of pain in general is ineffectual. Proper diagnosis and choice of therapy can change this and although the treatment of the most serious of the pain neuroses is a matter for experts, the general physician of any speciality is in a position to do a great deal of good and prevent a great deal of harm for these patients.

DIAGNOSIS

With such a heterogeneous population, the first thing that must be done is a careful diagnostic evaluation

of the pain complaint. The typical pain syndromes usually are not difficult to clarify. In the absence of an obvious physical diagnosis or in the presence of disability that seems more than would be expected from the physical abnormalities, it is necessary to carefully explore psychiatric and psychosocial factors that may influence the pain complaint. Psychiatric consultation is important, but any physician can ask the appropriate questions about marital status, social behavior, school record, military record, work history, and family history that will elicit clues regarding personality dysfunction. Depression, anxiety, and overuse of medications can occur in any patient with chronic pain and disability. They do not imply the presence of important psychiatric and psychosocial problems. The diagnostic evaluation must be thorough enough to convince the physician of the presence or absence of a potential ongoing physical cause of the disability. In the case of some diseases, such as trigeminal neuralgia, the history alone is virtually adequate. In the typical total body pain syndrome of the somatization disorder, the physician is usually certain within a few minutes about the diagnosis. However, it may take an exhaustive physical evaluation to be certain that the patient does not harbor some unusual rheumatologic or collagen vascular condition. There are no specific rules that can be given concerning the degree to which a physical diagnosis is pursued. This must be decided by the individual physician commensurate with the needs of the individual patient. The absence of an obvious physical diagnosis does not imply psychiatric or psychosocial problems, and the presence of a physical diagnosis does not guarantee that such factors are inconsequential. A complete physical and psychological evaluation is always the first step in pain therapy.

TREATMENT OF CHRONIC PAIN

Treatment of Depression and Anxiety. Depression, anxiety, and sleeplessness commonly accompany chronic pain and disability. They must be treated first in order to assess the patient's true status. A tricyclic antidepressant is usually satisfactory therapy. Amitriptyline, 50 to 100 mg given at bed time, usually restores normal sleep within 48 hours and produces rapid amelioration of symptoms of depression. Anxiety, when present, is best treated by a simple antianxiety agent, and Valium (diaze-

The reluctance to accept the fact that not all pain is generated from a physical cause is responsible for most of the errors in pain management.

The multimodal approach is very effective in reducing the iatrogenic component of

chronic pain Syndrome. That
is too many operations and
too much medication

Donlin Long, MD

pam) should be avoided because of its long-term propensity to augment depression.

Elimination of Harmful Drugs. Many patients with chronic pain are taking drugs inappropriate to their problem, using narcotics on a long-term basis and frequently in doses greater than should be taken. Nonnarcotic analgesics are used in excessive doses as well. It is not uncommon for these patients to be taking drugs that are not analgesics as if they were. True addiction is difficult to judge, but many patients are intoxicated from overuse of medication, and certainly some exhibit true drug-seeking behavior. It is mandatory that improper drug use be rectified. There are few instances in which the ongoing utilization of narcotics for the treatment of chronic pain of benign origin is warranted. Narcotic withdrawal is instituted immediately and carried out by gradual dose reduction of approximately 10 percent per day with the patient's understanding and cooperation. Valium is eliminated in the same way. Drugs without significant withdrawal symptoms are simply stopped. The so-called pain cocktail, which is used to hide from the patient the amount of drug being taken, is an alternative, but I prefer to simply withdraw the drug by gradually reducing the dose. Significant withdrawal symptoms, usually anxiety, sleeplessness, diaphoresis, extreme anxiety, and gastrointestinal disturbances, are relatively common. Patients must be warned about them and reassured. I find it necessary to carry out withdrawal on an inpatient basis in a controlled environment. Since there are no adequate analgesics that benefit most of these patients, I make no attempt to substitute non-narcotic analgesics. There are a few situations in which maintenance of a patient on long-term narcotic therapy is a viable alternative in a benign condition, but this decision really should be made by an expert after alternative therapies have failed.

Physical Rehabilitation. Virtually all patients incapacitated by the chronic pain syndrome have become sedentary. It is unusual for their pain to be truly increased by activity, and it is nearly always possible to dramatically increase their abilities without increasing pain. Patients require a complete physical assessment, appropriate physical therapy for muscle stretching, restoration of range of motion, and treatment of focal areas of myositis and fasciitis and similar symptoms. Transcutaneous electrical stimulation can be of great benefit in controlling these musculoskeletal symptoms. An adequate exercise program is mandatory, and the patient must be persuaded to resume the maximum physical activity commensurate with the actual physical disability.

Individualization of Treatment. The aforementioned basic measures are required in some degree for virtually all patients with chronic pain. Once these general measures are under way, it is necessary to individualize treatment. Patients for whom some specific interventional therapy is available should proceed to that treatment. Those who do not have significant associated psychosocial problems probably need nothing more than the general program and the appropriate intervention. Any physician willing to invest the time and effort can manage patients to this point. The real problem is the treatment of those patients with major psychosocial dysfunction and those without a treatable cause of pain. The therapy of these patients is so difficult that few physicians have the expertise to carry it out alone. Multimodal therapy through the utilization of many disciplines has proved effective. The basis of these so-called pain treatment centers must be psychotherapy. This therapy takes many forms and individual treatment should be available, but the most common technique now utilized is group therapy. Peer pressure is effective, and education of groups is more efficient than individual treatment. This therapeutic approach has several goals. Pain behavior that is detrimental to the patient's function must be eliminated. Pain control can be augmented through such techniques as biofeedback or relaxation. Education about pain, the underlying disease, and the resultant disability can be very useful. Vocational rehabilitation is not a goal of pain treatment, but is an extremely important adjunct. Most comprehensive pain treatment programs are arranged to provide patient understanding. It is this understanding that can lead to reduced utilization of health care services, reduction of dependence on physicians, and elimination of dependence on medication for the relief of symptoms.

The treatment of chronic pain at present does not offer a solution to the social problem of vocational disability. It cannot make the sociopathic patient function in a normal way. It has no secrets for the psychiatrically disturbed. However, the multimodal approach is very effective in reducing the iatrogenic components of the chronic pain syndrome. That is, too many operations and too much medication. Anxiety and depression can be effectively treated and physical abilities can be maximized. Unfortunately, most patients and many physicians fail to understand the great importance of psychosocial factors in the genesis of chronic pain syndromes and continue to rely on the medical model for diagnosis and treatment of all pain. The reluctance to accept the fact that not all pain is generated from a physical cause is responsible for most of the errors in pain management.

CONGENITAL DISORDERS

HYDROCEPHALUS

MEL H. EPSTEIN, M.D.

Hydrocephalus can result from many pathophysiologic entities. Hydrocephalus, by strict definition, is characterized by abnormal cerebrospinal fluid (CSF) accumulation within the head. It can result from loss of brain tissue (so-called hydrocephalus ex vacuo), from overproduction of CSF, or from blockage of normal drainage pathways. This disorder has been known since at least 400 BC and was first recognized by Hippocrates.

The advent of CT and MRI scanners has made the recognition of this disorder relatively simple. A determination of whether or not treatment is necessary is far more complex and requires sequential judgment decisions to determine the etiology of the hydrocephalus.

SIGNS AND SYMPTOMS

The spectrum of clinical presentation in patients with hydrocephalus is varied. In general, the initial sign of hydrocephalus in the infant with open sutures is a head that is enlarging faster than the normal growth pattern. As hydrocephalus progresses, the infant has difficulty elevating the eyes because of pressure on the tectal plate (sunset eyes). In end-stage hydrocephalus, rather sudden and frequently unexpected respiratory failure and secondary cardiac arrest can occur. In older children and adults, the presentation of hydrocephalus depends on the rate of obstruction of CSF pathways. If the obstruction is sudden, the patient becomes symptomatic rather quickly with severe headache, nausea, and vomiting, and, over a period of hours, lapses into coma and ultimately dies if the situation is not corrected. If the hydrocephalus occurs gradually over a long period of time, as with a minimal aqueduct of atresia, the hydrocephalus frequently is asymptomatic, without headache or any other symptoms, and the patient may first come to medical attention during routine eye examination when papilledema is found. Between those two extremes, there are variations in the degree of hydrocephalus which give a spectrum of symptoms from minimal headache to coma. Patients found to have papilledema should be given a high level of priority. Papilledema, if left untreated, can lead to optic atrophy and blindness. In addition, the compression of the posterior cerebral arteries from extreme hydrocephalus can lead to bilateral occipital infarctions and severe visual disorders. Transtentorial herniation is the ultimate complication of this disease and can occur without warning when pressure is severely elevated.

DIAGNOSTIC TESTS

The basis of diagnostic tests for hydrocephalus is now CT or MRI scanning. The presence of large ventricles alone does not indicate the need for surgery, since the hydrocephalus could be from atrophy. It is necessary to know more than the scan picture to understand the disease process.

The patient with a condition called low-pressure hydrocephalus, even with large ventricles and low pressure, might benefit from a shunt. This is particularly true in adults. One of the most useful methods for determining whether a patient with dilated ventricles and low pressure would benefit from shunting is to carry out chronic pressure measurements, either with an implantable pressure device or with a ventricular catheter placed in the ventricle overnight. Most of these patients who are shunt candidates demonstrate plateau waves, which are episodes of relatively high pressure superimposed on overall low pressure. Other means for looking at the dynamics of hydrocephalus involve putting an isotope in the lumbar spine or directly into the ventricular system. This isotope is usually bound to a large molecule such as albumin and can be seen on gamma cameras. If the isotope remains in the ventricular system or enters the ventricular system, this is a strong indication of transependymal absorption and hydrocephalus of a significant degree.

To make matters more complex, there is a group of patients who have had chronic CSF shunts and who developed what is known as the slit ventricle syndrome. They have small ventricles and yet have shunt failure with extraordinarily high pressure. Their increased pressure is manifested by cerebral edema and can lead to rapid decompensation and death. These are most difficult problems to manage.

CLINICAL ETIOLOGY

The causes of hydrocephalus can be classified as resulting from increased fluid production or impeded fluid absorption. Congenital malformations, infection, sterile inflammations, vascular malformations, trauma, and brain tissue destruction can be the causative agents in this disorder.

The only known cause of increased fluid production is tumor of the choroid plexus. These neoplasms may be malignant or benign, but most are well differentiated tumors that generate CSF. Impeded fluid absorption can occur from congenital abnormalities such as the Arnold-Chiari malformation, congenital atresia of the aqueduct of Sylvius, and absence of the foramina of Luschka and Magendie.

If hydrocephalus occurs in utero, the possibility for successful shunting is good. However, developmental abnormalities of the brain invariably lead to some degree of retardation. Occasionally even hydranencephaly is shunted because these children need to be institutionalized and most institutions require control of head growth for nursing purposes.

When neoplasms grow in critical areas, as do colloid cysts at the foramen of Monro and tumors blocking the fourth ventricle in the posterior fossa, CSF obstruction can occur. Tumor of the pineal gland, because the gland is located directly over the aqueduct of Sylvius, leads to hydrocephalus fairly quickly from compression of the proximal aqueduct. Infection within the ventricular system, such as ependymitis, and closure of the aqueduct or the outlets in the fourth ventricle are common causes of hydrocephalus. If the cisterns at the base of the brain are obliterated, this also causes hydrocephalic changes. Although vascular malformations do not usually cause hydrocephalus, the malformations that drain into the internal cerebral vein or the vein of Galen commonly compress the aqueduct of Sylvius from their mass effect. These relatively rare lesions can occur in the neonatal period, causing almost immediate heart failure, or can be more indolent problems that present later in life with slowly progressive heart failure. Trauma or injury to brain tissue can result in an obstruction of the arachnoid villi. By interfering with absorption, this can result in gradual dilatation of the ventricular system, which is a combined effect of loss of cerebral tissue and abnormal fluid accumulation. If trauma results in hemorrhage, such as subdural hematoma, absorption can be severely compromised and lead to significant hydrocephalus.

TREATMENT

Hydrocephalus is treated under standard conditions by diverting cerebrospinal fluid from the cavity from which it is accumulating to some other space. This can either be the blood stream or the peritoneal cavity. In general, peritoneal shunts are used in children because extra tubing can be placed to allow the child to grow. In adults, because of the long distance involved from the head to the peritoneal cavity and the shorter length of time the shunts will be in place, it is common practice to put in venous shunts through the common fascial vein into the jugular system with the shunt tip residing in the superior vena cava just above the right atrium. One of the most common complications of shunting operations is infection. However, recent studies have shown that proper use of prophylactic antibiotics pre- and intraoperatively can greatly diminish the incidence of infection in this group of patients. Siphoning of fluid is an important phenomenon. In infants, it is needed to drain the pliable cranial vault. In older children, it can result in overdrainage and the slit ventricle syndrome wherein patients have small ventricles, high pressure, and intermittent obstruction. In older patients with low pressure hydrocephalus, siphoning can result in collapse of the brain and subdural hematomas. The use of antisiphon devices must be carefully considered. At the time of this writing, there is a need to improve the "free flow" drainage concept of CSF shunts.

It is also possible to decrease CSF production by the use of the drug Diamox; however, this is only useful in marginal cases in which one would assume that CSF absorption would return to normal levels. Cases of hydrocephalus resulting from subarachnoid or intraventricular blood are most likely to respond to medical treatment. There are also forms of hydrocephalus that spontaneously arrest and do not require medication or shunting. In these cases, the increase in ventricular size places a slight increase in pressure on the absorptive mechanism; these patients tend to remain in a stable state with neither gradually increasing ventricular size nor increasing cranial size.

COMPLICATIONS

It is important to be aware that patients that have cerebrospinal fluid shunts are prone to a number of complications. There is a small ongoing risk of infection, especially in patients who have the catheters in their blood stream. Other complications include abdominal viscus perforations, abdominal abcesses and hygromas, and thromboembolic phenomena from embolization into the blood stream with pulmonary hypertension, chronic sepsis, and renal damage.

Overall, the prognosis for patients with hydrocephalus who are treated with shunts is favorable. The hardware that is used is constantly being improved and, together with a better understanding of CSF biochemistry and physiology, offers considerable hope for patients afflicted with this disorder.

MYELOMENINGOCELE

HAROLD J. HOFFMAN, M.D., F.R.C.S.(C)

The management of infants with myelomeningocele has remained a controversial topic for several decades. In the era prior to the development of modern techniques for treatment of hydrocephalus, the prognosis for a child born with an open neural tube defect was dismal. This pessimistic situation persisted until the mid 1960s, by which time, following the development of the valvular CSF shunt by Nulsen and Spitz in 1954, favorable experience had been amassed in the management of hydrocephalus. The group in Sheffield under the stewardship of the orthopaedic surgeon, Sharrard, began an aggressive approach to the treatment of the infant born with an open neural tube defect and published optimistic results. The pendulum then began to swing toward treatment of all myelodysplastic children.

However, a member of the original Sharrard team, John Lorber of Sheffield, began to look at the results of the treatment of all children with such defects and found that a group with "adverse criteria" fared badly. He then promulgated his criteria for the denial of treatment to specific children.

Some centers still adhere to Lorber's criteria, which were devised at a time when current techniques of management were not available. In view of these advances, many neurosurgeons again advocate treatment of all children born with an open neural tube defect.

In our own center, we suggest an aggressive approach to the newborn infant with spinal dysrophism. The early assessment of an infant with a myelomeningocele can give a misleading conception of the ultimate prognosis. The child with a small sacral lesion with excellent function at hip and knees and minimal weakness at the ankles can still suffer devastating harm from hydrocephalus and/or the Arnold-Chiari malformation and become an intellectual and physical cripple. Conversely, the child with overt hydrocephalus, a high thoracolumbar rachischisis, and no function below L1 at birth can, with adequate management, become a useful member of society and a joy to parents and family.

CLINICAL FEATURES

Hydrocephalus is common in infants with neural tube defects and occurs in over 80 percent of this population. It is more common with higher thoracolumbar lesions than with sacral lesions. However, unlike many forms of congenital hydrocephalus, the hydrocephalus associated with spina bifida tends to arrest spontaneously over the course of time so that eventually only half of the surviving children are shunt-dependent.

Although all infants with open neural tube defects have an Arnold-Chiari malformation, its symptomatology becomes evident in only 20 percent of these children.

It becomes manifest in 10 percent during the neonatal period, at which time it can pose a serious threat to the infant's life, impairing cranial nerve function, interfering with vital centers, and, if left untreated, producing paralysis of the vocal cords, of swallowing, and of all four limbs. Early recognition and treatment by surgical decompression can prevent these disastrous complications. In the older child, the Chiari malformation frequently leads to hydrosyringomyelia. Children with this condition present with a deteriorating neurological state consisting of increasing weakness in the legs and arms, cranial nerve dysfunction, a dissociated sensory loss, and a progressive scoliosis.

The neonate born with an open neural tube defect has an open exposed area of spinal cord in the midline. The lesion can be of variable size, but is rarely more than 3 or 4 cm in diameter. Attached to the open neural placode is stratified squamous epithelium applied to dura. This very thin membranous skin can vary in dimension from a few millimeters to 1 or 2 cm and is surrounded by relatively normal skin which is frequently discolored by a hemangioma. The neural placode is an open neural tube, and frequently the central canal can be seen at the cephalad portion of the open myelomeningocele leaking CSF.

The size of the lesion should not dismay the neurosurgeon. There is always sufficient skin available to close these lesions without resorting to extensive plastic surgical repairs. In a child with congenital kyphosis, as seen with thoracolumbar lesions, the laminae can be everted and protruding beneath the thin skin as bony spikes. These can further complicate treatment.

About 10 percent of children are born with a large head, a full fontanelle, and split sutures. The presence of hydrocephalus can be readily confirmed by an ultrasound scan. In such cases, it becomes imperative to treat the hydrocephalus concomitantly with repair of the myelomeningocele. In infants without overt hydrocephalus, the myelomeningocele can be repaired, and ventricular size can be monitored by ultrasound scan during the postoperative period in order to decide when and if a diversionary CSF shunt should be inserted.

ASSESSMENT

In initially assessing a newborn with an open neural tube defect, attention should be paid to the lesion. Occasionally, a bony spike may be evident on the surface; this denotes a diastematomyelia which will require repair. The state of neural function in the lower limbs should be accurately documented. Occasionally the trauma of birth impairs function of the exposed placode, and one can actually see improvement of function in a matter of hours after birth. Signs of hydrocephalus should be sought and a careful survey made for the possibility of other congenital lesions, the presence of which is unusual, but not impossible. Occasionally a cardiac defect may be found. Rarely, there may be some associated cerebral anomalies such as holoprosencephaly or an associated encephalocele.

MANAGEMENT

The myelomeningocele should be repaired within 24 to 48 hours of birth. Delay beyond this time incurs the risk of infection. There is no need to place the child on prophylactic antibiotics unless a shunt is inserted simultaneously with repair of the myelomeningocele. This is only necessary if overt hydrocephalus is present at birth. In such a situation, it is possible to have the myelomeningocele site and the sites for insertion of the shunt in the same operative field. The child is positioned prone with the body rotated slightly to one side and the head rotated in the same direction to allow the ipsilateral occipital region, neck, posterior chest, and flank to be in the same operative field as the back. The entire area is prepared and suitably draped. The area for the shunt is then covered with an adhesive transparent drape and the repair of the myelomeningocele is carried out in the fashion to be described. Once the myelomeningocele has been repaired, insertion of the shunt can proceed without re-prepping or re-draping. In the 15 patients in whom we have carried out this maneuver, we have not seen any incidence of shunt infection or any breakdown of the back repair.

In repairing a myelomeningocele, the entire back should be in the operative field. The incision should start out laterally at the junction between the thin epithelium and the neural placode. Care must be taken at the caudal and cephalad portions of the placode, as the spinal cord comes into and leaves the placode at these sites. Once the placode and the cord have been freed from dura and skin, the cord drops into the dural sac. With retractors in place, it is then possible to incise dura laterally where there is normal skin, and then to free up dura into the spinal canal. Using this maneuver, it is possible to preserve sufficient dura to encompass the neural placode and spinal cord completely in dural canal. If diastematomyelia is found, this must be repaired at the same time. If the end of the spinal cord is tethered to the end of the dural sac, it must be freed up. Care must be taken to avoid incorporating any of the squamous epithelium with the neural placode in the repair because any retained squamous epithelium will later give rise to an epidermoid cyst. There is no need to appose the pial surfaces except in rare situations in which there is extreme hypertrophy of the neural placode. By reconstituting the neural tube, as advocated by McLone and his colleagues, one can reduce the bulk sufficiently so as to get all of the neural tissue within the dural canal.

In patients with kyphosis and everted laminae, the paraspinal muscles on either side should be incised. This allows for fracture of the laminae. They can then be bent inward along with their attached musculature. These muscles should have been situated posteriorly and thus functioned as spine extensors. However, with an open neural tube defect, they are situated anteriorly and help to accentuate the kyphos. By means of this maneuver, initially described by Mustarde, it is possible to get the musculature posteriorly into an extensor position. If the dural repair is secure and the laminae are not everted, a fascial repair generally is not necessary, provided there is sufficient skin. The skin is closed in a single layer by means of absorbable vertical mattress sutures, with attention to good apposition of the epithelial elements.

The skin can always be approximated, usually vertically and occasionally transversely. Sometimes it is necessary to undermine the subcutaneous tissue widely, almost to the umbilicus, to allow one to pull the skin together without undue tension. Any size myelomeningocele can thus be closed directly without the need for extensive flaps and without the risk of necrosis that use of such flaps entails. A large bulky dressing is applied and is left in place with the child nursed prone for a minimum of 2 weeks, or until the problem of hydrocephalus has been resolved with either a shunt or a normal ultrasound scan.

It is imperative that CSF leakage through the skin be avoided because it contributes to poor healing. The bulky dressing and early use of a diversionary CSF shunt can do much to prevent such complications.

POSTOPERATIVE MANAGEMENT

The infant with a repaired myelomeningocele requires close and careful ongoing care by a team. The orthopaedic surgeon must deal with the orthopaedic deformities that many of these children have in their lower limbs and spine. The urologist must assess urologic function and instruct the parents in a proper protocol of intermittent catheterization and prevention of urinary tract infection. The physiotherapist is invaluable in carrying out assessments on these children and in detecting deterioration in function. The neurosurgeon continues to follow these children in regard to shunt function, cerebral function, and spinal cord function.

LATE DETERIORATION

A child with a repaired myelomeningocele can show evidence of late deterioration which can be multifactorial in etiology. With shunt obstruction, the first sign may be back pain and increasing neurological deficit. Shunt obstruction can lead to hydrosyringomyelia. Even with normal shunt function and normal ventricles, hydrosyringomyelia can still develop because of the Chiari malformation. Children with a Chiari malformation and hydroxyringomyelia respond very nicely to the operation initially described by Gardner, in which the Chiari malformation is decompressed and a plug of muscle is placed into the obex. With such treatment, the process of hydrosyringomyelia can be halted and its manifestations frequently reversed, particularly if the condition is treated early in its course.

Children with myelodysplasia can develop other problems which can lead to progressive neurological deterioration. They are prone to the development of midline cysts intracranially. These cysts arise either from septum pellucidum or from a cavum vergae and become an enormous isolated midline fluid space. They can stretch corticospinal tracts and produce progressive interference with lower limb function. The manifestations of an isolated fourth ventricle can be seen in the myelodysplastic child, leading to progressive dysfunction of brain stem. This can be easily remedied by shunting the isolated fourth ventricle.

If sufficient care has not been taken to remove all squamous epithelium at the site of the myelomeningocele repair, an epidermoid cyst can form and progressively compress neural tissue, producing neurological dysfunction. The site of the original neural placode can be tethered to dura, or if dural closure has been incomplete, the cord can be tethered to overlying soft tissues. Finally, diastematomyelia, particularly one with a spike that is attached to a laterally everted lamina may have been overlooked at the time of initial repair. This occurs especially in children with a hemimyelocele, in which one half of the cord has a neural placode and the other half of the placode is completely enclosed in dura with an overlying strut of bone. If this is not discovered at the time of initial repair, the child presents with tethering at the site of the laterally placed diastematomyelia spike, which must be untethered in order to prevent further deterioration.

COURSE WITHOUT TREATMENT

Without therapy, a child with an open neural tube defect can succumb to infection or hydrocephalus. How-

ever, the majority survive for at least 6 months or a year, during which time parents, social workers, and concerned individuals ensure that the child is brought back for treatment. One should therefore proceed with treatment early; the child treated early can have better preservation of neural and intellectual function than one left untreated for many months or years. Furthermore, examples of children have been reported who have been left untreated for many years and have survived, in whom the chronically draining back due to untreated hydrocephalus has led to chronic irritation and the development of squamous cell carcinoma at the site of the myelomeningocele. Thus, the withholding of treatment does not always cause the infant's demise. In my experience, the majority of untreated children survive for many months and some for many years.

Delay in treatment increases neurologic deficit and may produce irreversible harm to the brain because the untreated hydrocephalus stretches the cortical mantle. Early treatment, on the other hand, preserves neural function, prevents infection, and eases nursing care. Early treatment of the hydrocephalus prevents intellectual deterioration. Over 80 percent of well-treated children with open neural tube defects, regardless of location or size, have normal intelligence. This occurs despite the often-described abnormal architecture of their brain, namely, the Arnold-Chiari malformation, the beaking of the tectum, the large mass intermedia, and the uniquely shaped frontal horns.

CRANIOSYNOSTOSIS

JOHN A. PERSING, M.D.,
JOHN A. JANE, M.D.

Craniosynostosis refers to the abnormal skull development associated with premature closure of one or more cranial vault sutures. Clinically, premature fusion of an individual cranial vault suture is characterized by predictably abnormal skull shapes. For instance, premature fusion of the sagittal suture results in a long, narrow skull described as scaphocephaly, and premature fusion of the coronal suture bilaterally results in a broad, short skull, or brachycephaly.

Premature cranial vault suture fusion does not necessarily occur in isolation. Combinations of sutural stenoses, such as sagittal synostosis and unilateral coronal synostosis, occur frequently. Maldevelopment of the skull due to craniosynostosis also may be seen in association with facial maldevelopment, as in Crouzon's syndrome, and with extremity maldevelopment, as in Apert's syndrome.

GENERAL PRINCIPLES OF TREATMENT

Although skull deformities related to craniosynostosis may be quite varied, there are some generalizations which can be made about the surgical approach to all patients with craniosynostosis.

First, the most effective surgery in changing skull form is that which is performed early in life. This observation is based on the fact that brain enlargement is a major force in determining the overall shape of the skull. The brain mass doubles its birth mass by the age of 6 months and represents 47 percent of the total adult brain mass by the age of one year. The optimal date of surgery has yet to be determined, but in our practice, surgery is usually carried out 6 to 12 weeks after birth.

Second, simple extirpative surgery of the stenosed cranial vault suture usually is not sufficient to correct the abnormal skull shape. Although further growth of the brain and skull following extirpative surgery may ameliorate some of the cranial vault abnormalities due to craniosynostosis, there are usually significant retained deformities in the already developed vault bone that prevent achievement of a normal skull shape. These disfigured bones must be actively changed so as to achieve a satisfactory skull appearance.

Third, in addition to correcting the hypoplastic bony effects of the prematurely fused cranial vault suture in one region of the skull, one must also check for the need for correction of the compensatory enlargement of bone in other regions of the skull. This is particularly evident in patients with unilateral coronal synostosis, wherein frontal and parietal bones ipsilateral to the fused coronal suture have a less prominent than normal profile, but the contralateral frontal bone is excessively prominent and rounded. Both abnormalities must be addressed in order to achieve a normal skull shape.

SAGITTAL SYNOSTOSIS

The diagnosis of sagittal synostosis or scaphocephaly (from the Greek, *skaphe*, meaning skiff) is based in part on the clinical observation of a long narrow skull. There may be an accompanying frontal or occipital bone enlargement or bossing, and usually there is prominent ridging of the sagittal suture. Measurement of the head circumference is usually increased, and the cephalic index is low. Radiographically, the median basal angle is also reduced, resulting in an exaggerated cranial base kyphosis when compared to the normal.

Treatment

Premature closure of the sagittal suture generally results in a long narrow cranial vault. However, varying degrees of deformity of the skull result from premature closure of the sagittal suture, depending on the degree of sutural stenosis and the degree and direction of compensatory growth in the skull. A generalized or full stenosis of the sagittal suture results in restricted growth of bone perpendicular to the plane of the sagittal suture. Compensatory growth occurring parallel to the plane of the fused suture may occur as frontal bone bossing, occipital bone bossing, or both. Partial restriction of growth in only the anterior or posterior half of the sagittal suture may result in variable abnormalities of the anterior and posterior cranial vault skeleton. Particularly frequent is frontal bone bossing and posterior parietal narrowing associated with posterior sagittal synostosis. Anterior sagittal synostosis often is associated with a narrowed anterior biparietal dimension with frontal and occipital prominence. The operative procedures used for the three (full, anterior half, and posterior half stenosis) different abnormalities will be described.

For the partial or generalized sagittal suture stenosis with little or no occipital deformity, and significant anterior parietal and frontal abnormality, the child is placed in a semi-reclining supine position with the U-shaped cup head rest supporting the skull in the mastoid and low occipital areas. A bicoronal incision is then carried out, and anterior and posterior scalp flaps reflected in a supraperiosteal plane (to avoid increased blood loss when dissection is carried out in a subperiosteal plane). Parasagittal bur holes are then placed poste-

rior to the coronal suture. In patients without significant frontal or occipital bulging, a craniotome is then used to elevate a free bone segment in the shape of the Greek letter pi (π). The extent of bone removal includes the coronal suture and the lamboid suture in an anteroposterior direction, as well as the pterion laterally. Bone directly over the sagittal suture is allowed to remain so as to avoid the possibility of injury to the underlying sagittal sinus. In the region of the coronal suture, however, bone overlying the sagittal sinus is removed, to a distance of anticipated shortening of the cranial vault. The sagittal sinus in this region in the midline is separated from overlying bone for a distance of approximately 2 cm both anteriorly and posteriorly, to prevent buckling of the sinus with the shortening of the skull. A subtemporal decompression is then performed to allow the temporal region to bulge outward when the A-P shortening of the skull occurs. Two 28-gauge wires are passed first through the frontal bone and then through the strip of bone overlying the sagittal sinus posteriorly. Shortening of the skull, usually about 8 to 12 mm, is accomplished by slowly twisting the wires and approximating the bone edges. As this shortening occurs, bulging in the parietal and temporal regions develops. This bulging tends to further correct the deformity. The previously elevated π-shaped bone segment is then placed back over the dura, in the frontal and parietal regions, secured only by absorbable suture material through the center of the bone and the outer leaf of the dura. Individual tailoring of bone is done according to the appearance achieved by the compression and bone replacement. Ordinarily, some degree of bone reshaping using a Tessier rib bender is necessary. The scalp flap incisions are then closed.

In patients with complete or partial sagittal suture stenosis, but significant frontal bossing, the correction is similar to the previously described π procedure. The patient is placed supine, pressure points are padded, and a bicoronal incision is used to visualize the bony deformity. Parasagittal bur holes are then placed and a π-shaped segment of bone incorporating the coronal suture and parietal bone to the level of the lambdoid suture is removed. Additionally, in the region of bossing in the frontal bone, separate frontal craniotomies are performed bilaterally, leaving a midline strip of frontal bone. Inspection of the dura following shortening of the A-P dimension of the skull, as previously described, results in even more prominence of the frontal region. In these regions the dura is plicated to lessen the excessive roundedness of the region. The frontal bone itself is remodeled using the Tessier rib bender, then placed back on e dura and secured sturdily in all dimensions to surrounding bone.

The correction of the occipital bulging associated with synostosis is handled somewhat differently. The patient is placed in a padded head rest in a modified prone position, with the neck extended to allow visualization of the skull from the bifrontal region to the basiocciput. Again a bicoronal incision is used to expose the cranial bone. Bur holes are then placed approximately 1.5 cm from the midline and anterior to the lambdoid suture bilaterally. A π-shaped bone segment is then removed from the parieto-occipital region, with the transverse limb of the π including the lambdoid suture and the A-P limbs of the parietal bones, as previously described for complete sagittal synostosis. The dura overlying the sagittal sinus anteriorly and posteriorly is stripped from the overlying inner table of the skull. In patients with premature synostosis of the suture, this dissection is relatively bloodless. Wires (28-gauge) are then passed through drill holes in the occipital and posterior parietal bone overlying the sagittal sinus. A-P shortening is achieved by slowly twisting the wire to approximate the bone edges. The degree of shortening is determined by the degree of deformity, but may be safely approximately 8 to 12 mm. As the shortening occurs, parieto-occipital dural bulging again occurs, and plication of the dura is necessary to achieve the degree of prominence that is ultimately desirable. The parieto-occipital bone is remodeled to lessen its roundedness and then securely attached to adjacent posterior parietal and occipital bone.

METOPIC SYNOSTOSIS

Metopic synostosis or trigonocephaly (from the Greek *trionos*, meaning triangular) is characterized by a pointed forehead with narrowing of the frontal and temporal regions bilaterally. Frequent associated features are hypotelorism, elevation of the lateral canthus, and a prominent ridging of the metopic suture, particularly in the region of the glabella.

Radiographically, the diagnosis of metopic synostosis is supported by the triangular frontal bone shape seen on basal skull view, and hypotelorism on the posterior-anterior (P-A) projection.

Treatment

The treatment goals in most cases of metopic synostosis are to remove the midline prominence of the metopic suture, increase the projection of the lateral frontal and temporal regions, and increase the prominence of the supraorbital ridges bilaterally. The narrowed intercanthal distance usually is not addressed surgically.

The patient is placed supine in a padded head rest, and the cranium and face to the level of the mouth are prepped and draped. This allows intraoperative inspection of the "true" appearance of the periorbital region by reflecting the forehead scalp flap back and forth. A bicoronal incision is then placed. The frontal scalp is reflected forward in a supraperiosteal plane, to the level of the supraorbital ridge. A subperiosteal dissection in continuity with a subperiorbital dissection is then carried out, medially and laterally, in the superior orbit to permit visualization of the frontozygomatic suture, the glabella, and the frontonasal suture. A single bur hole is placed in the midline. Bilateral bur holes are then placed in a region of the pterion, and free frontal bone grafts are developed, leaving a segment of bone at the level of the

supraorbital ridge to form the new supraorbital margin. The bone paralleling the metopic suture is left as a strip, then cut off at the region of the glabella and freed from the dura. It is flattened with a shaping bur and Tessier rib bender. The frontal bone at the glabella is rongeured away to the level of the frontonasal suture. The supraorbital ridges, deficient laterally, are mobilized with a sagittal saw cut through the orbital roof and laterally through the temporal bone and frontozygomatic suture. Care must be taken to protect the orbital contents, and the temporal lobe in particular, from injury during the performance of these saw cuts. In young infants the mobilized supraorbital ridge is then advanced and remodeled by greenstick fracture techniques to shape it into a normal supraorbital contour. As the brain continues to grow, the supraorbital rim is further advanced, appropriate to the growth of the remainder of the craniofacial skeleton. In an adult or older child, in whom brain growth or expansion is an insignificant factor, the supraorbital ridges are secured in the advanced position by a strut of cranial vault bone harvested from the temporoparietal region. The dura in the midline or adjacent to the sagittal sinus is plicated to diminish the pointed projection of the midline frontal region. The bony strip from the metopic suture is replaced and secured to the dura. The frontal bone is remodeled to achieve a more rounded prominence in the lateral-frontal, and temporal regions. The temporalis muscle previously reflected is attached to the lateral orbit or frontal bone to prevent "hollowing" of the anterior temporal fossa.

UNILATERAL CORONAL SYNOSTOSIS

Unilateral coronal synostosis is characterized clinically by a ridging of one half of the coronal suture, particularly laterally in the suture, and a flattening of the ipsilateral frontal and parietal bone. The supraorbital margin ipsilateral to the fused half of the coronal suture is deficient as well. The diminished frontal and parietal bone prominence is often accompanied by bulging of the temporal bone ipsilateral to the fused suture. Contralateral to the fused coronal suture, in the frontal bone, excessive prominence also is seen. The supraorbital ridge contralateral to the fused suture is often displaced caudally resulting in vertical orbital dystopia.

Radiographically, increased bony density is appreciated at the level of the coronal suture. On the P-A view, an uplifting of the upper outer quadrant of the orbit is regularly seen and referred to as the harlequin deformity. On basal view and CT scan, the sphenoid ridge and petrous bones are seen anteriorly displaced, and the angle between the sphenoid wing and the petrous bone is reduced.

Treatment

The patient is placed supine on a padded head rest and a bicoronal incision is performed, followed by separate bifrontal craniotomies to include the coronal sutures bilaterally. A subtemporal decompression is then performed, and the region of the lateral coronal suture and pterion is radically removed. If the dura in the ipsilateral temporal or contralateral frontal region is excessively prominent, the dura is plicated to diminish its projection. The temporal region bone can be reversed so that the outwardly directed convex surface is directed intracranially, resulting in a less prominent temporal fossa.

The deficiency in projection of the supraorbital rim may be addressed in one of three ways: frontal bone overlay, modified lateral canthal advancement, or tongue-in-groove techniques.

The frontal bone overlay technique begins with extensive removal of orbital region bone, from the supraorbital notch medially to the frontozygomatic suture laterally. The orbital roof likewise is removed posteriorly to the level of the superior orbital fissure. The frontal bone (remodeled) is then attached laterally to the zygoma and medially to the supraorbital notch. The inferior border of the advanced frontal bone forms the new superior orbital margin. This technique is particularly useful in the very young infant (approximately 6 to 10 weeks of age).

The modified lateral canthal technique is performed following an anterior subperiosteal dissection of the frontal bone, in continuity with the periorbita. A frontal craniotomy is then carried out. The frontal lobe is gently retracted, and the supralateral orbital margin is mobilized by saw cuts in the region of the pterion and orbital roof. The extent of medial cut in the orbital roof is to the medial-most portion of the orbit; the lateral-inferior cut is at the frontozygomatic suture. The supraorbital segment is "greenstick" fractured forward. The supraorbital "bar" is remodeled to achieve normal orbital contour and secured forward in this anterior position by a strut of calvarial bone. This technique is particularly useful in the older infant or young child.

The tongue-in-groove technique is performed by completing the periorbital dissection and bifrontal craniotomies, then mobilizing the supraorbital bar as described in the modified lateral canthal advancement technique. The difference, however, is that a bone strut extending into the temporal bone region is left attached to the lateral frontal bone and supraorbital ridge. The length of the posteriorly directed limb is usually approximately 3 to 4 cm. At the distal end of the limb in the temporal bone region, an angular segment in the form of a triangle is cut in the temporal bone. This segment remains in continuity with the posteriorly directed limb of bone. The supraorbital ridge and this posterior limb are then advanced forward by greenstick fracture of the supraorbital bone, but the difference here is that the extent of the medial bone cut is across the midline. Dissection is carried across the midline in the correction of this anomaly because the deformity often extends beyond the midline in the form of a deficient prominence of the supraorbital ridge. The Tessier rib bender is used to reshape the supraorbital bar into a more normal form.

The advancement of the supraorbital ridge is usually approximately 1 to 2 cm. At the proposed site of advancement, a triangular cut is placed in the remaining temporal bone to allow the advanced supraorbital rim and attached limb of bone to be secured in that position. A wire loop is passed through the advanced supraorbital ridge bone and secured to the adjacent temporal bone. The temporalis muscle, which had been previously reflected, is advanced as well to attach to the lateral supraorbital margin to avoid the appearance of a hollow in the temporal fossa postoperatively. The frontal bone is then molded to achieve a symmetric forehead as before, with the bone flaps secured to the advanced supraorbital bar by wire suture. This technique is particularly useful in the older child with insignificant brain growth remaining and in whom the temporal region is not excessively rounded. This technique disallows a significant alteration of the temporal region bone profile as the temporal bone is used to secure the supraorbital bar. The squamous temporal bone therefore cannot be removed or significantly reshaped without losing its structural integrity.

BILATERAL CORONAL SYNOSTOSIS

Bilateral coronal synostosis is characterized by a flattening of the frontal bone bilaterally with ridging of the coronal sutures either ecto- or endocranially. The supraorbital ridges are deficient bilaterally, particularly supralaterally. The skull at its base is shortened in the anterior-posterior dimension and increased in height, resulting in a brachycephaly.

Radiographically increased sclerosis at the level of the coronal suture is seen, particularly laterally and bilaterally. Bilateral harlequin deformities are often seen in the supralateral orbit. The sphenopetrosal angle is diminished bilaterally compared to the normal.

Treatment

The treatment of bilateral coronal synostosis is similar to that for unilateral coronal synostosis in that the patient is placed in a supine position on a padded head rest, and a bicoronal incision is used to gain access to the skull. The skin flaps are reflected anteriorly and laterally to allow the placement of bilateral pterional region, as well as midline, low frontal bur holes. Separate bifrontal craniotomies are performed. One of the three techniques previously described for advancement of the supraorbital margins is then performed. The frontal bone, diminished in prominence and shortened in anterior posterior dimension, is then remodeled to give a rounder configuration. A generous removal of bone in the region of the pterion is frequently necessary to free the thickened and dense dural attachments to the bone. We believe that the dural attachments should be released to allow more satisfactory contouring of the dura. The frontal bone is remodeled again to give a more rounded configuration to the frontal region. This reshaping includes the coronal suture bone and the parietal bone as well as the bone anterior to the coronal suture. The frontal bone is loosely attached by silk sutures to the dura in the growing child, whereas in the older child, it is secured with wire to the adjacent frontal bone and supraorbital bone. However, no attempt is made to cover the gap of bone at the posterior margin of the frontal craniotomy in order to allow further A-P expansion with time. Additionally, we believe it is important to carry multiple parallel bone cuts back to the lambdoid suture. This allows for further growth of the skull to correct the brachycephaly.

UNILATERAL LAMBDOID SYNOSTOSIS

Clinically the diagnosis of unilateral lambdoid suture synostosis is made by the observation of unilateral occipital flattening and excessive prominence of the contralateral occipital region. Ridging of the lambdoid suture is infrequent. Often there is an accompanying ipsilateral frontal bone bossing with premature stenosis of one-half of the lambdoid suture. Lambdoid synostosis must be distinguished radiographically from postural flattening, which demonstrates increased density along both inner and outer margins of the lambdoid suture, particularly at the lateral border. The asymmetry of the posterior occiput is seen well on the basal view radiograph.

Treatment

Because many of these patients have relatively mild deformities and because the occipital region is an area in which hair growth can be expected to cover most of the abnormality, many mild abnormalities are not treated surgically. However, for patients who have severe flattening of the occipital region and significant frontal bone prominence, surgical correction is the rule. The affected patient is placed prone in a modified U-shaped head rest to allow visualization of the occipital region. A posteriorly located U-shaped incision posterior to the ears is carried down through the galea, and dissection in a supraperiosteal plane is carried out. Bilateral occipital bur holes are then placed and dissection carried out to free the sagittal and transverse sinuses from the surrounding parieto-occipital bone. Separate biparieto-occipital craniotomies are performed, and the bony removal includes the areas of increased and decreased prominence posteriorly. This usually requires reflection of the occipital musculature. The dissection of the ipsilateral occipital bone to the fused lambdoid suture needs to be carried down to the level of the rim of the foramen magnum. At this level, vertically directed struts appearing like "barrel staves" are developed by cuts in the bone down to the level of the foramen magnum. By means of a Tessier rib bender, the bone is then fractured outward to allow increased prominence posteriorly. In the contralateral occipital and parietal area, the dura is plicated to

achieve a lesser prominence of the dura. This decreases the roundedness of the bone in this region. The bone is then remodeled to achieve a symmetric contour. The bone is then replaced and, in a growing child, just secured with silk suture to the underlying dura. In the older child, a more secure fixation to the adjacent parietal occipital bone is achieved.

The child with significant frontal bone abnormalities is placed in a modified prone position that allows the simultaneous visualization of the supraorbital regions and the occipital region down to the level of the foramen magnum. In this situation the bicoronal incision is carried out with anterior and posterior scalp reflection. The same procedure is performed posteriorly, as just described, but in addition, in the frontal region, a unilateral frontal craniotomy is performed in the region of excess prominence of the frontal bone. The dura is plicated and the skull remodeled to achieve a form of diminished prominence and roundedness in that region. The bone is then securely fastened to the adjacent frontal and parietal bone.

BILATERAL LAMBDOID STENOSIS

A patient with bilateral lambdoid synostosis demonstrates occipital flattening bilaterally associated with bossing of the frontal regions bilaterally. The degree of bossing usually is not so prominent as that seen with unilateral coronal synostosis and usually is not associated with significant supraorbital bar abnormalities. The radiographic diagnosis is based on the observation of bilateral occipital flattening associated with increased bony density along the course of the lambdoid suture. There is no narrowing of the sphenopetrosal angle, and there is no demonstrated harlequin deformity of the supralateral orbits, as seen in coronal synostosis.

Treatment

The treatment of bilateral lambdoid synostosis is similar to that for unilateral lambdoid synostosis in terms of exposure and positioning. The patient is placed in a modified prone position on a padded modified head rest: a bicoronal incision is placed, and the bilateral separate occipital and parietal craniotomies are performed. The flattening of the frontal bone, which usually extends beneath the occipital musculature, is reflected posteriorly, and the dissection is carried down to the rim of the foramen magnum. Again the remainder of bone extending to approximately 4 to 5 cm from the foramen magnum is cut in a "barrel stave" configuration, allowing reshaping by greenstick fracture of the more caudally placed occipital bone. The occipital bones are then remodeled and secured to the underlying dura. If a frontal abnormality exists, separate bifrontal craniotomies can be performed through the same exposure, similarly, the dura may be plicated and the frontal bone remodeled to achieve a diminished prominence in this region.

TURRIBRACHYCEPHALY

The diagnosis of turribrachycephaly is made by observing clinically that the patient has a very short skull in the anterior-posterior dimension, but a very tall skull vertically. Normally the skull is also broad. The cranial base appears excessively shortened, and there may be accompanying midfacial abnormality. Radiographically this clinical abnormality is often associated with synostosis of both the coronal and the lambdoid sutures. Frequently there is associated hydrocephalus. Radiographically, the suture lines at the coronal and lambdoid sutures are increased in density, the skull is markedly increased in height, and the anterior cranial base, in particular, is shortened compared to the normal. The sphenopetrosal angle is often narrowed.

Treatment

The patient is placed in a modified prone position and well cushioned. Bicoronal incision is then placed, and the skin flaps are reflected anteriorly and posteriorly. Inspection of the cranium usually reveals that there is occipital flattening, increased prominence of the vertex of the skull, diminished supraorbital margins, and excessive prominence of the frontal regions with nearly vertical inclination of the forehead bone. For this abnormality, we perform what is described as a "barrel stave" osteotomy, which includes placement of bur holes in the bifrontal and occipital region, and bifrontal and biparieto-occipital craniotomies. We preserve a circular or oval skull plate on the vertex of the skull with four strutlike appendages at the anterior, posterior, and two lateral poles of the skull. Following removal of the fron-tal and parieto-occipital bone bilaterally, barrel stave osteotomies are then performed in the occipital region down to the level of the foramen magnum. The ring of bone surrounding the foramen magnum is preserved, however. The bone in the occipital region is then green-stick fractured posteriorly to allow posterior migration of the brain-dura envelope. The four polar struts are then severed at their caudal margin with the base of the skull and, depending on the amount of shortening desired, approximately 2 to 2.5 cm of bone may be resected from the caudal border of the struts. The height of the skull may be reduced by placing wire segments through the anterior and lateral bone struts, then through the adjacent basal vault bone, and gradually (over the course of 45 to 60 minutes) tightening these wires to achieve bony apposition. With superior-inferior compression of the skull, the brain dura envelope is then shifted posteriorly, to achieve A-P elongation of the skull. The frontal region, where there is excessive rounding of the dura, normally is reshaped by plicating the dura so that the excessive prominence in this region is reduced. The remaining frontal and parieto-occipital bone flaps are then remodeled by placing a series of radially directed pie-shaped cuts in the bone and shaping them with the Tessier rib bender. The frontal bone flaps are then secured to adjacent bone. In the occipital region, the occipital bone strut is *not* secured to the posterior occipital bone. A gap is purposely left between occipital bone segments to allow further migration of the brain-dura envelope posteriorly. The parieto-occipital bone flaps are attached securely only on their anterior border, allowing the posterior border to ride free. This method of attachment further promotes posterior migration of the brain-dura envelope and elongation of the A-P axis of the skull. Following the performance of these maneuvers, the skin flaps are returned and the incision sutured.

LIPOMA AND RELATED ABNORMALITIES SUCH AS DERMAL SINUSES

JOHN W. WALSH, M.D., Ph.D.

Lumbosacral lipoma, diastematomyelia, thickened filum terminale, dermal sinuses, and other forms of spina bifida occulta are usually considered under the terms "spinal dysraphism" or "the tethered cord syndrome". These are congenital disorders in which the spinal cord terminates at an abnormally low level because it has been prevented from ascending normally along with somatic and vertebral growth by persistent embryologic structures which tether it. This tethering leads to elongation and chronic stretching of the spinal cord, which then becomes more vulnerable to ischemia produced by repeated intermittent forceful flexions of the spine. Such flexions are a normal occurrence in childhood, and the cumulative effect of the ischemic injuries damages the spinal cord and leads to deficits of motor and/or sensory function in the lower extremities and/or impairment of bowel and/or bladder control.

Treatment is surgical and involves a release of the spinal cord from all abnormal attachments. Without surgical intervention, the loss of neurological function is generally progressive and inevitable.

CLINICAL PRESENTATION

The age at which these patients come to neurosurgical attention varies considerably, but is most concentrated in the years before age 14. The occurrence is about equal in males and females, the notable exception being that diastematomyelia occurs almost exclusively in females.

Diagnosis centers around two major features: (1) cutaneous and subcutaneous anomalies over the lumbosacral spine, such as a tuft of hair, hemangioma, nevus, dimple, dermal sinus, cicatrix (atretic meningocele), sacral appendage, or subcutaneous lipoma, and (2) neurological impairments of lower extremity, bowel, and bladder function. At birth, patients can present with any combination of these features, but often are apparently normal.

The cutaneous and subcutaneous anomalies are a most useful indicator of the diagnosis; they are rarely seen in the absence of spinal dysraphism. Several may be seen in a given patient, and their size varies from pinpoint, as with some dermal sinuses, to massive, as with many subcutaneous lipomas.

The neurological impairments generally develop with a rostrocaudal dermatomal distribution, and this gives rise to two distinctly different clinical pictures, the so-called orthopaedic syndrome and the urologic syndrome. With the orthopaedic syndrome, lesions affecting the spinal cord at mid or lower lumbar levels produce, as their initial and most severe deficit, disturbances of lower extremity motor and sensory function in distributions corresponding to the specific cord level impaired. In this pattern, bowel or bladder dysfunction occurs only at a later stage. In contrast, with the urologic syndrome, lesions that compromise spinal cord function at sacrococcygeal levels (conus medullaris) initially produce disturbances of bowel or bladder function and only years later produce mild-to-moderate L5 or S1 motor and sensory dysfunction.

Orthopaedic Syndrome

Except for one or more cutaneous anomalies over the lower spine, these patients are usually normal at birth or have only very slight abnormalities of lower extremity development, such as equinovarus or calcaneovalgus posturing in one or both feet or shortening of one leg. If the cord is not released in the next few months, severe impairments of motor and sensory function generally develop. If the lesion is not repaired by 5 or 6 years of age, the patient will have developed a marked weakness of ankle dorsiflexion and inversion and severe muscle wasting. At this time, some disturbance of urinary tract function also begins to appear. Thus, these children, who had normal or near normal neurological function at birth, now resemble those unfortunate ones we see more often with lumbosacral myelomeningoceles and severe neurological deficits for whom we have so little to offer. If the condition still goes untreated, more extensive paraparesis and bladder dysfunction ensue, and fecal incontinence is also seen. This increase in the extent and severity of impairment of neurological function varies markedly according to the particular type of dysraphism present, extent of cord involvement, level of the conus and degree of tethering.

Urologic Syndrome

These patients are noted at birth or shortly thereafter to have urinary dribbling and/or an absent anal wink, but motor and sensory function in the lower extremities and perineal sensation are usually normal. If the cord is not released in the next 2 or 3 years, urinary incontinence becomes more severe, and they develop frequent urinary tract infections. Toilet training may be completely unsuccessful or achieved and then lost, and pharmacologic agents, such as Ditropan or Urecholine, and/or intermittent catheterization are usually required. A few years later, fecal incontinence usually develops. In some patients, impairments of motor and sensory function in the L5 or S1 distribution become apparent, but only very late in the course of deterioration.

Myelomeningocele and Tethered Cord

Recently, I have seen a number of children with fixed impairments of lower extremity and bowel and bladder function who had undergone repair of a myelomeningocele or myelorachischisis shortly after birth. Months to years later, they experienced a further deterioration of neurological function and were found to have fibrous bands or other abnormally persistent embryologic structures which caused spinal cord tethering. Such dysraphic structures may be proximal or distal to the site of previous surgery and must be divided if continued neurological deterioration is to be prevented. Most often the deterioration of function in these patients has involved bowel and/or bladder function.

RADIOLOGIC AND LABORATORY DIAGNOSIS

Roentgenograms of the spine and computed tomography (CT) scan are most useful in demonstrating the level and extent of spina bifida in these children. If diastematomyelia is present, a median bony septum may also be displayed and the degree of scoliosis and/or kyphosis established. Sacral agenesis, hemivertebrae, and block vertebrae, when present, are also well seen.

Myelography is the procedure of choice for preoperative evaluation because the level and position of the spinal cord, conus medullaris, and exiting nerve roots can be determined with accuracy and because the exact site(s) of attachment to the cord of tethering bands or structures can often be shown. For years, myelography was performed with iophendylate (Pantopaque), an oil base dye which did not outline the lower cord and filum very well. More recently, Amipaque (metrizamide) has been used because it is water-soluble and resorbs spontaneously from cerebrospinal fluid (CSF) into the blood stream, because it makes detailed imaging of the subarachnoid space and all its contents possible, and because it can be visualized with both fluoroscopy and CT scanning.

CT scanning without Amipaque does not distinguish individual intradural components (spinal cord, roots, and filum) from one another or from surrounding leptomeningeal structures, but with Amipaque it demonstrates each structure very well.

With myelography and CT scanning, it is essential to determine (1) the level of the conus, (2) the dorsal or ventral position of the cord within the spinal canal, (3) the extent of lateral displacement or rotation of the conus and its roots, (4) the size of the caudal subarachnoid space, (5) the extent of any intraspinal or intramedullary mass, such as a dermoid tumor or abscess, and (6) the location and course of any other secondary structures, such as a thickened filum terminale, that restrict normal ascent of the cord with growth.

Over the past 3 years, several reports of the usefulness of ultrasonography for imaging tethered cords in infants have been published. The method is attractive because its resolution is only slightly less than that achieved with myelography and because it is noninvasive and does not require the use of radiation. The level of the conus is easily established, as are the sites of attachment of lipomas and other intraspinal dysraphic structures. However, the specific course of individual nerve roots cannot always be determined.

Magnetic resonance imaging (MRI) is also still in its infancy, but preliminary studies in our center show that exceptionally good localization of the conus and its attachment to tethering structures can be obtained.

Since most patients exhibit some compromise of urinary tract function, an intravenous pyelogram (IVP) and voiding cystourethrogram (VCUG) should be carried out as part of the initial evaluation, and at scattered intervals prior to surgery. Urodynamics or cystometrography is also necessary in order to determine whether the child has a neurogenic bladder; whether the dysfunction is spastic, flaccid, or mixed in type; and whether the deficit is minor or severe. With urodynamics, urethral pressure profile and rectal sphincter tone are also determined.

INDICATIONS FOR SURGERY

The most commonly accepted indication for surgery is the development of progressive neurological deficits. Surgery is principally aimed at preventing further loss of function, but may also make some recovery possible. Recently, surgery at an earlier date on children without neurological impairment or with only very slight deficits has been advocated because a loss of neurological function is most often inevitable and because the extent to which recovery of function, once lost, can be obtained is usually limited.

Ideally, the diagnosis should be made within the first few months of life and surgery carried out at that time. Unfortunately, however, the condition often goes unrecognized for many years until severe and irreversible neurological deficits become evident. Even when the diagnosis is established early, surgery is often postponed, sometimes for months or years, because the progressive nature of the disorder is not appreciated. Early diagnosis and treatment can make the difference between a normal or nearly normal life and one limited by immobilization and incontinence. If the child is otherwise clinically normal and has no progressive loss of neurological function, I operate as early as possible after the child reaches 3 months of age. Before that, there are increased risks associated with being a neonate, such as enterocolitis, and surgery is appropriate and essential during this period only when a further loss of function is observed.

Occasionally, surgery is necessary for alleviation of pain or appropriate for cosmetic reasons. Dermal sinuses require complete excision to prevent meningitis or deficits from associated intraspinal abscesses or dermoid tumors. Some patients with diastematomyelia and kyphoscoliosis require removal of a median bony or fibrous septum before corrective orthopaedic surgery in order to prevent spinal cord injury and postoperative paraplegia.

TREATMENT

Laminectomy under general anesthesia, intradural exploration, and division or resection of all tethering structures is the treatment of choice for most children with these disorders. A midline vertical incision is made throughout the extent of the spina bifida and 1 or 2 segments above and below it. Dermal sinuses, subcutaneous lipomas, atretic meningoceles, and other lesions associated with a tract or stalk that passes intraspinally are freed from surrounding fascia and other tissue and followed circumferentially to the underlying vertebrae. One or two laminae rostral to the stalk or spina bifida are then removed so that normal dura and spinal cord can be exposed. Using these normal structures as a plane of reference, dissection can then safely and with maximum orientation be extended in a caudal direction, lamina by lamina, until the entire dysraphic lesion is exposed. Under increased magnification, lipomatous or other fibrous stalks are divided just above their attachment to the posterior cord surface, conus, or roots of the cauda equina, and all tethering fibers or bands are sectioned. Continuous intraoperative monitoring during this portion of surgery using somatosensory evoked potentials, cystometrography, or recording of anal sphincter tone is often of considerable help. A watertight closure of the dura is essential to prevent postoperative complications such as CSF leak, wound infection, and/or meningitis. In order to eliminate dead space produced by the resection of the dysraphic tissue, a meticulous closure of muscle, fascia, subcutaneous tissue, and skin layers must be carried out. After surgery, patients should be kept flat for 7 to 10 days to minimize the risk of CSF leak and its deleterious effect on wound healing.

SPECIFIC TYPES OF SPINAL DYSRAPHISM

Congenital Lipomas of the Lumbosacral Spine

These lesions include lipomyelomeningocele, intradural lumbosacral lipoma, intrafilar lipoma, and lipoma associated with diastematomyelia or neurenteric cyst.

Lipomyelomeningocele generally presents as a large midline or paramedian subcutaneous lipoma which attaches extradurally within the spinal canal to the posterior cord surface. The spinal cord itself is generally dorsally displaced within the canal; but if the lipoma and fibrolipomatous stalk are eccentrically situated, it may also be pulled laterally. A meningocele sac of variable size is usually seen just caudal to the fibrolipomatous stalk, and a thickened filum terminale may also be present. At surgery, the fibrolipomatous stalk is divided just posterior to the dorsal root entry zones or caudal to the conus, and the filum and all accompanying abnormal tethering bands and nerves are released.

Intradural lumbosacral lipomas may be totally intradural or intradural with an eccentric sacral subcutaneous extension. The lipomatous tissue is attached to the conus and extends caudally adjacent to nerve roots of the cauda equina or around them. A thickened filum terminale may also be present, passing through the lipoma and through the end of the dural sac to the overlying dimpled skin. Surgery involves a generous decompressive laminectomy, subtotal resection of the intradural fat, and a division of the filum and any other tethering bands.

Intrafilar lipomas are usually incidental and directly removable. Lipomas associated with diastematomyelia or neurenteric cyst are removed along with the primary dysraphic anomaly.

Diastematomyelia

In this disorder, a portion of the spinal cord in the lower thoracic or midlumbar region is congenitally divided longitudinally into two segments by a fibrous or bony septum. Caudal to this, the two cord segments reunite to form a single abnormally low conus medullaris. Normal upward migration of the cord is arrested when the reunited portion of neural tissue reaches and comes in contact with the septum. The resulting compression and ischemia produce impairments of lower extremity, bowel, and bladder function. Aberrant nerve roots and arachnoid bands may extend from the two segments of the cord along their medial surfaces, attach to the overlying dura, bone, or fascia, and thus contribute to spinal cord tethering. A thickened filum terminale

is usually present. Treatment requires laminectomy over the involved cord segments, circumferential opening of the dura around the bony or fibrous septum, and removal of the septum and surrounding dural sheath. Tethering bands, aberrant nerve roots, and the filum terminale are then divided.

Thickened Filum Terminale

Occasionally this is the only anomaly present. In these cases, the conus medullaris, unlike its normal counterpart, gradually tapers and almost imperceptibly becomes the filum. An intrafilar lipoma is frequently present. The patients usually present with impairments of bladder and/or bowel function. Treatment involves section of the filum, but this must be carried out at as caudal a level as possible in order to ensure the integrity of the conus.

Dermal Sinus

In these cases the cord is tethered by a sinus or tract which opens onto the skin. The cutaneous opening is frequently missed because it may be very small, and patients often initially present with a series of bouts of meningitis. Excision of the tract is essential to prevent further infection and to release caudal spinal cord structures. All epithelial tissue must be removed because residual intradural remnants of epithelial tissue may lead to formation of a dermoid tumor which would adhere densely to adjacent neural structures and therefore would not be totally resectable.

RESULTS

The long-term results of surgery for this group of patients, as reported in the literature, varies considerably with the case mix, the age of the patients, the number of patients with preexisting and/or progressive neurological deficits, the severity of these deficits, and the operative experience of the surgeon with disorders of this type.

I have a series of just over 100 patients with rather encouraging results. All those who were neurologically normal before surgery remained normal. Those with diastematomyelia and fixed neurological impairment, retained their preoperative neurological status after removal of a midline bony or fibrous septum prior to surgery for correction of scoliosis. Of the patients with progressive neurological deterioration, approximately 30 percent regained normal motor and sensory function in their lower extremities or experienced recovery sufficient to enable them to walk without braces. Another 30 to 40 percent improved significantly, but to a lesser extent. Complete continence of both bowel and bladder function was regained in about 12 percent, and an improvement in function sufficient to keep previously wet patients dry with the aid of pharmacologic agents and intermittent catheterization was obtained in another 25 to 30 percent. Three patients required reexploration 3 to 5 years later for division of an unrecognized thickened filum terminale. Two patients sustained slight additional impairment after surgery.

PERIPHERAL NERVE DISORDERS

CARPAL TUNNEL SYNDROME AND ULNAR NEUROPATHY AT THE ELBOW

GEORGE EHNI, M.D.

Median nerve entrapment in the carpal tunnel and ulnar involvement at the elbow are less frequent than radiculopathy due to arthrosis with discal prominences compressing roots in the intervertebral foramina, and feature subjective complaints of numbness and sleepiness in appropriate parts of the hands rather than severe shoulder and arm pain, limitation of neck motion, and the pareses and reflex changes characteristic of radiculopathy. The median and ulnar entrapments occur with much greater frequency than thoracic outlet syndromes and are not accompanied by any of the arterial or venous compressive phenomena associated with the latter.

CARPAL TUNNEL SYNDROME

The carpal tunnel syndrome is most frequently idiopathic in middle-aged women, who describe onset and aggravation during sleep, during the finger activities required in sewing or use of scissors, or while gripping a steering wheel. A clear relationship to biomechanical activity, especially flexion of the wrist and use of the fingers in a wrist-flexed position, is much more frequent than causation by a specific disorder such as a dislocated semilunar bone, fracture of the scaphoid bone, hematoma, ganglion, neurofibroma, lipoma, or other tumors of the nerve or of the tendons and sheaths. It is occasionally found secondary to tuberculosis, amyloid or other type of tenosynovitis, acromegaly, myxedema, rheumatoid arthritis, gout, and multiple myeloma. As a rule the sufferer is otherwise healthy, and search for obscure causation unfruitful.

The initial manifestations are subjective, consisting of paresthesias in the median nerve distribution, which may be described as stinging, burning, bursting, tingling, and even outright painful. Sometimes discomfort extends up the arm and, in rare instances, above the elbow or into the shoulder, causing confusion with radiculopathy. The

reason for the occasional upward extension is unknown. Sometimes the whole hand, including the ulnar aspect, feels affected.

Biomechanical effects are suggested by the presence of paresthesias when the patient awakens from sleep and with its disappearance with change of position and with daytime activities involving use of the hand and, particularly, wrist flexion. Avoidance of provocative activities and adoption of a neutral position, particularly in sleep by use of a splint or clamping the affected hand between the thighs while lying on one side or the other, generally gives relief at first. The diagnostic impression is strengthened if characteristic symptoms are evoked by maintained passive flexion of the wrist for approximately one minute and if tingling in a characteristic distribution is evoked by finger percussion over the nerve at the wrist. Median nerve conduction velocity is slowed and a latency in excess of 4.7 msec after delivery of a standard stimulus is confirmatory, but not invariably present. In more advanced cases, light touch and pinprick sharpness may be reduced on the tip of the index and adjacent fingers and two-point discrimination lost. The abductor pollicis brevis, the flexor pollicis brevis, and the opponens pollicis may atrophy and weaken, so that the thenar eminence flattens. Buttoning and other tasks requiring fine finger coordination become clumsy, often more so on awakening in the morning, when the subjective symptoms are most intense. Once begun the condition is likely to be slowly progressive, generally in the dominant hand, though it often becomes bilateral unless provocative activities can be avoided and a neutral position of the wrist enforced during sleep.

The therapeutic options include, obviously, treatment of primary conditions to which the carpal tunnel symptomatology may be secondary, such as fracture fragments, tenosynovitis, acromegaly, and myxedema, but for the vast majority of sufferers from this condition, there is no discernible etiology to eradicate, and the treatment options narrow to those locally applicable. Corticosteroid injections into the carpal tunnel may as easily worsen the condition as benefit it, and anti-inflammatory and antiarthritic remedies are not regularly helpful. Strict avoidance of provocative activity, particularly involuntary prolonged wrist flexion in sleep, gives the best chance of nonsurgical relief. A splint may be applied for sleep, or the patient may be advised to sleep on one side or the other with the underarm extended outward and the wrist kept neutral under a pillow, while the uppermost hand is clamped between the thighs. Most patients are able to readopt the favored position every time they wake up with the hand numb, and they get used to sleeping in this position, with benefit to their symptoms.

If this fails, the flexor retinaculum, which has no known useful function, should be cut from its proximal through its distal edge along the ulnar side of the median nerve. This may be done through a palmar skin crease incision extending down to the wrist and then transversely for a short distance in the transverse flexion crease of the wrist. Incision through the palmar fascia to the ulnar side of the flexor palmaris longus tendon exposes the flexor retinaculum. The distal forearm aponeurosis, which fuses with the flexor retinaculum, and the flexor retinaculum are then cut, always staying along the ulnar border of the median nerve. This procedure thoroughly decompresses the nerve and affords almost 100 percent satisfaction.

An alternative and more refined method, but only for those who have practiced it on a cadaver, is to make a short transverse incision in the distal flexor crease of the wrist, centered over the palmaris longus tendon or placed 1 cm ulnarward of the flexor carpi radialis tendon. Through the very superficial incision (to spare the twig to the palmar skin), blunt dissection exposes the forearm aponeurosis. Vertical incision of the forearm aponeurosis exposes the median nerve for an inch into the distal forearm, after which it is sectioned down to its point of fusion with the proximal edge of the flexor retinaculum. Then an artificial tunnel is created with a spreading scissors or other instrument between the palmar fascia and the flexor retinaculum, to receive the end of a Senn retractor. This exposes the superficial surface of the flexor retinaculum. Along the ulnar side of the median nerve, a ballpoint probe may be gently passed to gauge tightness with the wrist in extension. Then, under direct vision the flexor retinaculum is cut from its proximal edge through its distal edge with snips of a very stout Mayo-type scissors. The direction of this cut should be toward the ring finger and should not deviate radially. No fibers of the ligament should be left uncut.

Complications of surgery include failure to relieve symptoms because of incomplete section of the flexor retinaculum, particularly its distal edge, damage to the median nerve by wandering radially in making incisions, section of an anastomotic branch with the ulnar nerve, and damage to the superficial palmar arterial arch by incision beyond the distal edge of the flexor retinaculum.

Most surgeons prefer the palmar incision exposure of the flexor retinaculum because it affords a better view of the entire surface of the structure to be cut, with less risk of damage to the median nerve and the artery by the inexperienced. Anyone interested in carrying out the operation through a limited wrist incision should first practice the operation in the morgue or anatomy laboratory. If the palmar arch is wounded and arterial bleeding results, the artery should be ligated if the palmar incision has been employed. Firm compression with a sponge wad under an Ace bandage applied for 3 hours, if such bleeding results in connection with the short transverse wrist incision, is effective.

Properly carried out, either technique reliably relieves the median nerve compressive symptoms. Recovery of muscle bulk in case of severe atrophy is long delayed. Some sensory impairment may be permanent if sensory loss has been severe. If the palmar incision is used and if the palmar aponeurosis and skin are not closed carefully, the scar may be unsightly.

ULNAR NEUROPATHY AT THE ELBOW

The ulnar nerve at the level of the elbow, where it runs behind the medial epicondyle of the humerus and under the muscle aponeurosis bridging between the olecranon and the medial epicondyle, is vulnerable to traction, compression, and percussion. The first description of ulnar neuropathy to the French Academy of Medicine in 1878 included patients with old fracture leading to cubitus valgus deformity, a sesamoid bone lying against the nerve at the level of the medial collateral ligament, compression by arthritic spurs, and onset with an anatomically normal elbow after strenuous rowing. Unfavorable biomechanical activity or external compression while resting on the elbow in bed after other illness or injury figures prominently in the etiology of patients' complaints nowadays. Sometimes innocent-seeming trauma initiates or triggers an ulnar disorder, which proceeds to get worse rather than better, though the initiating incident is not repeated or recurrent. Occupation is sometimes suspected, but infrequently proved. Elbow flexion, asleep or at work, appears to be a prominent biomechanical agent in initiating and perpetuating this condition. The nerve passes behind the medial epicondyle in a groove where it is surrounded by light fibrous and fatty tissue, which allows a certain degree of gliding motion. Just distal to the epicondyle, the nerve passes between the two origins of the flexor carpi ulnaris and the aponeurosis, bridging the two. In flexion the nerve becomes taut around the epicondyle while the aponeurosis, also called the cubital ligament, tightens. In some cases the nerve does not stay in the groove, but dislocates over the prominence of the medial epicondyle with additional opportunity for traction and compression trauma. Contraction of the flexor carpi ulnaris muscle when the hand is used in strenuous activity also tightens the aponeurosis, contributing to ulnar nerve compression.

The diagnosis of ulnar neuropathy at the elbow depends on finding both local and acral manifestations. Only infrequently does pain extend above the elbow, but there may be great tenderness on manipulation or percussion of the nerve, with paresthesias running into the ulnar fingers. Occasionally the nerve may be felt to be thickened or swollen or to ride up over the prominence of the medial epicondyle. Distal manifestations may include ulnar paresthesias, sensory loss, weakness of the intrinsic hand muscles innervated by the ulnar nerve, and atrophy of these muscles, particularly the adductor pollicis and dorsal interossei. The hand often displays a *griffe* deformity, with the ring and little fingers extended at the metacarpal phalangeal joint and flexed at the interphalangeal joints. The ulnar border of the hand may be flattened instead of convex owing to atrophy of abductor digiti quinti. The flexor carpi ulnaris muscle is infrequently involved because its motor branch departs from the ulnar parent in a position favorable for escape from compression. Two eponymic tests are associated with this condition: (1) Tinel's sign on percussion of the nerve at the elbow or below, and (2) Froment's sign, consisting of unnatural flexion of the terminal phalanx of the thumb when the subject grasps folded paper between the thumb and the flexed proximal interphalangeal joint of the index finger in an attempt to keep it from being pulled from his grasp.

Radiography of the elbow is prudently requested if there is any question of the existence of an old fracture, osteoarthritic spurs, or sesamoid bones, but generally this is uninformative. The principal ancillary examination is that of ulnar nerve conduction velocity, with the principal action potential slowed to 30 meters per second or even less, instead of travelling at 50 to 55.

This condition, once in evidence, has little disposition to spontaneously improve or disappear because the anatomic surround of the nerve remains the same and avoidance of elbow flexion and strenuous use of the hand is not often possible. One useful conservative measure is changing one's sleep habit so that the arm is not lain upon or kept in a flexed position, but rather fully extended out to the side or downward with the hand between the thighs. Splinting of the elbow in extension has limited patient acceptance. In the face of advancing symptomatology or abnormality, effective (surgical) treatment should be offered without great delay because the ulnar nerve has a limited capacity to regenerate after wallerian degeneration is under way.

The choices of operative therapy include (1) actual transposition of the nerve to a new path anterior to the medial epicondyle, and (2) section of the cubital ligament with or without medial epicondylectomy. For transposition of the nerve, a fair length of it must be dissected free, and the nerve ends up in a superficial or intramuscular (depending on the technique employed) location, where subsequent fibrosis may initiate additional irritative changes which are frequently irreversible. Furthermore, the transposed nerve may sometimes be placed in unfavorable tension on elbow extension. Cubital ligament section does not result in much exposure of the nerve or damage to its freely gliding investment, and is much to be preferred. Medial epicondylectomy may contribute to a good result in some individuals undergoing cubital ligament section, and medial epicondylectomy has been found effective by itself, without division of the cubital ligament. Cubital ligament section carries little or no risk of making the situation worse. Medial epicondylectomy, if too radical, may result in detachment of the collateral ligament of the elbow with resultant elbow instability and possible need of ligamentous reconstruction at a later date. If medial epicondylectomy is to be done, the anatomy of the medial side of the elbow, and especially the site of attachment of the collateral ligament to the medial epicondyle, must be kept firmly in mind. Cubital ligament section alone may be carried out under local anesthesia, but medial epicondylectomy takes somewhat longer and is best done under general anesthesia.

Ulnar nerve transplantation, the most frequently performed operation for this condition because medial epicondylectomy and cubital ligament section are neglected in many teaching programs, has a failure rate due to persistence or worsening of symptoms in the neighborhood of 5 to 10 percent. Medial epicondylectomy, with or without cubital ligament section, has so far never failed me, but faultless technique with respect to the collateral ligament is essential. After medial epicondylectomy and cubital ligament section, the patient can be expected to return to work as soon as sutures are removed, but with the transplantation operation, several weeks' to a month's convalescence may be needed.

ROOT AND NERVE INJURY

DAVID G. KLINE, M.D.
ROGER D. SMITH, M.D.

While not all nerve injuries require operation, undue delay or reluctance in offering operative treatment may result in unnecessary permanent loss of function and associated major disability. Thus, timing and selection of appropriate cases for operation are critical factors in the treatment of nerve injuries. To appropriately treat their patients, neurosurgeons should be informed as to the indications for operation, the various procedures done, and anticipated results of treatment.

Recognizing that considerable controversy exists concerning nerve injuries, we will outline our method of evaluation and management, using the experience gained in treatment of these lesions over the last 20 years.

CATEGORIES OF NERVE INJURY

Nerve injuries can be generally divided into two groups: those in which the nerves are presumed to be "in continuity", and those which are presumed to be "not in continuity". In more complex injuries, there may be a mixture of these two lesion types, particularly when the mechanism of injury is relatively sharp, e.g., glass or metal (Table 1). Plexus injuries, or injuries to both median and ulnar nerves at the elbow or wrist frequently show such a mixture of lesions. Continuity of the injured nerve is one of the primary determinants as to selection for and timing of operation and type of surgery to be performed.

A second important determinant is whether the loss of function in the distribution of the injured nerve distal to the lesion is complete or incomplete. Injuries with partial or incomplete loss usually, although not always, improve with time, especially when the mechanism of injury is blunt rather than sharp. Partial injury caused by a sharp object may involve a portion or certain fascicles of the nerve. Decision to operate in such a setting, therefore, will depend on whether the loss in the distribution of the nerve is to functionally important muscles or sensory zones. Occasionally, the entire cross-section of a nerve will be partially involved; this type of injury invariably improves with time unless complicated by entrapment or mass lesions.

The third important consideration in nerve injury is whether the lesion is focal or nonfocal, with reference to the length of the nerve involved in the lesion. A sharp injury to any segment of nerve or blunt injury over a bony prominence may involve only a few millimeters of the nerve, while a severe stretch injury to the brachial plexus may involve several inches of many elements. Most focal lesions have a better chance for spontaneous recovery than do nonfocal lesions; at operation, prognosis for recovery is better when either direct repair or short rather than lengthy grafts can be employed. Lesions associated with fractures, low caliber gunshot wounds, injections, and some iatrogenic injuries tend to be focal, while stretch injuries, high velocity gunshot and shotgun wounds, massive soft tissue injuries, and irradiation plexitis are usually diffuse and thus nonfocal in nature.

Nerve Injuries in Continuity

When a nerve injury is presumed to be in continuity, the patient is followed for 2 to 3 months before a

TABLE 1 **Gunshot Wounds and Focal Contusions with Severe Deficit**

Lesions with incomplete distal loss may recover without operation while those with complete loss usually require operation.

Obtain baseline clinical evaluation of the entire limb. Begin physical therapy early.

Baseline EMG at 2 to 3 weeks

Clinical and electrical follow-up carried out periodically over next 2 to 3 months

If function does not improve, exploration is necessary.

Evaluate the lesion in continuity by stimulation and stimulation plus recording (NAP) studies.

If there is no operative electrical evidence of regeneration, resection and repair by suture or grafts is necessary.

Some lesions in continuity with NAPs may require split repair where a portion of the cross section of fascicles receives neurolysis and another portion, suture or graft repair.

decision to operate is made. A baseline examination is necessary shortly after injury and includes thorough testing of the muscles innervated by the nerve in question and a good assay of sensory function, especially in areas supplied only by that nerve (autonomous zones). Electromyography (EMG) is performed 2 to 3 weeks after injury and involves a complete sampling of electrical activity in muscles in the distribution of the nerve as well as nerve conduction studies. Muscle sampling is important to determine the pattern and extent of denervational changes including fibrillations, denervation potentials, and changes in insertional activity. Clinical examination and EMG are repeated over the next 2 to 3 months looking for early return of function due to reversal of neuropraxic injury or, in an occasional case when injury has been relatively close to a muscle recording site, early reversal of denervational changes. If the patient has shown no improvement in this time period, operative exploration is recommended. With nonfocal lesions such as those due to stretch, an additional 1 or 2 months are allowed to elapse before operation. Between the time of injury and operation, mobilization of the paralyzed portion of the limb is of paramount importance and often requires the assistance of physical and occupational therapy.

At operation, intraoperative electrophysiological studies help to further clarify the nature of the lesion and the potential for recovery. An adequate monitoring system is capable of both direct stimulation studies and the recording of nerve action potentials (NAP) above, below, and across the lesion. Bipolar electrodes are constructed of stainless steel or platinum-coated iridium #18 wire, bent like a shepherd's crook at the bottom and hand held with Delrin rod holders. Direct nerve stimulation is used proximal and distal to the injury site, looking for distal muscle contraction. To measure an NAP, a Grass S-55 stimulator with a stimulus isolation unit (SIU) is used for output, and response is measured by a differential amplifier and oscilloscope and recorded with a Polaroid camera. An NAP is recorded by placing both sets of electrodes proximal to the injury and stimulating and recording. Once an NAP is recorded, the distal electrodes are moved through the lesion and on distally, to see if the NAP is conducted through the injury site to distal nerve and how far down the distal stump it can be traced.

If an adequate NAP can be recorded, the nerve has good potential for further regeneration and, usually, the type of recovery which is functional in nature. In this case, only external neurolysis—freeing of the nerve from adjacent scar tissue—will be done. If no NAP is recorded across the lesion in continuity, the damaged portion of nerve is resected between two preplaced, lateral 6–0 nylon sutures which help maintain some degree of fascicular orientation. The ends are drawn together under as little tension as possible, and the nerve stumps joined with fine, closely spaced epineurial sutures. Fascicular dissection or repair is usually not necessary unless grafts need to be interposed. In some cases, an adequate NAP will be conducted across the lesion, but it is noted that one portion of the nerve is more severely damaged than the rest. This portion of the nerve is split away from the remainder and an attempt made to record NAPs from each portion. If an NAP can be recorded from one portion but not another, the latter's injured segment is resected and a "split" repair is done by either end-to-end suture or interposition of grafts.

Tension on a suture line is extremely deleterious to successful nerve repair. Length may be obtained by mobilizing the nerve well proximal and distal to the lesion site, taking care to preserve as much epineurium and longitudinal vasculature as possible. With ulnar, and to some extent radial lesions in the lower upper arm and forearm, more length can be made up by transposing the ulnar nerve volar to the elbow or transposing the radial nerve from its humeral groove and lateral lower arm to a position beneath the biceps brachialis muscle so that repair is done on the medial side of the upper arm. If more length is necessary, the surgeon must turn to nerve grafts. Sural nerves make excellent grafts since the resulting sensory deficit is small and in a nonfunctional area involving the side of one or both feet. If sural nerves are not available because of lower leg injury and one is operating on the upper extremity, the lateral and medial antebrachial cutaneous nerves provide good grafts. If the radial nerve at the elbow or the posterior interosseous nerve in the forearm needs replacement, the superficial radial sensory nerve provides a satisfactory graft.

Nerve Injuries Not in Continuity

Where continuity is suspected to be lost, primary repair is recommended for those nerves that are sharply and nearly transected. Laceration of the median and/or ulnar nerves at the wrist or elbow by knife or glass would be a typical example. Occasionally, a sharp injury to the brachial plexus is seen, and there is special benefit to primary repair in this situation, for at secondary operation, elements will be retracted and scarring will be heavy, particularly if a primary vascular and/or orthopaedic procedure has been required. A similar argument can be advanced for sciatic transections, where, without acute repair, retraction of the stumps will be significant and secondary repair without grafts difficult.

If at acute exploration, an element is found to be partially divided, but in a clean, neat fashion, suture of the divided portion is aided by dissecting it longitudinally away from the nondivided portion. Often, the remaining, nondivided portion may be severely contused and imposible to assess acutely. If clinical and/or electrical recovery does not occur over the next few months and the loss is significant and important from a functional standpoint, reexploration and intraoperative NAP recordings may be necessary, to see if the incontinuity portion needs resection and repair. At that time, the suture line of the repaired portion of the nerve can be checked also for electrical conductivity.

Where the soft tissue wound is inspected acutely, either because of the need for vascular or orthopaedic repair, or because of suspected sharp transection of the nerve, and blunt or ragged transection of the nerve is found, it is best to tack each stump down with a single suture to different but adjacent tissue planes, in order to maintain length. The nerve is then reexplored several weeks later, at which time the degree of injury to each stump can be easily delineated, and the extent of resection necessary to gain healthy fascicular structure both proximally and distally will be more obvious. The keys to successful nerve repair of any type are trimming the stump back to healthy tissue and avoiding distraction of the suture line by reducing tension as much as possible. In this regard, the decision whether to attempt end-to-end repair or to turn to grafts is a very important one.

UPPER EXTREMITY NERVE INJURY

Since radial nerve innervates large bulky muscles located at relatively short distance from the injury site, both spontaneous regeneration and surgical repair have a high order of success. Injuries at midhumeral level with complete loss are followed and, if there is no recovery, explored at 2 to 3 months after injury, a time when intraoperative recording can be used to document the need for resection. Repair often requires transposition of the distal stump of the nerve beneath the biceps brachialis so that suture or graft placement is completed on the medial side of the upper arm. Surgery at the elbow level for injury involving the posterior interosseous nerve is more complex than that for more proximal radial nerve involvement; but response to repair is also good, although recovery of extensor pollicus longus function is difficult to obtain. Dorsal forearm injury often involves the branches of the posterior interosseous nerve, making their surgical identification and repair difficult but not prohibitive.

Most serious median injuries should be repaired, even at a proximal level, so that some degree of sensation can be recovered in thumb and forefinger. Even with proximal injury, restoration of the pinch mechanism is possible because innervational sites for the flexor pollicis longus and flexor profoundus of forefinger are relatively proximal in the forearm. Thenar intrinsic return is less certain but is partially substituted for by ulnar innervated thumb intrinsic muscles. Forearm and wrist level repair is almost always worthwhile, even if the injury involves a segment of the nerve, because regenerative potential for this nerve is good.

The situation is not as encouraging for the ulnar as for the median nerve. With serious proximal injury, recovery of hand intrinsics is seldom obtained unless the injury can be shown to be regenerating by operative electrical recordings; then, some degree of hand function is possible. Nevertheless, ulnar injuries at the elbow level or below should be operated upon; enough return may be gained to avoid an ulnar claw, and even partial recovery of ulnar distribution sensation in the hand is worthwhile. Such a procedure is often accompanied by transposition of the nerve volar to the olecranon notch and burial beneath pronator teres and flexor carpi ulnaris in order to make up length. A similar transposition procedure is used for ulnar entrapment or the cubital tunnel syndrome. Although function lost is only regained in one-third of entrapments, the progressive loss of hand intrinsic function seen with most such ulnar neuropathies can usually be halted. The compressed ulnar nerve must be dissected and manipulated with great care, or ulnar distribution hyperesthesia and hyperpathia will be increased and any potential recovery of motor function obviated.

LOWER EXTREMITY NERVE INJURIES

Injury to the femoral or sciatic nerve presents a particularly difficult problem, in that distance between the site of injury and the innervated muscle is long, and unless functional regeneration can be obtained, loss in function is considerable. Femoral nerve lesions are, unfortunately, often iatrogenic. Causes include ill-advised and poorly executed resection of pelvic tumor including benign tumors such as neurofibromas and inadvertent injury during hip replacement. Less frequently encountered causes include damage during femoral-popliteal bypass or high varicose vein stripping including saphenous vein ligation. Noniatrogenic causes include laceration by knife and glass, the occasional gunshot wound where major vascular injury does not take the patient's life, and acute compression of the nerve by hematoma secondary to anticoagulants or coagulopathy.

Paralysis of the quadriceps muscle leads to severe functional deficit; this loss is compounded if proximal femoral nerve or its lumbar plexus origins are involved. Under such circumstances, iliopsoas and sartorius function will be impaired; therefore, hip flexion will be lost as well as the ability to extend the lower leg and to lock the knee while walking. We favor a relatively aggressive approach to these lesions, planning repair as soon as it can be proven necessary. Since the femoral nerve has an unimportant sensory distribution to the anteromedial thigh, efforts are directed toward reestablishing femoral nerve motor input to quadriceps and, if necessary, hip flexor muscles. Thus, transecting injuries are explored as soon as possible; those suspected to be in continuity are explored at 2 to 3 months after injury unless there is either early clinical or EMG evidence of return of function in the quadriceps.

Sciatic injury can be equally devastating because of loss of foot function and plantar sensation. The long distances over which the nerve must regenerate to reach the calf musculature and lantar skin allow a long period of denervation and associated end-organ atrophy. Those injuries associated with hip fractures and/or dislocation or inadvertent injury during hip repair are particularly frustrating because of the very proximal and often presciatic notch or pelvic locus of the injury. Operative

repair under these circumstances is difficult and spontaneous regeneration poor, for new axons have to grow 3 or more feet before innervating functionally important structures. Nevertheless, if repair is indicated and can be done in a timely fashion, some recovery of the more important sciatic functions, such as those in the tibial distribution which provide plantar flexion and sensation on the weight-bearing portion of the foot, can sometimes be achieved. Peroneal loss is difficult to reverse by repair at this level as well as at distal levels, except in some children, but can be compensated for with a foot brace.

Some sciatic injection injuries, which usually occur at the buttock level, require surgical intervention. If loss is complete in one or both divisions and persists, exploration, intraoperative recordings, and resection and/or repair are necessary. Another indication for early operation in injection injury is pain of a noncausalgic nature that does not respond to one or two months of medical treatment including amitryptiline and carbamazepine. Sometimes, external or internal neurolysis will help the pain; sympathetic block and sympathectomy seldom do.

Lacerated sciatic nerves are best repaired primarily, before retraction and scarring make replacement of the gap with grafts a necessity. Those best repaired primarily are due to guillotine-like injury from glass or a knife. Such injuries have relatively neatly transected epineurium and minimal contusion and therefore benefit from immediate end-to-end repair. Transection due to propellor blades, shark or dog bites, or more blunt mechanisms such as auto metal penetration of the thigh, are best operated upon 2 to 4 weeks after the incident. Unfortunately, end-to-end repair cannot always be achieved under these circumstances, and grafts become necessary.

Sciatic palsy is an occasional complication of fracture of the femur at the midthigh level or treatment of such fracture. These sciatic injuries are usually in continuity and if there is no early clinical or electrical evidence of recovery, exploration and intraoperative recordings should be done 2 to 3 months after injury. If an intraoperative NAP is obtained, the nerve is split into its two divisions and each evaluated independently. If an NAP is obtained from both, then only an external neurolysis is done. If one division does not have an NAP, then resection followed by repair of that division's lesion is done, and neurolysis of the other. If no NAP is obtained from the whole sciatic nerve, then it is still split into its two divisions and each repaired separately. If grafts are used, the proximal and distal stump ends are split into 4 or 5 groups of fascicles so that a "grouped interfascicular graft repair" can be achieved.

Especially frustrating to manage have been most of the contusive stretch injuries to peroneal nerve at the knee level. The length needing replacement is usually great; functional, regenerative results even with focal lesions are poor except in children. Fortunately, a spring-loaded or plastic splint, kickup device substitutes nicely when surgery has not restored spontaneous func-

TABLE 2 Stretch Injuries to the Brachial Plexus with Severe Deficit — Unfavorable Findings:

Complete loss in the distribution of all five roots

Serratus anterior, rhomboid, and/or diaphragmatic paralysis

Spinal cord injury and/or vertebral column fracture(s)

Widespread paraspinal deinnervation by EMG

Positive sensory NAPs from multiple nerves and/or somatosensory abnormalities consistent with preganglionic injuries. Absence of sensory NAPs can mean both pre- and post-ganglionic injury.

Meningoceles at multiple levels especially if at C4-5 and C5-6. Myelographic changes at a root level does not necessarily mean that damage has occurred to the same proximal segment of root where such changes are absent but does suggest this. Occasionally, roots at levels where there are myelographic abnormalities can regenerate spontaneously or be successfully repaired.

Plexus lesions involving only lower roots, lower trunk, or medial cord seldom recover unless partial to begin with or unless they can be spared resection because of absence of intraoperatively, recorded NAPs.

Horner's syndrome usually stands against successful spontaneous regeneration or effective repair of lower elements.

tion. Although less frequently seen than either the carpal or cutibal tunnel syndrome, peroneal entrapment at the fibular level does occur and is readily documented by conduction studies. Treatment is straightforward and includes releasing the nerve as it crosses the fibular head and runs beneath the lateral fascia of the peronei. The posterior half of the fibular head is then resected to provide a less angulated course for the nerve.

Pelvic plexus injuries are often partial and improve with time. Some are due, however, to penetrating wounds or inadvertent surgical injury; these do require exploration and repair, particularly the elements contributing to femoral nerve. Several such patients have had successful outcomes.

BRACHIAL PLEXUS INJURIES

A challenging group of lesions to manage are those injuries affecting the brachial plexus. This relates both to the difficulty in regaining innervation of musculature often quite distal to the lesion site(s) and to the severity and length of some injuries, particularly those due to stretch and contusion of the plexus (Table 2). It is important to be aware of not only the distribution of injury by plexus level but of the specific elements involved at that level, such as C6 root, middle trunk, or posterior cord. In deciding the need for and timing of operation, continuity of the lesion, completeness of loss and how focal the injury is, must be considered for each element at each level of the plexus. Sharply transected plexus elements fare best with acute repair; those bluntly divided merit secondary repair. For gunshot wounds or inadvertent surgical injury involving the plexus, the patient is followed clinically and by EMG for several months. If recovery does not begin, exploration and intraoperative NAP evaluation are undertaken. Contusive stretch inju-

ries result in nonfocal lesions and are followed for a longer period, usually 4 to 5 months, since evidence of spontaneous recovery will take longer to appear by clinical and EMG examination, as well as by intraoperative electrical study.

It is important to recognize those situations where operation is not fruitful for plexus injuries (Table 3). Studies need to evaluate whether there is root involvement and, particularly, whether the lesion is preganglionic or postganglionic referable to the dorsal root ganglion. Findings of proximal root involvement and therefore probably irrepairable damage, at least with regard to reinnervation of muscles, include paraspinous denervation, serratus anterior paralysis (C5, C6, C7, long thoracic nerve), rhomboid paralysis (C5, C6, dorsal scapular nerve), and paralysis of the diaphragm (C2, C3, C4, phrenic nerve). Horner's syndrome usually indicates proximal preganglionic injury at D1 and sometimes C8 as well and suggests, but does not prove, that injury to other roots has occurred at the same level. Presence of sensory potentials from median, ulnar, and radial nerves when sensory function is absent in those distributions indicates preganglionic injury. Unfortunately, if such sensory potentials are absent, injury that has involved preganglionic as well as postganglionic elements is not excluded. In addition, there are no equivalent sensory potential studies for assessing the C5 and C6 roots and their outflow. Finally, lesions involving the C8 and D1 roots, lower trunk, or medial cord are less likely to benefit from exploration than are those involving upper elements. Thus, if lower element loss is unassociated with upper element loss, surgical exploration is usually not indicated.

TABLE 3 Stretch Injuries to the Brachial Plexus with Severe Deficit — Favorable Findings:

Incomplete loss in the distribution of all elements

Some, but unfortunately not all, infraclavicular lesions

Those with complete loss but only in the distribution of a few, usually upper roots, Many of these patients still need, however, operative repair.

Reversal in the early few months post injury of deinnervational changes in supraspinatus, deltoid, and/or biceps muscles

Negative myelogram, absence of proximal muscle paralysis, and absence of sensory NAPs and/or somatosensory responses all of which suggest but do not prove postganglionic lesion(s).

Tinel's sign on tapping supra- or infraclavicular space is only a relatively favorable sign, since only a portion of one root needs to have postganglionic injury to have a Tinel's sign. Other roots may all have pre- and postganglionic injury.

If gross continuity of roots and trunks is found at operation, as it is in the majority of cases, and if NAPs can be recorded distal to the injury and/or muscle contraction is stimulated

C5 and C6 root, upper trunk, lateral and posterior cord repairs fare better than C8 and D1 roots, lower trunk, and medial cord repairs unless NAPs indicating regeneration can be recorded and lower elements spared resection.

Operations for brachial plexus injuries are lengthy, very demanding, and highly technical. In addition to using magnification either with the operating microscope or magnifying loupes, intraoperative recording of NAPs is necessary to establish the extent of the injury and the need for resection versus neurolysis, since many plexus injuries leave the elements with some degree of gross continuity.

PAINFUL PERIPHERAL NERVE SYNDROME

JAMES N. CAMPBELL, M.D.

Painful sequelae of nerve injuries represent common, yet difficult, challenges to the practitioner. They include problems with neuromas, reflex sympathetic dystrophy, entrapment neuropathies, and stump and phantom pain.

We begin by considering the case of nerve section followed by repair either by direct suture or cable grafts. As sensory regeneration proceeds, sensory aberrations are noted. These may involve unpleasant dysesthesias, which are merely annoying, or may involve ongoing pain and intermittent electric shocks. Hyperpathia, the exaggerated, sometimes delayed, dysesthesia or pain which accompanies moderate intensity stimuli of the involved skin, may also occur. This normal occurrence of pain associated with sensory regeneration must be distinguished from other sequelae of pain, such as causalgia.

A major aspect of treatment is reassurance. As the regenerating receptors mature, the dysesthesias abate. Further surgery can only interrupt this process. The diagnosis is established by noting steadily progressive regeneration. Many practitioners find "desensitization" to be a helpful therapy. This treatment, normally conducted by physical therapists, consists of manipulation of the skin and involved joints. It has been noted that patients often protect the affected limb, which can in turn lead to progressive stiffness of the joints. The stiff joints subsequently become more painful. This vicious cycle can be interrupted by vigorous physical therapy directed at maintaining normal motion through passive exercises.

NEUROMAS

As long as the cell body of peripheral nerve fibers, located in the dorsal root ganglia, is intact, the severed end of nerve fibers form sprouts. These sprouts grow in different directions in a search for Schwann cell guides that will facilitate regeneration. When regeneration fails, the regenerating sprouts form a tangled mass, which is termed a neuroma. After months to years the bulbous mass fades as the regenerating sprouts eventually spread into the adjoining tissues. Overall, it is probably only the occasional neuroma that causes pain, but this varies with location. Neuromas involving the distal extremities, in particular the hand, often cause significant pain.

The characteristics of neuroma pain are sometimes difficult to distinguish from other painful sequelae of nerve injury. Pain associated with neuromas is focal, and tenderness is usually evident at the neuroma site. Occasionally, the neuroma can be felt with palpation, but usually it is too matted to the tissues to be easily discerned. If the patient permits, percussion may evoke paresthesias in the region normally innervated by the nerve. If the neuroma is embedded near moving structures such as a joint, pain may be evoked by that movement. This, more than focal tenderness, is probably the greatest source of distress to patients. Although it may be possible for the patient to avoid contact of the tender skin with objects, joint movement may be nearly impossible to avoid. This movement may evoke pain by stretching the regenerated sprouts.

Another hallmark feature of neuroma pain that distinguishes this condition from other painful nerve injuries is that, generally, neuroma pain develops gradually over time. If severe pain is a problem from the start, other conditions should be considered, such as causalgia. Another diagnostic feature of neuroma is that infiltration of the neuromatous region with a local anesthetic promptly relieves the pain. Pain from joint stiffness may remain, of course, and it is important to distinguish this pain from the neuroma pain in order to interpret the results of the block correctly. Time and observation, with early emphasis on preserving joint motility, are the mainstays of initial treatment. If the nerve normally innervates an important area such as the hand, every effort should be made to facilitate regeneration by use of nerve suture and, if necessary, graft. Usually, pain from an untreated neuroma gradually recedes over several months to a year or more. The once bulbous neuroma grows into adjacent tissue and becomes less tender.

From time to time, operative intervention is necessary to treat neuromas. There is little in the way of established procedures to treat this condition satisfactorily. The following principles are generally agreed to be important. The nerve end should be placed in well-vascularized tissue, away from scar. Perhaps, most importantly, the nerve should be placed away from pressure areas. Muscle tissue of limited excursion or holes placed in bone may be suitable locations for the nerve ending.

Another treatment that should be seriously considered in cases in which there is a need to temporize, or in which surgery has been of little help, is to use transcutaneous nerve stimulation (TNS). Some of the most dramatic successes of TNS are in cases of nerve injury. Principles of using TNS will be described subsequently. Implanted peripheral nerve stimulators may often provide even greater pain relief.

NERVE ENTRAPMENT

The most common nerve entrapment syndromes, carpal tunnel syndrome and ulnar nerve entrapment at the elbow, are generally accompanied by little in the way of pain. There are other syndromes, however, such as thoracic outlet syndrome and suprascapular nerve entrapment, in which pain is the hallmark. One of the notable manifestations of nerve entrapment is hyperalgesia, a painful condition that is manifested by striking hypersensitivity of the skin. Light touching of the skin evokes marked pain. It is important to realize that hyperalgesia can be a manifestation of nerve entrapment since the treatment consists merely of releasing the entrapment. Sometimes the patient is mistakenly diagnosed as having causalgia or reflex sympathetic dystrophy.

The key to therapy is recognition. Decompression generally is the easiest of rehabilitative nerve operations and should always be attempted before trying more serious interventions if there is any chance that entrapment is the culprit. In many cases, an electromyogram and nerve conduction studies are helpful in diagnosing entrapment. Local nerve blocks at or proximal to the nerve entrapment relieve the pain, and also may be helpful in diagnosis.

CAUSALGIA

There is confusion in the literature concerning causalgia relating to disagreements over its definition. Some diagnose a case as causalgia only if the pain remits with interruption of sympathetic innervation to the affected area. It seems ill-advised, however, to define a clinical entity in terms of response to treatment. Here we shall refer to causalgia as a painful sequela of nerve injury in which there is traumatic injury to a peripheral nerve associated with cutaneous hyperalgesia. If the skin innervated by the affected nerve is touched lightly, marked pain is evoked. In some cases, there are signs of marked sympathetic overactivity. In these cases, the affected limb is cold and sweaty. Osteoporosis ensues with time, and is due either to disuse or decreased blood supply to the bone. The subcutaneous tissue often becomes atrophic, and the skin shiny. The patient keeps the limb in a protected position. Often the patient discovers that keeping the affected part covered, perhaps by wearing a glove on the hand, is helpful in keeping objects from lightly brushing the skin. Covering the affected area may possibly help by warming the skin. Warming helps in some cases, but in other cases the opposite holds true. In time, adhesive capsulitis ensues, the joint stiffens, and further function is lost.

Cases characterized by signs of marked sympathetic overactivity respond to sympathectomy. In these cases the affected part may be 2°C (or more) cooler than the corresponding part. There seems to be a predilection in these cases for large nerves such as the median, ulnar, and sciatic nerves, perhaps because of the large number of sympathetic fibers in these nerves. Temporary blockade of the appropriate part of the sympathetic chain is useful in terms of predicting success. During the block, the hyperalgesia dramatically abates. If hyperalgesia persists during the block, sympathectomy will not be helpful. Too many surgical sympathectomies are done in cases of causalgia in which there has been no clear indication that this treatment would be of value.

The traditional approach to sympathectomy is to surgically excise the sympathetic chain. There is some preliminary evidence that a chemical sympathectomy may be effected by arterial injection of guanethidine to the affected limb. More experience is needed before its use can be advocated as a treatment of causalgia.

As noted, we have chosen also to diagnose as causalgia cases that do not respond to sympathetic blockade and seem not to be due to nerve entrapment. Though missile injuries are the classic cause of causalgia, this condition can result from a wide variety of lesions, most, but not all, of which involve nerve trauma. Beyond the occasional case in which nerve entrapment may play a role, these disorders are unlikely to be helped by surgical intervention. Nerve transection, dorsal rhizotomy, injection of toxic chemicals such as alcohol, cordotomy, nerve transection with grafting, and other destructive procedures are more likely to make the condition worse than better. Undoubtedly, central changes occur which cause these conditions to be resistant to destructive procedures.

Nevertheless, there are treatments that should be considered which, in the context of a carefully guided therapeutic approach, prove useful in reducing the patient's suffering. Tricyclic antidepressant therapy is sometimes partly effective. The effect seems to derive from the analgesic, not the antidepressant, effects of the drug. The pain relief occurs early in therapy, unlike the effects on depression, which may take weeks to evolve. As with many drug therapies, blood levels should be monitored in order to ensure that therapeutic blood levels are obtained. Agents such as amitriptyline and imipramine, when taken at bedtime, have the added advantage of facilitating sleep, for which the causalgic patient is most grateful.

If the patient has not discovered that covering the affected part is helpful, this also can be tried. Use of sympathetic antagonists such as phenoxybenzamine or propranolol have not proved helpful for long-term treatment.

Early in therapy, transcutaneous nerve stimulation (TNS) should be tried. TNS is particularly useful if the affected nerve is close to the skin so that it can be readily stimulated. Electrodes may be directly applied temporarily to the nerve via insertion of needles proximal to the site of trauma. If stimulation applied in this manner induces pain relief, a peripheral nerve stimulator may be implanted on a permanent basis. Patients often describe nearly complete pain relief from this technique. The pain relief, unfortunately, generally is obtained only while the stimulator is in use. A major advantage of this technique is that it is nondestructive. If it proves to be ineffective, little is lost. Electrodes are available that can be applied to the nerve under local anesthesia so that the actual parts of the nerve stimulated may be adjusted intraoperatively to optimize pain relief. It is also possible to avoid strong stimulation of motor fascicles in favor of maximizing stimulation to the involved sensory fascicles. The ideal configuration is that which maximizes paresthesias referrable to the painful part at the lowest amplitude of stimulation. Stimulation frequencies of 30 to 100 Hz generally are favored by patients.

Sometimes electrical stimulation does not work, or perhaps more than one nerve is involved in the injury, as with trauma to the brachial plexus. These cases pose a difficult therapeutic dilemma. When the lower extremity is involved, spinal cord stimulation should be tried. For technical reasons, spinal cord stimulation is not as effective for upper extremity problems. Deep brain stimulation has also been advocated. Whether this therapy works in cases in which electrical stimulation of other parts of the neural axis have failed has not been well established, but deserves consideration.

In certain carefully selected cases, narcotic therapy should be tried. The narcotic of choice is methadone. Methadone is well absorbed when taken orally and may have a longer "analgesia half-life" than other narcotics. The serum half-life is greater than 12 hours, but patients nevertheless need to take the drug three to four times a day to obtain sustained relief. Methadone should not be taken on a *prn* basis because the patient may spend much time in pain before taking the medication. It seems that if methadone is going to work, doses of 40 mg per day or less will prove sufficient. The well-advertised tachyphylaxis of narcotics does not often prove to be a problem. There are now many patients who have taken methadone for several years and still obtain effective pain control. Nausea and drowsiness are occasional adverse side effects early in therapy, but these tend to decrease in severity with time. Obviously the lowest effective dose should be used. It may be useful to supplement methadone therapy with a nonsteroidal anti-inflammatory drug. Constipation is a common complication of narcotic therapy and should therefore be treated expectantly. Close supervision of methadone therapy is mandatory. A close rapport between patient and physician is of inestimable value and should be achieved before this therapy is begun.

There are certain types of nerve injury associated with pain that deserve special mention. A nerve entrapped in the scar tissue, particularly where the skin is adjacent to the scar, often proves to be very painful. Whether this is a causalgic state or better considered in the category of neuroma pain is moot. An example of this injury is the situation in which the median nerve is partly or completely severed at the wrist. There is little soft tissue available to provide protection of the wrist. Innovative operations such as rotating vascularized muscle flaps to cover the nerve may prove to be efficacious. TNS or an implanted nerve stimulator is usually of great help, though not curative.

PHANTOM LIMB PAIN

This fascinating perplexing entity has resisted a surfeit of therapies to persist in remaining a major clinical problem. The natural history of phantom pain is quite variable. Phantom sensation is a normal outcome of amputation of a major body part such as a finger, arm, or leg. With time, phantom sensation usually telescopes, then disappears. For example, the phantom arm gradually shortens until the hand is felt to be near the shoulder, and then phantom sensation may disappear altogether. Phantom pain may be present with phantom sensation and abate as the phantom sensation abates. Phantom pain seems to occur more often in cases of traumatic amputation. Perhaps this relates to the specific nature of how the nerves are sectioned and traumatized. In some cases, phantom pain develops after an interval of a year or more after injury. Patients afflicted with pain often perceive the amputated part to be in a contorted posture. Paroxysms of increased pain are associated with a perception of further distortion of this posture.

Phantom pain and stump pain, though occasionally seen together, are separate entities. Fortunately, phantom pain often remits with time. This is particularly true if the phantom pain occurs early after amputation. Thus, the first line of treatment is to reassure the patient that odds favor spontaneous remission of pain.

When remission does not occur over a 1- to 3-year period, the patient unfortunately may be faced with a longstanding affliction. Regardless of the duration of pain, two lines of therapy should be used with little reservation. The first is tricyclic antidepressant therapy. The effects at therapeutic levels can be dramatic. The pain subsides to tolerable levels soon after therapy is begun. TNS should also be tried early because it is a safe and sometimes effective therapy. Little is lost if the procedure proves to be ineffective. More effective still, as with causalgia, is treatment with an implanted peripheral nerve or spinal cord stimulator.

Destructive nervous system procedures may only complicate phantom pain. Proximal nerve resection may help in the treatment of a tender stump, but usually does not relieve phantom pain. Dorsal rhizotomy, cordotomy, sympathectomy, and other CNS destructive lesions rarely provide long-term relief.

Occasionally, anticonvulsants such as phenytoin and carbamazepine may decrease the paroxysms of pain. Therapeutic blood levels should be attained before deeming this therapy a failure. Whether combination anticonvulsant therapy or therapy with baclofen is useful, as has been proposed in trigeminal neuralgia, has not been well demonstrated. As in causalgia, narcotic therapy in a carefully supervised program may warrant consideration.

REFLEX SYMPATHETIC DYSTROPHY

Reflex sympathetic dystrophy (RSD) usually occurs after minor trauma. Soon after injury, patients develop marked pain in the injured area. The chief clinical feature, as in causalgia, is hyperalgesia. Sympathetic overactivity is prominent. The skin temperature is ordinarily 2°C (or more) cooler than the corresponding part on the opposite side. The appearance of the skin and other features are similar to those of causalgia, in which sympathetic overactivity is prominent. RSD, unlike causalgia, does not entail a major nerve injury. As the syndrome persists, weakness and muscle atrophy may occur, but this is due to disuse, not denervation. Thus, the distribution of the hyperalgesia generally does not follow the innervation patterns of a given nerve. In many cases, the hyperalgesia follows a stocking-glove distribution.

The pain begins soon after injury. The injury itself may be trivial. A hairline fracture, a ligamentous tear, or other soft tissue injury may be all that occurs. The pain from the onset is out of proportion to the injury. Patients often describe an initial period of swelling of the affected area. In time, osteoporosis, marked sweating, cold clammy skin, hyperalgesia, and other symptoms in common with causalgia become manifest. The distinction from causalgia may in certain cases be moot.

Fortunately, RSD almost invariably responds to sympathectomy. It has been claimed that sympathectomy works only if done early in the course of the disease. This has not been our experience, as we have seen dramatic pain relief in patients who have had the disease as long as 10 years. If therapy is delayed, secondary complications become established such as "frozen joints", which, after sympathectomy is performed, may require extensive physical therapy, manipulation, and occasionally further surgery. In some cases, failure of sympathectomy results from lack of attention to these secondary complications of joint disease.

BRACHIAL PLEXUS AVULSION

Special mention of pain resulting from brachial plexus avulsion is warranted because of a new, highly effective therapy developed by Nashold of Duke University. Avulsion of the plexus occurs typically from injuries in which the shoulder is forced downward and the head is forced to the other side. The resulting traction on the plexus leads first to a stretch injury to the plexus, and finally avulsion of the roots from the spinal cord. A typical accident leading to this injury is one in which the victim riding a motorcycle is thrown over the handle bars. All or part of the plexus may be avulsed, the extent of which can be determined by clinical examination. Myelography may reveal a pseudomeningocele involving some, but usually not all, of the avulsed roots.

More than half of these patients develop severe problems with pain in the denervated arm. The constant pain is compounded by paroxysms of added pain. The victims are often incapacitated by the pain. Until recently, this problem was resistant to nearly all forms of therapy. Based on the rationale that the pain resulted from ectopic discharges of pain-related neurons in the superficial part of the dorsal horn, superficial radiofrequency heat lesions were made in the zone where the dorsal roots once entered the spinal cord. It is now established that this DREZ operation (from dorsal root entry zone), when performed by experienced surgeons, can usually lead to complete pain relief with minimal if any adverse side effects. The lesions are placed in the region between the posterior columns on one side and the corticospinal and spinocerebellar tracts on the other, and thus there is a danger that these and other tracts may be damaged in the operation. When done precisely, however, these tracts are spared, and little neurologic dysfunction occurs. The lesions are spaced at intervals of about 2 mm throughout the length of the avulsed area.

Patients awake from the anesthesia pain-free, save for the incisional pain. There are many patients who have now been followed for years who remain pain-free. Thus, the problem of return of pain, which occurs so often with other destructive nervous system procedures, does not seem to apply here. Furthermore, the length of time from injury to time of surgery does not appear to be critical. Patients with injuries over 30 years old have responded with complete pain relief.

Because of the success of the DREZ operation in relieving pain resulting from brachial plexus avulsion, its use has been advocated for numerous other conditions including causalgia, phantom pain, and postherpetic pain. The results, however, have been mixed. There are several cases in which the pain, if anything, has gotten worse after the DREZ operation. At this time, therefore, the DREZ operation cannot be advocated for conditions other than brachial plexus avulsion.

ELECTRICAL STIMULATION

In this chapter, there have been many allusions to use of TNS and other types of nervous system electrical stimulation. Since this therapy is particularly effective in treating painful sequelae of nerve injury, it is worthwhile to review principles of its use. In using TNS, the electrodes should be placed as near as possible to the affected nerve in a region either overlapping or proximal to the site of injury. The closer the nerve is to the electrodes the better. To be effective, patients should perceive paresthesia in the painful area. The patient should adjust the amplitude so that he perceives strong but not unpleasant paresthesia. The frequency on most commercially available units can be adjusted over a wide range, but most patients choose 30 to 100 Hz as the ideal setting. The pulse width can be adjusted to the comfort of the patient, but ordinarily this is not a critical parameter. It does not seem to matter greatly whether the anode or cathode is placed proximally.

Skin irritation is a major factor limiting use of TNS. Alternate types of available electrode pads may sometimes be tried if this is a problem. The sites of stimulation can be varied to some extent. The electrodes and underlying skin should be carefully cleaned between uses, and use of the stimulator should be limited to 12 hours or less a day.

TNS often is not effective because insufficient current is delivered to the relevant neural structures. This problem has been solved by the availability of implantable devices. Electrodes are placed on the peripheral nerve or, in some cases, the spinal cord. These in turn are connected to a receiver that is placed in the subcutaneous tissue. The power supply is carried by the patient and is about the size of a cigarette package. Current is delivered to the system via an antenna leading from the power supply to a lead taped over the subcutaneous receiver. Patients can vary the current, pulse width, and frequency of stimulation. Paresthesias must be felt in the region of pain, and the stimulation must be applied proximal to the source of pain.

CRANIAL RHIZOPATHY

PETER J. JANNETTA, M.D.

It has become established in recent years that a number of apparently disparate cranial nerve disfunction symptoms are a direct reflection of the aging process and are caused by vascular compression, usually cross-compression of the root entry zone of the appropriate cranial nerve. The aging process phenomena primarily responsible for this are: (1) arterial degeneration, which is presumably the deterioration of collagen and arteriosclerotic in nature, so that arteries around the base of the brain elongate minimally or significantly; and (2) hind brain "sag", a well-known phenomenon whereby the hind brain sags a bit caudally in the posterior fossa. The combination of these two processes, arterial elongation and hind brain "sag", causes abnormal contacts between blood vessels and the junctional areas of cranial nerves as they leave the brain stem in the cerebellopontine angle. At the junctional area, or root entry zone, defects in myelination exist. At this junction or proximal to it (i.e., the brain stem non-fascicular nerve side of the junctional area), pulsatile, arterial, or venous compression interferes anatomically with myelination and axis cylinder integrity and interferes physiologically with nerve conduction.

Precise physiologic mechanisms involved in the malfunction, although studied extensively in experimental models and occasionally in humans over the years, have not been precisely clarified in most hyperactive cranial nerve dysfunction syndromes. Thus the theories of mechanism remain quite theoretical except perhaps in hemifacial spasm in which delays in transmission, ephaptic transmission, and after-discharge have been clearly and cleanly demonstrated. It is probable, however, that further work in progress will show that the mechanisms are the same in the other nerves.

A number of investigators, epecially Dandy and Gardner, found abnormalities in the cerebellopontine angle in certain cases of trigeminal neuralgia and/or hemifacial spasm. However, the idea that abnormal vascular contacts were globally causal of these problems could not be proved until advanced technology enabled surgeons to operate safely in the cerebellopontine angle and magnification techniques allowed precise delimination of the pathology, even when subtle, in the vast majority of cases. Ideas that come before their time lie fallow until technology is available to prove or disprove them. Treatment of the hyperactive cranial nerve dysfunction syndromes, including trigeminal neuralgia, hemifacial spasm, glossopharyngeal neuralgia, tinnitus and vertigo, consisted, over the years, of replacing the hyperactive symptoms (i.e., pain) with loss of function in the area of distribution that was symptomatic (i.e., a trade-off of numbness in the area of the pain). Denervation as treatment has side effects that are considerable, carries a progressive recurrence rate, and affects quality of survival. However, such treatment was the best and often the only operative treatment available for patients who had failed on medical therapy. These operations were also safe since they were generally not intrusive into the central nervous system. During an era when neurosurgery was striving for recognition as a specialty, it was important that procedures with a high morbidity or mortality rate be avoided. It is my opinion that denervation procedures can now be considered the last rather than the first surgical procedure for an intractable condition such as lumbar disc disease or the "failed back syndrome".

In the pages that follow, the major problems due to vascular compression of four cranial nerves in the cerebellopontine angle will be discussed. These include trigeminal neuralgia; hemifacial spasm; vertigo, disequilibrium, and tinnitus; and glossopharyngeal neuralgia.

TRIGEMINAL NEURALGIA

Trigeminal neuralgia consists of lancinating facial pain of sudden onset and offset located more commonly on the right side of the face (3 to 2), in the lower and central face (>95%), in the V_1 distribution (<5%), and more commonly in women than in men (3 to 2). The diagnosis is easily made. The only real confusion is with dental problems as patients often feel that their pain is a toothache early in the syndrome. Furthermore, patients who have had trigeminal neuralgia for many years frequently have constant burning pain and/or mild numbness. Indeed, one-third of patients have mild but reproducible numbness in the pure trigeminal distribution on the side of their pain. Pain may occur spontaneously or is precipitated by chewing, talking, and stimulation of evanescent trigger points, which are usually located around the snout. As in all cranial nerve problems, plain skull films and CT scans are performed mainly to try to rule out benign extra-axial tumor as a cause of the syndrome. Tumors, when present, usually cause the syndrome by causing vascular compression.

Therapeutic options after a patient has failed on medication such as phenytoin (Dilantin) and carbamazepine (Tegretol) include microvascular decompression via a retromastoid craniectomy, or a destructive procedure. In our institution, we have discontinued the use of radiofrequency lesions and now use stereotactic glycerol rhizotomy as our destructive procedure. We have eliminated age considerations as a factor in the decision making for microvascular decompression. We consider only the general health of the patient. If a patient can undergo a general anesthetic and is expected to have a 5-year survival, microvascular decompression is our procedure of choice for trigeminal neuralgia. Microvascular decompression following recurrent pain after a destructive procedure on the trigeminal nerve has been shown to be much less effective than in those patients who have not had such a prior procedure.

The operation is performed with the patient under general endotracheal anesthesia in the lateral decubitus position, although some surgeons prefer the prone or supine position. A small (3 cm in diameter) retromastoid craniectomy is performed using microsurgical techniques. The trigeminal nerve is exposed via a supralateral exposure over the ala of the cerebellum and the vascular-neural relationships established. A rather precise clinical correlation exists between the location of the pulsatile compression on the trigeminal nerve and the location of the pain. The superior cerebellar artery is causal of tic douloureux in approximately 80 percent of cases. This artery, usually having bifurcated, loops downward and then upward along the pons, compressing the rostral and anterior aspects of the root entry zone of the trigeminal nerve and causing lower facial tic. The most common cause of isolated V_2 trigeminal neuralgia is a blood vessel, usually an aberrant bridging vein, on the lateral aspect of the nerve. The rare V_1 tic is caused by a blood vessel on the caudal side of the nerve. The junctional area of myelin in the portio major extends quite a distance along the nerve. Therefore, lateral and caudal vessels causative of classic trigeminal neuralgia can be quite distal on the nerve. Treatment consists of mobilization of arterial loops, holding them into a new position away from the nerve by means of small permanent implants of shredded Teflon felt. Large veins can also be decompressed in this fashion. Smaller veins are coagulated and divided.

The most common cause of recurrent pain in our series at present is recollateralization of intrinsic pontine veins, which occurs about 4 months postoperatively. The major specific risks of the procedure include ipsilateral hearing loss, which has been eliminated to a large degree by the use of intraoperative brain stem auditory evoked potential monitoring. Disorders of sensation in denervated areas do not occur since the nerve is not sectioned in this procedure. Cerebrospinal fluid leaks, infection, cerebellar hematomas, and infarctions are rare, but do occur. I have had one case of postoperative infection in over a thousand microvascular decompression procedures since utilizing Malis' antibiotic regimen. If the patient awakens with pain as severe as it was preoperatively, and it does not begin to recede within 5 days or so, re-exploration should be carried out since a blood vessel may have been missed (multiple blood vessels are common) or the decompression of an involved vessel may be inadequate. Many patients develop some mild postoperative pain, but this is usually relieved by phenytoin (Dilantin), which is discontinued after a few weeks. In general, complete permanent relief of pain can be expected in 80 percent of patients, with another 10 percent having some pain, usually relieved by Dilantin. There is a 10 percent failure rate. If the patient is well for 6 months to a year, he will probably remain free of pain, with a 1 percent late recurrence rate. Bone chips are replaced in the craniectomy, creating a solid cranial vault. This further adds to the quality of life of the patient, who should have no reminders of his prior disabling pain.

HEMIFACIAL SPASM

Hemifacial spasm consists of spasmodic contractions in the muscles of facial expression on one side of the face. It can develop bilaterally, sequentially. It is easily differentiated from nervous tics or habit spasms, blepharospasm, and facial myokymia. Spasms usually start in the orbicularis oculi muscles and gradually work their way down the face to include the platysma. In time, rather sustained contractions of the muscles occur which cause eye closing and grimacing (the tonus phenomenon). The problem is economically, socially, and psychologically disabling. Hemifacial spasm is caused by vascular compression of the root entry zone of the facial nerve. In typical hemifacial spasm, with the rostral-to-caudal sequence as described above, the causal blood vessel is located anterior or caudal on the root entry zone and may be as caudal as the pontomedullary junction in front of the ninth nerve, where the facial nerve actually starts its external course. Less than 10 percent of the patients have their spasms begin in the buccal muscles and progress rostrally. Although the end result may be the same, this atypical variety of spasm is different in that the blood vessel is usually located rostral to the seventh nerve or actually between the seventh and eighth nerves. Decompression in this situation is a technically more difficult procedure and carries a greater risk of neurological disability (hearing loss).

The procedure of choice is microvascular decompression via a low lateral retromastoid craniectomy with the patient under general anesthesia in the lateral decubitus position. Using microsurgical techniques, the cerebellum is allowed to fall away, elevated off the ninth and tenth nerves, and the facial nerve root entry zone inspected. The offending blood vessel (may be multiple) is mobilized from the root entry zone and held away with an implant, as already described. Small veins are coagulated and divided. If the patient has atypical spasm, it is important that the rostral side of the facial nerve and the area between the seventh and eighth be inspected. In addition to brain stem auditory evoked potentials, we use direct auditory compound action potential monitoring intraoperatively. With increased experience and utilization of these techniques, our ipsilateral hearing loss percentage has dropped from 10 percent to 1 percent over the years. Lateral-to-medial retraction of the cerebellum is injurious to the eighth nerve. Therefore, the direction of retraction of the cerebellum is primarily caudal-to-rostral in the lower cranial nerve problems. Patients who have had a prior destructive procedure generally do not have the same capacity for improvement as those patients who have not undergone such procedures. Morbidity consists of ipsilateral hearing loss and immediate or delayed facial weakness or palsy. Complete relief can be expected in about 95 percent of patients. Permanent facial palsy is rare (less than 0.25% of the patients).

AUDITORY NERVE

The auditory nerve, a special sensory nerve concerned with hearing and balance, is also subject to vascular compression in the cerebellopontine angle. The central myelin in the auditory nerve extends to the region of the internal auditory meatus. Peripheral vessels in the cerebellopontine angle, therefore, can cause problems. Again, a precise clinical-pathologic correlation exists. Tinnitus is caused by compression from blood vessels anywhere on the cochlear portion of the auditory nerve from the pontomedullary junction to the internal auditory meatus. Vertigo, in our experience, has been caused only by blood vessels on the vestibular portion of the nerve at the brain stem. Disequilibrium is frequently seen in combination with vertigo. If it occurs without vertigo, the blood vessel is just adjacent to the brain stem on the vestibular portion of the nerve. Prior destructive procedures to the eighth nerve (e.g., labyrinthectomy) are a contraindication to microvascular decompression. We believe that these destructive procedures should be done as a last resort for a patient with intractable symptoms.

Indications for operation are positional vertigo or tinnitus, which is generally exacerbated by putting the head down on the ipsilateral side, and abnormalities in the brain stem auditory evoked potentials on the side of the syndrome. We may liberalize these indications in time. Again, age is no real contraindication to operation, although we have not performed this procedure on patients over the age of 70. Operative exposure is similar to that for hemifacial spasm. The procedure is more difficult and tedious, and carries a somewhat higher risk of hearing loss than the other cranial nerve decompression procedures. Monitoring of both brain stem auditory evoked potentials and direct auditory compound action potentials is mandatory. Veins are more commonly causal than in hemifacial spasm or trigeminal neuralgia, and one can coagulate and divide them, making certain that they are elevated away from the nerve so that current does not spread to the auditory nerve. Major complications include ipsilateral hearing loss. The patients may have exacerbation of the preoperative symptoms postoperatively, during a period that the physiologic studies show recovery of function from the preoperative status. Hearing may improve. Vestibular function does improve. It may take weeks to months for full recovery from vertigo or disequilibrium and many months for recovery from tinnitus. The more prolonged the tinnitus and the greater the hearing loss, the less likely it is that the tinnitus will be improved. However, many patients have such a decrease in their tinnitus that they are happy, although it is not completely gone. Relief of vertigo and disequilibrium can be expected in 90 percent of patients, and of tinnitus, in 60 percent.

GLOSSOPHARYNGEAL NEURALGIA

The lancinating pain of trigeminal neuralgia occurring in the tonsillar region, which is exacerbated by swallowing and frequently accompanied by deep ear or throat pain, is the hallmark of glossopharyngeal neuralgia. Mildly decreased palatal function and gag reflexes on the side of the pain are common. Glossopharyngeal neuralgia is a rare entity. Indication for operation consists of recurrence after a course of phenytoin (Dilantin) and/or carbamazepine (Tegretol) or toxic reactions to the drugs. We have also operated on a number of patients with trigeminal neuralgia and glossopharyngeal neuralgia who have, for one reason or another, never taken carbamazepine (Tegretol).

The operative exposure of the ninth and tenth nerve is similar to that for the seventh and eighth nerves, except that the medulla must be seen both rostral anterior and posterior to the root entry zone of the ninth and the upper fascicles of the tenth nerves. Arteries are mobilized and held away with an implant of shredded Teflon felt. Intrinsic veins are coagulated and divided. Morbidity consists primarily of temporarily decreased palatal function and decreased gag reflex. There is a risk, on the left side, of postoperative hypertension which is more profound than that generally seen in other patients, and this must be monitored carefully and treated.

These operative procedures for cranial nerve vascular compression syndromes appear to be definitive and are well tolerated by patients. We have had a 0.2 percent mortality rate in our microvascular decompression series and have a virtually zero infection rate. Nevertheless, patients must be forewarned of the potential for postoperative problems. It is incumbent upon the neurosurgeon to learn the nuances of these procedures before attempting to do them. It is recommended that any microneurosurgeon who would perform microvascular decompression of the cranial nerves spend some time observing, and scrubbing if possible, at operations performed by an expert. He will save himself, and especially his patients, considerable grief by doing so.